PRINCIPLES OF ANATOMY AND PHYSIOLOGY

Study Guide for Health Professionals

TONY FARINE

Specialist Leader in the Biological Sciences,
Mid–Trent College of Nursing and Midwifery, UK

DAVID McCAUGHERTY

Biology Theme Leader,
Bath and Swindon College of Health Studies, UK

KATHLEEN PREZBINDOWSKI

Professor of Biology,
College of Mount St. Joseph, USA

HarperCollins*Publishers*

Adaptation (Principles of Anatomy and Physiology: Study Guide for Health Professionals) copyright © 1995 by HarperCollins Publishers Ltd, UK.

Learning Guide for Tortora and Grabowski: Principles of Anatomy and Physiology, 7th Edition, copyright © 1994 by Kathleen Prezbindowski and Gerard Tortora.

Adaptation published by arrangement with HarperCollins Publishers, Inc, USA.

This edition first published in 1995 by
HarperCollins College Division
An imprint of HarperCollins Publishers Ltd, UK
77-85 Fulham Palace Road
Hammersmith
London W6 8JB

Tony Farine and David McCaugherty assert the moral right to be identified as the authors of the adapted material.

British Library Cataloguing in Publication Data
A catalogue record for this book is available from the British Library.

ISBN 0-00-499003-X

Typeset by Dorchester Typesetting Group Ltd, Dorchester, Dorset, England
Printed and bound by Bath Press, Bath
Cover design: The Senate

CONTENTS

PREFACE

The completion of the Study Guide for students in the health care profession (especially those undertaking the P2000 Diploma in Nursing) has been achieved following many months of discussion and consultation with senior educational managers/teachers from various nursing colleges.

It is as well to mention from the outset that the Study Guide is not another textbook of anatomy and physiology. Whilst its content, in terms of body systems, is based upon the popular textbook, *Principles of Anatomy and Physiology, 7th Edition*, by Gerard Tortora and Sandra Grabowski (HarperCollins, 1993), its approach is quite different.

The Study Guide has been designed in the firm belief that it will assist students in their learning of anatomy and physiology – and to integrate this theory into practice. One of the main aims is to enhance students' understanding of applied physiology, so that they are able to develop into critical, analytical thinkers, and therefore able to relate theory into practice in most fields of health care, particularly in nursing and midwifery. The Study Guide does this by presenting patient scenarios, and guides the student in relating relevant patient problems to the underlying anatomy and physiology. Thus, practice (patient problems) will be seen to link to anatomy and physiology.

The other aims of the Study Guide are:
- To stimulate and motivate students – especially those who enter courses with little or no previous knowledge in the basic sciences – to study and appreciate the biological sciences.
- To provide an alternative approach in the learning and teaching of anatomy and physiology through self-directed learning methods.
- To underpin the depth and level in the biological sciences appropriate for the P2000 Diploma in Nursing programme.

The Study Guide tries to address what is perhaps the greatest challenge faced by both teachers and students – what content of biological sciences is appropriate for diploma level nursing studies?

The United Kingdom Central Council for Nursing, Midwifery and Health Visiting (*Project 2000: A New Preparation for Practice*, 1988) states that the Project 2000 preparation for practice should include 'life sciences relevant to nursing practice, normal and disordered structure and function; the nature and causation of disease; aspects of microbiology and pharmacology and their application to care and provision'. These guidelines have been interpreted widely and inevitably biological science programmes have varied in the UK. Another factor to be considered since the introduction of the P2000 programme, is that of clinical placement. Much of what is taught is meant to be related to practice, but if this is lacking or takes place haphazardly, the notion of transfer of theory to practice is lost. This all had to be borne in mind in the preparation of the Study Guide, and a serious attempt has been made to incorporate these theoretical and practical needs.

We would like to thank the following people for their advice and help in preparing the Study Guide: Raj Bally (University of North London), Desmond Cornes (Glasgow College of Nursing and Midwifery), Rita Crafer (University of Portsmouth), Patrick Saintas (Sussex University) and Norma Stride (Bloomsbury and Islington College). Thanks also to Peter Hart for producing some of the figures.

Tony Farine
David McCaugherty

TO THE STUDENT

To gain maximum benefit from this Study Guide, you will need to use it in conjunction with the textbook, *Principles of Anatomy and Physiology, 7th Edition* (HarperCollins, 1993) by Gerard Tortora and Sandra Grabowski. What follows is advice on using this textbook and Study Guide, helping you to make the best of both books.

Chapter topics and lay out

Each chapter in the Study Guide links to a specific chapter or group of chapters in the *Principles of Anatomy and Physiology* textbook, and this is noted at the beginning of each chapter by the symbol 📖. In addition, there are references to specific pages of the textbook, and these are indicated by the same symbol 📖 within the Study Guide text.

You will find that each chapter of the Study Guide provides a link to the textbook in the following ways:

1. Through the use of questions, which will prompt you into thinking and finding out about anatomy and physiology in the textbook. This encourages so-called 'active learning'.
2. Most chapters contain a patient scenario, which is designed to promote the link between anatomy and physiology (theory) and practical patient care. The scenario is followed by questions which will prompt you into considering the link between anatomy and physiology and the patient's problems, together with the associated nursing care and treatment.

These are the two main features of each Study Guide chapter. In addition, the chapters have the following features to help you in your study and understanding of the subject:

3. Overview and key terms: this provides an overall picture of the topics that are to be covered in the chapter.
4. Learning outcomes: these explain the learning aims of the chapter.
5. Checkpoint exercise: this comprises a set of questions, and provides a summary of the main points that the chapter has covered. If you wish, you can attempt these questions first before working on the chapter to give you an indication of your level of knowledge.
6. Discussion points: these are designed to take you beyond the chapter, but still into areas that are relevant to the patient scenario. They can be used for individual study or group work and discussion.
7. Answers to questions: at the end of each chapter, full answers to the questions posed in the chapter are given.

The questions

The questions are a central learning feature of this Study Guide. They are there to motivate you and to encourage you to think critically – as opposed to being the passive recipient of a lecture. You do not have to work through chapters on your own; some of you may find it beneficial to work with fellow students.

The questions fall roughly into two categories. Those which precede the scenario are mostly testing your knowledge and comprehension of specific topics covered in the textbook. Other questions – mostly those that link to the scenario – are designed to test your ability in applying knowledge of anatomy and physiology to an understanding of the patient's problems; and in analysing and recognising how biological principles apply to patient care.

'Applying' and 'analysing' are abilities that are somewhat more difficult than just recalling facts. However, they are necessary skills if a full understanding of a patient's problems and care is to be developed. Should you get stuck on a question, turn to the answers at the end of the chapter. But we urge you to attempt the question before resorting to the answer section.

In summary, the questions are the main tools for promoting thought. As you progress through a chapter, it should provide you with reassurance and confidence that your capabilities are increasing, from pure recall of facts to 'applying' and 'analysing' in the context of patient care.

Questions for discussion

There are about six of these in each chapter, following the patient scenario. Their purpose is to stimulate you into considering important topics that are related to the scenario, and in particular, to look in more depth at aspects of the patient's care and treatment.

For this reason, the questions are probably best tackled after working through the chapter. They need not be undertaken on an individual basis – each question could form the basis for small group work.

A final note

We would like to wish you every success with this Study Guide and hope that it offers you the opportunity to learn at your own pace those topics that are relevant to your particular course. And in so doing, we hope your understanding of anatomy and physiology will improve in relation to patient care.

Tony Farine
David McCaugherty

Overview and key terms

An introductory tour of the human body

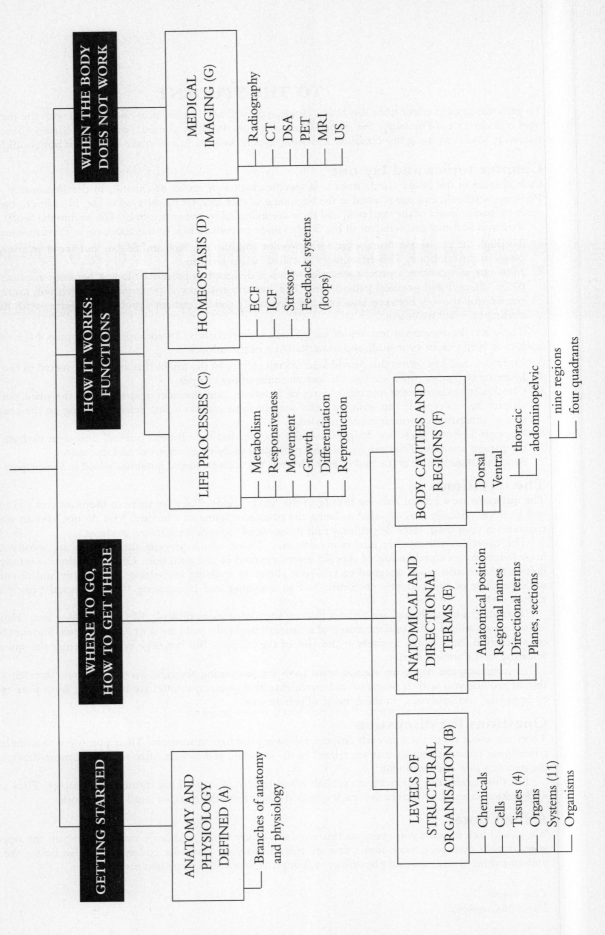

GETTING STARTED

ANATOMY AND PHYSIOLOGY DEFINED (A)
- Branches of anatomy and physiology

WHERE TO GO, HOW TO GET THERE

LEVELS OF STRUCTURAL ORGANISATION (B)
- Chemicals
- Cells
- Tissues (4)
- Organs
- Systems (11)
- Organisms

ANATOMICAL AND DIRECTIONAL TERMS (E)
- Anatomical position
- Regional names
- Directional terms
- Planes, sections

BODY CAVITIES AND REGIONS (F)
- Dorsal
- Ventral
  - thoracic
  - abdominopelvic
    - nine regions
    - four quadrants

HOW IT WORKS: FUNCTIONS

LIFE PROCESSES (C)
- Metabolism
- Responsiveness
- Movement
- Growth
- Differentiation
- Reproduction

HOMEOSTASIS (D)
- ECF
- ICF
- Stressor
- Feedback systems (loops)

WHEN THE BODY DOES NOT WORK

MEDICAL IMAGING (G)
- Radiography
- CT
- DSA
- PET
- MRI
- US

1. Organisation of the Human Body

Learning outcomes

1. To define such terms as: chemical, cellular, tissue, organ, system.

2. To list the main body systems and to describe their functions.

3. To define several important life processes of humans.

4. To define homeostasis and explain the effects of stress on homeostasis.

5. To differentiate between negative and positive feedback mechanisms.

6. To define the anatomical position and compare common and anatomical terms used to describe various regions of the human body.

7. To define several directional terms and anatomical planes used in association with the human body.

8. To list the principal cavities and the organs contained within them.

9. To outline the techniques of medical imaging and their uses.

Chapter 1

INTRODUCTION

The first section of this study will be an attempt to familiarise you with the different levels of organisation of the body. You will also be introduced to some aspects of chemistry that are essential for proper functioning of the body.

Many of you may already be familiar with the study of *anatomy* (structures of the body) and physiology (functions of the body structures), if you have been undertaking a course in *Biology* or other allied subjects. If you have not studied *Biology*, the first section here will serve as an introduction to the study of anatomy and physiology. The human is a very complex organism and to appreciate the functions of the body fully, you would also need to be able to grasp the basics of *Chemistry, Biochemistry* and *Microbiology*.

It is recognised that if you are studying anatomy and physiology for the first time, you may find some areas difficult, especially with *terms* that are difficult to pronounce. However, you are strongly advised to persevere, as you will eventually become familiar with them.

As a nurse or midwife, if you are to plan and deliver care of a high standard, you do need to understand the normal functions of the body, in order to be able to understand altered body functions later. It is hoped that through studying this chapter on the organisation of the human body, you will discover some of the basic principles governing the existence of all living organisms.

LEVEL OF STRUCTURAL ORGANISATION 📖 *Pages 5–6*

Q1.   **Arrange the terms below in order from highest to lowest in level of organisation.**

Cell, Chemical, Organ, System, Tissue, Organism.

_____

Q2.   **List four basic types of tissue.**

_____

_____

UNDERSTANDING BODY SYSTEMS 📖 *Page 8*

The body is like a factory and therefore has many specific parts that undertake specific functions. We refer to these parts as **body systems**. Each system can function by itself, but for the smooth running of the whole body, systems do interact with each other. Q3 will introduce you to some of the body systems. Take your time when working on this question, as you will need to grasp the essential body components and their functions. This will assist you later when you study the specific system in more depth.

Q3.   **Complete the following table describing systems of the body. Name two or more organs in each system. Then list one or more functions of each system.**

System	Organs	Functions
	Skin, hair, nails	
Skeletal		
Muscular		
		Regulates body by nerve impulses
	Glands that produce hormones	
	Blood, heart, blood vessels	
Lymphatic		
		Supplies oxygen, removes carbon dioxide, regulates acid–base balance
		Breaks down food and eliminates solid wastes
	Kidney, ureters, urinary bladder, urethra	
Reproductive		

LIFE PROCESSES 📖 *Pages 6–9*

The body is different from non-living things, and performs many functions that are vital to its existence. These functions can be called life processes. When you have worked through questions 4–5, you should have a better understanding of life processes.

Q4. **Six characteristics distinguish you from non-living things. List these characteristics below and give a brief definition of each.**

a. _____

b. _____

c. _____

d. _____

e. _____

f. _____

Q5.   Check your understanding of life processes by placing the appropriate term (number 1–6) in the box next to the letter of the correct definition.

> **1. Anabolism 2. Catabolism 3. Metabolism 4. Differentiation 5. Responsiveness 6. Reproduction**

☐   a. Chemical processes which involve the breakdown of large, complex molecules into smaller ones with release of energy.

☐   b. Energy-requiring chemical processes which build structural and functional components of the body.

☐   c. Sum of all the chemical processes in the body.

☐   d. Formation of new cells for growth, repair or replacement, or for production of a new individual.

☐   e. Changes that cells undergo during development from unspecialised ancestor cells to specialised cells such as muscle or bone cells.

☐   f. Ability to detect and respond to changes in the environment, e.g. production of insulin in response to elevated blood glucose level.

Homeostasis 📖 *Pages 9–12*

One of the most important biological principles that has led to the success of higher living organisms colonising the world is the ability of these organisms to maintain their body's internal environment constant despite changes in the external environment. This relative stability is known as **homeostasis**. This is a term that you need to remember, as most of what will be discussed throughout your study will in one way or another be related to homeostasis. There are many homeostatic control mechanisms, e.g. the maintenance of the body temperature, body fluids and blood pressure. You will first be introduced to homeostasis of body fluids.

Q6.   Describe the types of fluid in the body and their relationships to homeostasis by completing the statements and Figure 1.1.

Figure 1.1.
Internal environment of the body: types of fluid.

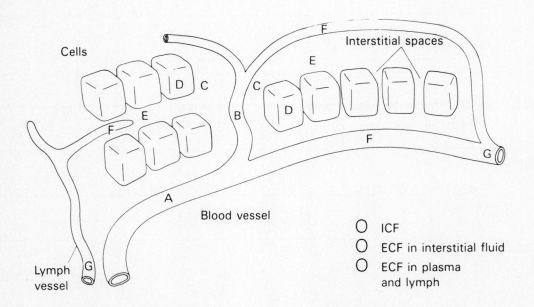

Cells

Interstitial spaces

Blood vessel

Lymph vessel

○ ICF
○ ECF in interstitial fluid
○ ECF in plasma and lymph

Fluid inside cells is known as (a)_____. You may colour those areas containing this type of fluid yellow. Fluid in spaces between cells is called (b)_____. It surrounds and bathes cells and is one form of (c)_____ fluid. You may colour the spaces containing this fluid light green. Another form of extracellular fluid is that located in (d)_____ _____ vessels and (e)_____ vessels. Colour these areas in dark green. The body's internal environment (that is, surrounding cells) is (f)_____. The condition of maintaining extracellular fluid in relative constancy is known as (g)_____.

Q7. **Refer to Figure 1.1 and show the pattern of circulation of body fluids by drawing arrows connecting letters in the figure in alphabetical order (A → B → C, etc.) Now fill in the blanks below describing this lettered pathway:**

A (arteries and arterioles) → B (capillaries)
→ C (_____) → D (_____)
→ E (_____) → F (_____)
→ G (_____).

Q8. **List six qualities of your extracellular fluid that are maintained under optimal conditions when your body is in homeostasis.**

_____

_____

_____

Q9. **From what you have studied so far on body fluids, identify as many factors as you can that could affect the homeostasis of body fluids.**

_____

_____

_____

Q10. **List, according to the systems mentioned below, the changes your body would probably make in order to maintain homeostasis, if you were to run a quarter of a mile at top speed.**

a.   Nervous.

_____

_____

_____

b.   Endocrine.

_____

_____

_____

c.   Cardiovascular.

_____

_____

_____

d.   Muscular and skeletal.

_____

_____

_____

e.   Skin.

_____

_____

_____

Feedback system (loop) 📖 *Pages 10–11*

In order for any system to be regulated, it needs to receive information continuously and act accordingly. This efficient monitoring mechanism is referred to as a feedback system. When you have read this section and answered questions 11–13, you should have grasped the essentials of the feedback system.

Q11.   List three compartments of a feedback system.

_____

Q12. **Name the two feedback systems.**

_____

Q13. **Check that you have understood the feedback system by completing the exercise below.**

After a good night's rest, as you wake up in the morning, your blood pressure needs to be readjusted. During sleep the blood pressure is usually reduced, but as you stand up there is a resetting of blood pressure, and if you are healthy, you do not notice anything, i.e. you are unaware of any readjustment in blood pressure. If there was no readjustment in blood pressure, you would probably faint.

Match the terms in the box (numbers 1–8) with factors and functions that help maintain your blood pressure when you stand up on waking.

---

1. Control centre 2. Controlled condition 3. Effector 4. Input 5. Output 6. Receptors
7. Response 8. Stimulus

☐ a. Your blood pressure: a factor that must be maintained homeostatically.

☐ b. Standing up; blood flows by gravity to lower parts of your body.

☐ c. Pressure sensitive nerve cells in large arteries in your neck and chest.

☐ d. Nerve impulses bearing the message 'blood pressure is too low' (since less blood was in the upper part of your body as you were standing).

☐ e. Your brain.

☐ f. Nerve impulses from your brain to your heart, bearing the message 'beat faster'.

☐ g. Your heart (which beats faster).

☐ h. Elevated blood pressure.

Nursing application

As a nurse, you will be caring for the elderly, the malnourished and individuals with certain neurological disorders and you may observe in these patients that their blood pressure may drop as they suddenly change position (from lying to sitting or sitting to standing). This is referred to as **postural hypotension**. It may also occur in patients who are taking medication for the control of high blood pressure.

Q14. **As a nurse, what should you do when you are moving elderly patients, e.g. from bed to chair, bearing in mind the possible problem of postural hypotension?**

_____

_____

_____

DIRECTIONAL TERMS 📖 *Pages 14–15*

It is essential that as a nurse you are familiar with some of the terms that are often used to locate different parts of the body. These are commonly used in anatomy to describe the precise position of specific structures within the body. Questions 15 and 16 relate to some of the directional terms.

Q15. **Complete the table relating common terms to anatomical terms. (For help, refer to Figure 1.5 on page 13 of PAP.)**

Common term	Anatomical term
	Axillary
Fingers	
Arm	
	Popliteal
	Cephalic
Mouth	
	Inguinal
Chest	
	Cervical
	Lumbar
Buttock	
	Plantar

Q16. **Write the correct directional term(s) to complete each of the statements below.**

a.   The liver is _____ to the diaphragm.

b.   Fingers (phalanges) are located _____ to wrist bones (carpals).

c.   The skin on the dorsal surface of your body can also be said to be located on your _____ surface.

d.   The great (big) toe is _____ to the little toe.

e.   The little toe is _____ to the great toe.

f.   The skin on your leg is _____ to muscle tissue in your leg.

g.   Muscles of your arm are _____ to the skin of your arm.

h.   When you float face down in a pool, you are lying on your _____ surface.

i.   The lungs and heart are located _____ to the abdominal diaphragm.

j.   Since the stomach and the spleen are both located on the left side of the abdomen, they could be described as _____.

k.   The _____ pleura covers the external surface of the lungs.

Q17. **Match each of the following planes with the terms that describe how the body would be divided by such a plane.**

| 1. Frontal (coronal) 2. Parasagittal 3. Transverse 4. Midsagittal (median) |

☐   a.   Into superior and inferior portions.
☐   b.   Into equal right and left portions.
☐   c.   Into anterior and posterior portions.
☐   d.   Into right and left portions.

BODY CAVITIES, REGIONS 📖 *Pages 16–22*

The body can be divided into four main **cavities** and they are: cranial, thoracic, abdominal and pelvic cavities.

Each of the cavities contains different organs. Question 18 should help you to understand body cavities.

Q18. **Study Figures 1.9, 1.10 and 1.11 of PAP (📖 *Pages 18–21*) and then complete the exercise below, which relates to body cavities. Underline the correct answer in each statement.**

a.   The (dorsal? ventral?) cavity consists of the cranial cavity and the vertebral canal.

b.   The viscera, including such structures as the heart, lungs, and intestines, are all located in the (dorsal? ventral?) cavity.

c.   Of the two body cavities, the (dorsal? ventral?) appears to be better protected by bone.

d.   Pleural, mediastinal and pericardial are terms that refer to regions of the (thorax? abdominopelvis?).

e.   The (heart? lungs? oesophagus and trachea?) are in close contact with in the pleural cavities.

f.   The division between the abdomen and the pelvis is marked by (the diaphragm? an imaginary line from the symphysis pubis to the superior border of the sacrum?).

g.   The stomach, pancreas and small intestine, and most of the large intestine are located in the (abdomen? pelvis?).

h.   The urinary bladder, rectum, and internal reproductive organs are located in the (abdominal? pelvic?) cavity.

Regions of the ventral body cavity 📖 *Pages 20–1*

Now that you are aware of body cavities, you can check your progress by completing question 19, which relates to Figure 1.2.

Q19. **Figure 1.2 shows regions of the ventral body cavity.**

a.   Label each organ on the diagram (A–K). You may colour each organ if you wish. Select your labelling from the list of structures given.

b.   Draw lines dividing the abdomen into **nine** regions, and note which organs are in each region.

Figure 1.2.
Regions of the ventral
body cavity.

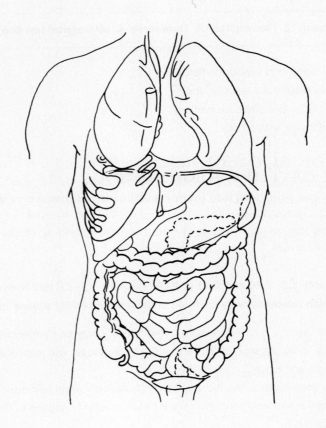

○ Appendix   ○ Lungs

○ Diaphragm   ○ Pancreas

○ Gallbladder   ○ Small intestine

○ Heart   ○ Spleen

○ Large intestine   ○ Stomach

○ Liver

Q20. **Using the names of the nine abdominal regions and quadrants, complete these statements. Refer to the figure that you have just completed and to** 📖 *Pages 20–1,* **Figure 1.11.**

a. From superior to inferior, the three abdominal regions on the right side are _____ , _____ and _____ .

b. The stomach is located primarily in the two regions named _____ and _____ .

c. The navel (umbilicus) is located in the _____ region.

d. The region immediately superior to the urinary bladder is named the _____ .

e. The liver and gallbladder are located in the _____ quadrant.

MEDICAL IMAGING 📖 *Pages 21–5*

Although you are not expected to know the details of medical imaging procedure, as a nurse you may be called upon to give simple explanations to patients if they are undergoing any of these procedures. You should therefore be aware of the basic principles and the reasons that these procedures are undertaken. When you have read the section on medical imaging in PAP, and completed question 21, you should have gained some useful knowledge on this topic.

Q21. **Match the radiographic anatomy techniques listed in the box with the correct descriptions.**

> **1. Conventional radiograph 2. Computed tomography 3. Ultrasound 4. Positron emission tomography 5. Magnetic resonance imaging 6. Digital subtraction angiography 7. Dynamic spatial reconstruction**

☐ a. A recent development in radiographic anatomy, this technique produces moving three-dimensional images of body organs.

☐ b. This method provides a cross-sectional picture of an area of the body by means of an X-ray source moving in an arc. Results are processed by a computer and displayed on a video monitor.

☐ c. This technique produces a two-dimensional image (radiograph) via a single barrage of X-rays. Images of organs overlap, making diagnosis difficult.

☐ d. A method used to study blood vessels by comparing a region before and after injection of a contrast substance (dye).

☐ e. Utilises injected radioisotopes that assess function as well as structure.

☐ f. Two techniques that are non-invasive and do not utilise ionising radiation (two answers).

You have now completed this study. We hope that you enjoyed this very first chapter. Well done! If you wish to check your progress, try the Checkpoints Exercise.

CHECKPOINTS EXERCISE

Q22. **In a negative feedback system, when blood pressure decreases slightly, the body responds by causing a number of changes which tend to:**

a. Lower blood pressure.

b. Raise blood pressure.

Q23.   Which one of the following structures is not located in the ventral cavity?

a.   Spinal cord.

b.   Urinary bladder.

c.   Heart.

d.   Gallbladder.

e.   Oesophagus.

Q24.   Which is most inferiorly located?

a.   Abdomen.

b.   Pelvic cavity.

c.   Mediastinum.

d.   Diaphragm.

e.   Pleural cavity.

Q25.   Which system comprises the following organs: spleen, tonsils and thymus?

a.   Nervous.

b.   Lymphatic.

c.   Cardiovascular.

d.   Digestive.

e.   Endocrine.

Q26.   Which one of the following structures is located totally outside the upper right quadrant of the abdomen?

a.   Liver.

b.   Gallbladder.

c.   Transverse colon.

d.   Spleen.

e.   Pancreas.

Q27.   Which one of the following is not a true statement?

a.   Stress disturbs homeostasis.

b.   Homeostasis is a condition in which the body's internal environment remains relatively constant.

c.   The body's internal environment is best described as extracellular fluid.

d.   Extracellular fluid consists of plasma and intracellular fluid.

Q28.   The system responsible for providing support, protection, leverage, storage of minerals and for production of most of the blood cells is:

a.   Urinary.

b.   Skin.

c.   Reproductive.

d.   Skeletal.

e.   Muscular.

Q29.   Which is most proximally located?

a.   Ankle.

b.   Hip.

c.   Knee.

d.   Toe.

Q30.   Circle T (true) or F (false) for each of the statements below.

T   F   a. Anterior and ventral are synonymous.

T   F   b. The appendix is usually located in the left iliac region of the abdomen.

T   F   c. Anatomy is the study of how structures function.

T   F   d. In a negative feedback system, the body will respond to an increased blood glucose level by increasing blood glucose to an even higher level.

T   F   e. The right kidney is located mostly in the right iliac region of the abdomen.

T   F   f. The study of the microscopic structure of cells is cytology.

T   F   g. The term homeostasis means that the body exists in a static state.

Answers to questions

Q1.   Organism, system, organ, tissue, cell, chemical.

Q2.   Epithelial tissue, muscle tissue, connective tissue and nervous tissue.

Q3.   If you had problems with this question, refer to 📖 Page 8, Exhibit 1.2.

Q4.   a. Metabolism: provides energy for the building of the body's structures and functional components.
b. Responsiveness: the ability to detect and respond to changes.
c. Movement: many types of cell move to various destinations, to promote co-ordination of the body system.
d. Growth: increase in size and complexity.
e. Differentiation: ensures cell specialisation and specific functions.
f. Reproduction: both cell reproduction and reproduction of the species.

Q5.   2a, 1b, 3c, 6d, 4e, 5f.

Q6.   a, intracellular; b, interstitial; c, extracellular; d, blood; e, lymph; f, extracellular; g, homeostasis.

Q7.   C, interstitial; D, intracellular; E, interstitial; F, blood or lymph capillaries; G, venules.

Q8.   Concentration of gases (such as oxygen or carbon dioxide), nutrients (such as proteins, fats and glucose), ions (such as sodium and potassium), water, blood volume and temperature.

Q9.   Sweating in hot weather, during exercise or fever, vomiting, diarrhoea, haemorrhage, severe burns, intestinal obstruction (this is because fluid stagnates in the intestine and there is failure of absorption by the intestinal mucosa).

Q10.   *Nervous* – co-ordination of all body systems through nerve impulses. There is an increase in respiratory rate, thus an increase in oxygen uptake and offload of carbon dioxide. This causes the heart to pump more blood in the circulation (increase in cardiac output), due to increased demand for oxygen by the muscles. Heart rate and blood pressure are increased.
Endocrine – Release of hormones such as adrenaline, noradrenaline and glucagon. They can all promote the conversion of glycogen to glucose and therefore the body is provided with an immediate source of energy. Do not worry at this stage, if you have not met these terms before. You will meet them when you study the digestive system and metabolism.
Cardiovascular – Increase in force of contraction, so as to deliver more blood and hence more oxygen to the muscles. This is also explained above under *Nervous*.
Muscular and skeletal – Increase in blood supply due to increase in metabolic activity, increase in oxygen consumption, and production of excess carbon dioxide and also lactic acid.

Skin – Dilatation of blood vessels, allowing heat to dissipate much quicker, and increased sweating, which, through evaporation of latent heat, cools the body. All these processes are to assist the body in maintaining homeostasis of body temperature.

Q11. Control system, receptor and effector.

Q12. Negative and positive feedback systems.

Q13. 2a, 8b, 6c, 4d, 1e, 5f, 3g, 7h.

Q14. Always ensure that the patient's position is changed gradually. Allow the patient to sit on the side of the bed and observe whether he/she feels all right and not dizzy. Ask the patient how he/she feels before carrying on with the procedure. The patient may complain of feeling faint or light-headed and sometimes this may also be accompanied by sweating.

Q15. Refer to  Page 13, Figure 1.5.

Q16. a, inferior; b, distal; c, posterior; d, medial; e, lateral; f, superficial; g, deep; h, anterior/ventral; i, superior; j, ipsilateral; k, visceral.

Q17. 3a, 4b, 1c, 2d.

Q18. a, dorsal; b, ventral; c, dorsal; d, thorax; e, lungs; f, an imaginary line from the symphysis pubis to the superior border of the sacrum; g, abdomen; h, pelvic.

Q19.

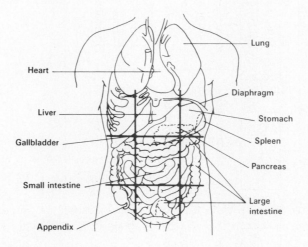

Q20. a, right hypochondrium, right lumbar and right iliac/inguinal; b, left hypochondrium and epigastric; c, umbilical; d, hypogastric/pubic.

Q21. 7a, 2b, 1c, 6d, 4e, 5 and 3 for f.

Q22. b.   **Q23.** a.   **Q24.** b.   **Q25.** b.   **Q26.** d.   **Q27.** b.   **Q28.** d.   **Q29.** b.   **Q30.** a, T; b, F; c, F; d, F; e, F; f, T; g, F.

Overview and key terms

The chemical level of organisation

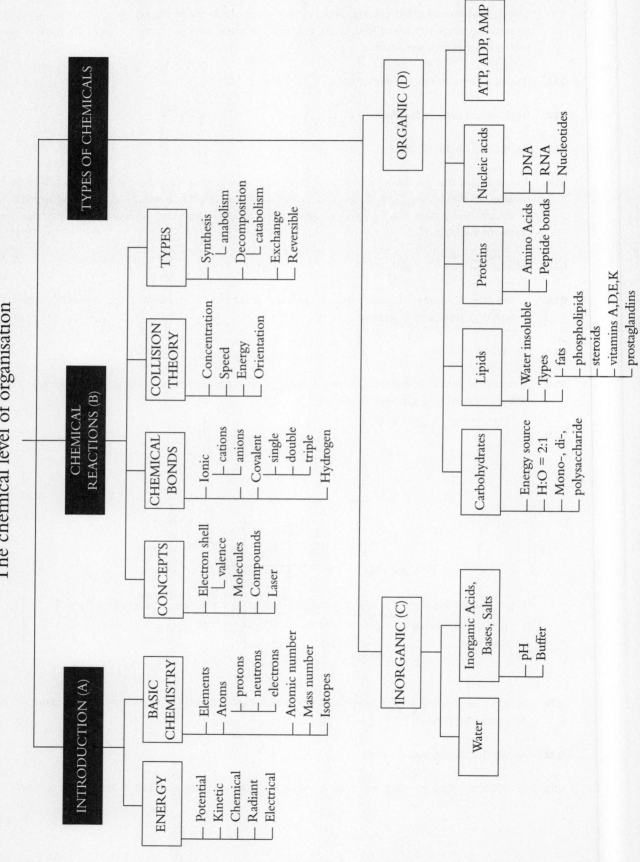

2. The Chemical Level of Organisation

Learning outcomes

1. To distinguish between matter and energy.

2. To describe the structure of an atom.

3. To identify by name and symbol the principal chemical elements of the human body.

4. To explain how ionic, covalent and hydrogen bonds form.

5. To define a chemical reaction and explain the basic differences between synthesis, decomposition, exchange and reversible chemical reactions.

6. To list and compare the properties of water and inorganic acids, bases and salts.

7. To define pH and explain the role of a buffer system as a homeostatic mechanism that maintains the pH of a body fluid.

8. To compare the structure and functions of carbohydrates, lipids, proteins, deoxyribonucleic acid (DNA), ribonucleic acid (RNA), adenosine triphosphate (ATP) and cyclic adenosine monophosphate (cyclic AMP).

9. To describe the characteristics and importance of enzymes.

Chapter 2

INTRODUCTION

To many students, chemistry is often seen as a daunting subject, and yet the many substances that surround us in nature and the composition of our own bodies is all to do with chemistry. All our foods are chemicals, e.g. carbohydrates, lipids, proteins, minerals and vitamins.

Chemical substances fall into two classes: organic and inorganic compounds. Organic compounds include all the food components mentioned above and also other substances such as the energy-storing compound adenosine triphosphate (ATP).

It is hoped that when you have studied this chapter, you will be able to see the relevance of chemistry and its application to nursing practice.

We will begin by looking at matter and energy.

MATTER AND ENERGY *Pages 29–31*

When you have read this section, complete the following exercises.

Q1.   **Complete this exercise about matter and energy.**

Matter exists in three states: solid, (a) _____ or (b) _____.
When you are on a mountain top, your (c) _____ (mass? weight?) is less than when you are standing on an ocean beach at sea level. (d) _____ is the capacity to do work. Inactive or stored energy is known as (e) _____ energy, whereas the energy of motion is (f) _____ energy. (g) _____ energy is the energy released or absorbed as chemicals are either broken apart or formed. An action potential in a nerve or muscle cell is an example of (h) _____ energy. Energy that travels in waves, such as microwaves, ultraviolet rays or X-rays, is classified as (i) _____ energy.

Chemical elements

There are over 109 elements and these are placed in a table known as the **periodic table** (Figure 2.1) according to their chemical properties. You only need to be familiar with some of the common elements occurring in the body, e.g. oxygen, hydrogen, potassium, phosphorus, carbon, calcium, iron and iodine.

Q2.   **Refer to figure 2.1, which shows the periodic table, and then write the chemical symbols for the following elements: magnesium, iodine, chlorine, sulphur, lithium and cobalt.**

_____

_____

Q3.   **Refer to *Page 30, Exhibit 2.1*. Match the elements listed in the box with descriptions of their functions in the body. When you have done that, locate each of the elements in the periodic table (opposite) and write the atomic number of each element after its description.**

Figure 2.1.
Periodic table.

Key:

Atomic number	2
Chemical symbol	He
Mass number	4.00

Periodic table (Periods 1–7):

Period	1A	2A	3B	4B	5B	6B	7B	8	8	8	1B	2B	3A	4A	5A	6A	7A	0 (Noble gases)
1	1 H 1.0079																	2 He 4.00260
2	3 Li 6.941	4 Be 9.01218											5 B 10.81	6 C 12.011	7 N 14.0067	8 O 15.9994	9 F 18.998403	10 Ne 20.179
3	11 Na 22.98977	12 Mg 24.305											13 Al 26.98154	14 Si 28.0855	15 P 30.97376	16 S 32.06	17 Cl 35.453	18 Ar 83.80
4	19 K 39.0983	20 Ca 40.08	21 Sc 44.9559	22 Ti 47.90	23 V 50.9415	24 Cr 51.996	25 Mn 54.9380	26 Fe 55.847	27 Co 58.9332	28 Ni 58.70	29 Cu 63.546	30 Zn 65.38	31 Ga 69.72	32 Ge 72.59	33 As 74.9216	34 Se 78.96	35 Br 79.904	36 Kr 83.80
5	37 Rb 85.4678	38 Sr 87.62	39 Y 88.9059	40 Zr 91.22	41 Nb 92.9064	42 Mo 95.94	43 Tc (98)	44 Ru 101.07	45 Rh 102.9055	46 Pd 106.4	47 Ag 107.868	48 Cd 112.41	49 In 114.82	50 Sn 118.69	51 Sb 121.75	52 Te 127.60	53 I 126.9045	54 Xe 131.30
6	55 Cs 132.9054	56 Ba 137.33	57 *La 138.9055	72 Hf 178.49	73 Ta 180.9479	74 W 183.85	75 Re 186.207	76 Os 190.2	77 Ir 192.22	78 Pt 195.09	79 Au 196.9665	80 Hg 200.59	81 Tl 204.37	82 Pb 207.2	83 Bi 208.9804	84 Po (209)	85 At (210)	86 Rn (222)
7	87 Fr (223)	88 Ra 226.0254	89 †Ac 227.0278	104 Unq (261)	105 Unp (262)	106 Unh (263)	107 (262)	108 (265)	109 (266)									

* Lanthanide series:

58 Ce 140.12	59 Pr 140.9077	60 Nd 144.24	61 Pm (145)	62 Sm 150.4	63 Eu 151.96	64 Gd 157.25	65 Tb 158.9254	66 Dy 162.50	67 Ho 164.9304	68 Er 167.26	69 Tm 168.9342	70 Yb 173.04	71 Lu 174.967

† Actinide series:

90 Th 232.0381	91 Pa 231.0359	92 U 238.029	93 Np 237.0482	94 Pu (244)	95 Am (243)	96 Cm (247)	97 Bk (247)	98 Cf (251)	99 Es (254)	100 Fm (257)	101 Md (258)	102 No (259)	103 Lr (260)

> 1. Carbon 2. Calcium 3. Chlorine 4. Iron 5. Iodine 6. Potassium 7. Sodium 8. Nitrogen
> 9. Oxygen 10. Phosphorus.

☐   a. Found in every organic molecule.

☐   b. Component of all protein molecules and DNA and RNA

☐   c. Vital to normal thyroid gland function

☐   d. Essential component of haemoglobin

☐   e. Constituent of bone and teeth; required for blood clotting and for muscle contraction

☐   f. Constituent of water; functions in cellular respiration

☐   g. Most abundant positively charged ion in intracellular fluid

☐   h. Most abundant cation in extracellular fluid

☐   i. Most abundant negatively charged ion (anion) in extracellular fluid.

☐   j. Component of DNA, RNA, ATP; found in bone and teeth.

Atomic structure 📖 *Pages 29–31*

When you have read this section, complete the exercises below.

Q4. **Complete this exercise about atomic structure.**

An atom consists of two parts: the nucleus and (a) .

Within the nucleus are positively charged particles called

(b) and uncharged particles called (c) .

Electrons bear (d) charges. The number of electrons forming a charged cloud around the

nucleus is (e) (greater than? equal to? smaller than?) the number of protons in the nucleus of

the atom.

Q5. **Refer to Figure 2.1 above and Figure 2.2 in PAP, page 32, and complete this exercise about atomic structure.**

The atomic number of potassium (K) is (a) _____. Locate this number above the

symbol K in figure 2.1. This means that a potassium atom has (b) _____ protons and

(c) _____ electrons.

Identify the number located immediately under the K in Figure 2.1. This number is (d) and it

represents the mass number of the potassium atom. This indicates the total number of protons

and neutrons in the potassium nucleus.

Compound 📖 *Page 33*

You have met the terms **element** and **atom**. Two other important terms are **molecule** and **compound**.

Q6. **Giving an example of each, define the terms molecule and compound.**

_____

_____

_____

Q7.   Circle the molecules that are classified as compounds.

a.   H

b. H_2

c. H_2O

d.   Glucose.

e. N_2

Isotopes 📖 *Page 31*

Read the section on isotopes and then complete the following exercise.

Q8.   Complete this exercise about isotopes.

If you subtract the atomic number from the mass number, you will identify the number of neutrons in an atom. Most potassium atoms have (a) _____ neutrons. Different isotopes of potassium all have 19 protons, but have varying numbers of (b) _____.

The isotope ^{14}C differs from ^{12}C in that ^{14}C has (c) _____ neutrons. Radioisotopes have a nuclear structure that is unstable and can decay, emitting (d) _____. Each radioactive isotope has its own distinctive (e) _____, which is the time required for the radioactive isotope to emit half of its original amount of radiation.

A radioactive form of iodine, ^{131}I, is most often used to indicate the size, location and activity of the (f) _____ gland.

Chemical reactions 📖 *Pages 32–7*

Chemical reactions are essential for life processes, and electron interactions are the basis of all chemical reactions. In the continuation of this study, you will meet the terms: electron shell, valence, electron donor, electron acceptor, covalent, ionic and hydrogen bond.

Q9.   The type of chemical bonding that occurs between atoms depends on the number of electrons of the bonding atoms. Complete this exercise about electrons and bonding.

Electrons are arranged in electron shells. The electron shell closest to the nucleus has a maximum capacity of (a) _____ electrons, whereas the second shell holds a maximum of (b) _____ electrons.

The combining capacity (or (c) _____) refers to the number of extra or deficient electrons in the outermost shell (or (d) _____ shell).

Write the chemical symbols of several atoms in the periodic table that have only one electron in the valence shell.

_____.

Potassium has one (e) _____ (extra? missing?) electron in its valence shell. It is therefore more likely to be an electron (f) _____ (donor? acceptor?). When it gives up an electron, it becomes more (g) _____ (positive? negative?); in other words potassium forms K^+, which is a (h) _____.

Chlorine has a valence of (i) (+1? –1?), indicating that it has one (j) (extra? missing?) electron in its valence shell. As potassium chloride is formed, chlorine (k) (accepts? gives up?) an electron and so becomes the (l) (anion? cation?) Cl^-.

Certain elements have completely filled outer shells and therefore do not tend to gain or lose electrons. These elements, which do not participate in chemical reactions, are known as (m) _____ elements.

Q10.   Refer to Figure 2.2 and complete this exercise.

a.   Write atomic numbers in the parentheses, under each atom. Hint: if you count the number of electrons or protons, this is in fact the same as the atomic number.

b.   Write the name or symbol for each atom on the line under that atom. Hint: when you know the atomic number, you can refer to the periodic table.

c.   Based on the number of electrons that each of these atoms is missing from a complete outer electron shell, draw the number of covalent bonds that each of the atoms can be expected to form. Note that this is the valence, or combining capacity, of these atoms. One is done for you.

d.   Draw the atomic structure of an ammonia molecule (NH_3). Note that ammonia is a covalently bonded compound.

Figure 2.2.
Atomic structure of four common atoms in the human body.

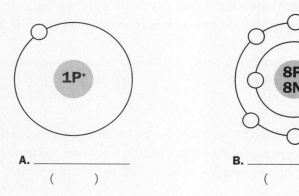

A. _____
( )

B. _____
( )

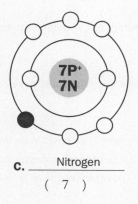

C. ____Nitrogen____
(7)

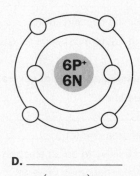

D. _____
( )

Chemical bonds 📖 *Pages 33–4*

Q11. Define the term chemical bond.

_____

_____

Q12. Name the two main types of chemical bonds.

_____

Q13. Why are hydrogen bonds important for molecules such as proteins?

_____

_____

Q14. Match the description with the types of bonds listed in the box.

1. Covalent 2. Hydrogen 3. Ionic

☐   a. Atoms lose electrons if they have just one or two electrons in their outer orbits; they gain electrons if they need just one or two electrons to complete the outer shell, as in potassium chloride.

☐   b. This bond is a bridge-like, weak link between a hydrogen atom and another atom such as oxygen or nitrogen.

☐   c. This type of bond is most easily formed by carbon (C), since its outer orbit is half filled.

☐   d. These bonds are only about 5% as strong as covalent bonds and so are easily formed and broken. They are vital for holding large molecules like proteins or DNA in proper configurations.

☐   e. Double bonds, such as O=O (O_2) or triple bonds, such as N≡N (N_2).

☐   f. These bonds may be polar, such as H_2O (H-OH), or nonpolar, such as O_2 (O=O).

Chemical reactions in the body 📖 *Pages 36–7*

In chemical reactions, bonds are broken and formed. All the chemical reactions occurring in the body are referred to as **metabolism**, a term that you have already met. When you have completed question 15, you should be familiar with all the types of chemical reactions that take place in the body.

Q15. Identify the kind of chemical reaction described in each statement below.

1. Decomposition reaction 2. Exchange reaction 3. Reversible reaction 4. Synthesis reaction

☐   a. The end product can revert to the original combining molecules.

☐   b. Two or more reactants combine to form an end product; for example, many glucose molecules bond to form glycogen.

☐   c. Such a reaction is partly synthesis and partly decomposition.

☐   d. All chemical reactions involve the making or breaking of bonds. This type of reaction involves only the breaking of bonds.

☐   e. This type of reaction is catabolic, as in the digestion of foods, such as starch digestion to glucose.

Inorganic and organic compounds 📖 *Pages 37–40*

Chemical compounds belong to two classes: inorganic and organic compounds. In the study to follow, you will first be introduced to inorganic compounds and then to organic compounds.

Q16.   Write 'inorganic' after statements that describe inorganic compounds and 'organic' after those that describe organic compounds.

a.   Held together almost entirely by covalent bonds: _____ .

b.   Tend to be very large molecules which serve as good building blocks for body structures: _____ .

c.   The class that includes water, the most abundant compounds in the body: _____ .

d.   The class that includes carbohydrates, proteins, fats and nucleic acids: _____ .

Q17.   Answer these questions about the functions of water.

Water is normally a (a) _____ (solute? solvent?). Water requires a (b) _____ (large? small?) amount of heat in order to increase its temperature and change it into a gas. As a result, for each small amount of perspiration evaporated during heavy exercise, a (c) _____ (large? small?) amount of heat can be released. This is fortunate since dehydration is less likely to occur with such heat loss. Name a location where water functions as a lubricant (d) _____ .

Q18.   Match the descriptions below with the answers in the box.

1. Acid 2. Base 3. Salt

☐   a. A substance that dissociates into hydroxide ions (OH^-) and one or more cations. Example: NaOH

☐   b. A substance that dissociates into hydrogen ions (H^+) and one or more anions. Example: H_2SO_4

☐   c. A substance that dissolves in water, forming cations and anions neither of which is H^+ or OH^-. Example: $CaCl_2$.

Q19.   Draw a diagram showing the pH scale. Label the scale from 0 to 14. Indicate by arrows increasing acidity (H^+ concentration) and increasing alkalinity (OH^- concentration). Now answer the following questions about pH.

a. Which pH is most acid ? (4? 7? 10?)

b. Which pH has the highest concentration of OH^- ions? (4? 7? 10?)

c. Which solution has pH closest to neutral? (Gastric juice? Blood? Lemon juice? Milk of magnesia?)

d. A solution with pH 8 has 10 times (more? fewer?) H^+ ions than a solution with pH 7.

e. A solution with pH 5 has (10? 20? 100?) times (more? fewer?) H^+ ions than a solution with pH 7.

Q20. **Outline how buffers help to maintain homeostasis.**

_____

_____

_____

More about organic compounds 📖 *Pages 40–53*

When you have worked through the following questions, you should have grasped the essentials of organic compounds.

Q21. **Define the term 'organic compound'**

_____

Q22. **State two reasons why carbon is an ideal element to serve as the primary structural component of living systems.**

_____

_____

Q23. **a. State the principal functions of carbohydrates.**

_____

b. State two secondary roles of carbohydrates.

_____

More about carbohydrates 📖 *Pages 41–2*

Q24. **List four groups of substances that are carbohydrates.**

(For more detail on carbohydrates, you can refer to question 11 in Chapter 17.)

_____

Q25.   Contrast carbohydrates with lipids in this exercise. Write 'C' next to any statement true of carbohydrates, and 'L' next to any statement true of lipids.

☐   a. These compounds are insoluble in water (hydrophobic).

☐   b. These compounds are organic.

☐   c. These substances have a hydrogen:oxygen ratio of about 2:1.

☐   d. Very few oxygen atoms (compared to the numbers of carbon and hydrogen atoms) are contained in these compounds. (Refer to 📖 *Page 44, Figure 2.9*).

For more information on types of lipids, refer to question 68 in the Checkpoints Exercises, Chapter 17.

Q26.   Complete this exercise about fat-soluble vitamins.

a. Name **four** fat-soluble vitamins. (Check 📖 *Page 43, Exhibit 2.3* for help).

_____

b. Since these four vitamins are absorbed into the body along with fats, any problem with fat absorption is likely to lead to _____.

c. The fat-soluble vitamin that helps with calcium absorption and so is necessary for normal bone growth is vitamin _____.

d. Vitamin _____ may be administered to a patient before surgery in order to prevent excessive bleeding, since this vitamin helps in the formation of clotting factors.

e. Normal vision is associated with an adequate amount of vitamin _____.

f. Vitamin _____ has a variety of possible functions, including the promotion of wound healing and prevention of scarring.

Q27.   List five main functions of proteins.

_____

_____

Q28.   Match the types of proteins listed in the box with their functions given below.

1. Catalytic 2. Contractile 3. Immunological 4. Regulatory 5. Structural 6. Transport

☐   a. Haemoglobin in red blood cells.

☐   b. Proteins, such as actin and myosin, in muscle tissue.

☐   c. Keratin in skin and hair; collagen in bone.

☐   d. Hormones, such as insulin.

☐   e. Defensive chemicals, such as antibodies and interleukins.

☐   f. Enzymes, such as lipase, which digests lipids.

To differentiate between proteins and other organic compounds, refer to question 71 in the Checkpoints Exercise, Chapter 17.

Q29.   This question will demonstrate to you the importance of the sequence of amino acids in a protein.

There are _____ different kinds of amino acids forming the human body, much like a 20-letter alphabet that forms protein 'words'. It is the specific sequence of amino acids that determines the nature of the protein formed. In order to see the significance of this, do the following activity. Arrange the five letters listed below in several ways so that you form different five letter words. Use all five letters in each word.

EILMS

_____ _____ _____ _____ _____   _____ _____ _____ _____ _____

_____ _____ _____ _____ _____   _____ _____ _____ _____ _____

Note that although all of your words contain the same letters, the sequence of letters differs in each case. The resulting words have different meanings, or functions. Such is the case with proteins, too, except that protein 'words' may be thousands of 'letters' (amino acids) long, involving all or most of the 20 amino acid 'alphabet'. Proteins must be synthesised with accuracy.

When you study enzymes, you will see how important it is for proteins to maintain their three-dimensional structure, if there is to be any chemical reaction.

Q30.   What is the name given to the type of diet that excludes meat, eggs and dairy products?

_____

Q31.   List three groups of foods that, in combination, are likely to provide an adequate intake of all essential amino acids.

_____

Q32.   List two or more vitamins and two or more minerals that are common in animal products and are more difficult to obtain on a vegan diet.

_____

_____

Q33.   Match the description below with the four levels of protein organisation in the box.

1. Primary structure 2. Quaternary structure 3. Secondary structure 4. Tertiary structure

☐   a. Specific sequence of amino acids.
☐   b. Twisted and folded arrangement (as in spirals or pleated sheets).
☐   c. Irregular three-dimensional shape.
☐   d. Two or more tertiary patterns bonded together.

Q34. Describe changes in protein structure by completing this activity.

Replacement of one amino acid (valine) with another (glutamate) at two locations in the protein portion of haemoglobin results in a condition known as (a) _____.

Cooking an egg white results in destruction or (b) _____ of the protein albumin. Extreme increases in body temperature, for example caused by (c) _____, can denature body proteins, such as those in skin and blood plasma.

Q35. Define the term 'enzyme'.

_____

Q36. Match the terms in the box with correct descriptions related to enzymes.

1. Apoenzyme 2. Cofactor 3. Coenzyme

☐ a. Protein portion of an enzyme.

☐ b. Non-protein portion of an enzyme; may be organic molecule or metal ion (inorganic), such as calcium, magnesium or zinc.

☐ c. Organic cofactor.

Enzyme specificity, efficiency and control 📖 *Pages 49–50*

Check that you understand enzyme functions by completing questions 37 and 38.

Q37. Write one or more sentences to explain the terms: specificity, efficiency and control with regard to enzymes.

_____

_____

_____

Q38. Explain the functions of the following enzymes: lipase, protease, oxidase, hydrolase, isomerase and transferase.

_____

_____

_____

NUCLEIC ACIDS AND ADENOSINE TRIPHOSPHATE

The last section of this study will deal with three of the most important chemical compounds in nature, and they are: deoxyribonucleic acid (DNA), ribonucleic acid (RNA) and adenosine triphosphate (ATP).

DNA forms the genetic code inside each cell. What is commonly referred to as a 'gene' is, in fact, a segment of a DNA molecule. Genes determine the traits (characteristics) we inherit, and by controlling protein synthesis, they regulate most of the activities that take place in our cells throughout a lifetime. To develop your understanding of DNA, refer to questions 1 to 14 in Chapter 21, and when you have completed the exercises, return to this chapter and continue with the rest of the study.

Q39. Describe the structure and significance of ATP by completing these statements.

ATP stands for adenosine triphosphate. Adenosine consists of a base that is a component of DNA, that is (a) _____, along with the five-carbon sugar named (b) _____. The 'TP' of ATP stands for (c) _____. The final (d) _____ (one? two? three?) phosphates are bonded to the molecule by high-energy bonds. When the terminal phosphate is broken, a great deal of energy is released as ATP is split into (e) _____ plus (f) _____. ATP, the body's primary energy-storing molecule, is constantly re-formed by the reverse of this reaction, as energy is made available from foods we eat. Write this reversible reaction.

_____

Q40. A compound similar to ATP, but with only one phosphate, is named (a) _____. A cyclic form of this molecule can be made with the help of the enzyme (b) _____. Cyclic AMP has important regulatory functions and will be discussed in Chapter 17.

This completes the study on the chemical level of organisation and we hope that you have enjoyed it. To check your progress, you may wish to attempt the Checkpoints Exercise below.

CHECKPOINTS EXERCISE

Q41. Which one of the following statements is not true?

a. A reaction in which two amino acids join to form a dipeptide is called a dehydration synthesis reaction.

b. A reaction in which a disaccharide is digested to form two monosaccharides is known as a hydrolysis reaction.

c. About 65 to 75% of living matter consists of organic matter.

d. Strong acids ionise more easily than weak acids.

Q42. Choose the one true statement.

a. A pH of 7.5 is more acidic than a pH of 6.5.

b. Anabolism consists of a variety of decomposition reactions.

c. An atom such as chlorine (Cl), with seven electrons in its outer orbit, is likely to be an electron donor (rather than electron acceptor) in ionic bond formation.

d. Polyunsaturated fats are more likely to reduce cholesterol level than are saturated fats.

Q43.   In the formation of an ionically bonded salt such as NaCl, Na⁺ has :

a.   Gained an electron from Cl⁻.

b.   Lost an electron to Cl⁻.

c.   Shared an electron with Cl⁻.

d.   Formed an isotope of Na⁺.

Q44.   Over 99% of living cells consist of just six elements. Choose the element that is not one of these six.

a.   Calcium.

b.   Hydrogen.

c.   Carbon.

d.   Iodine.

e.   Nitrogen.

f.   Oxygen.

g.   Phosphorous.

Q45.   Which one of the following describes the structure of a nucleotide?

a.   Base–base.

b.   Phosphate–sugar–base.

c.   Enzyme.

d.   Dipeptide.

e.   Adenine–ribose.

Q46.   Which of the following groups of chemicals includes only polysaccharides?

a.   Glycogen, starch.

b.   Glycogen, glucose, galactose.

c.   Glucose, fructose.

d.   RNA, DNA.

e.   Sucrose, polypeptide.

Q47. $C_6H_{12}O_6$ is most likely the chemical formula for:

a.   Amino acid.

b.   Fatty acid.

c.   Hexose.

d.   Polysaccharide.

e.   Ribose.

Q48. **All of the following answers consist of correctly paired terms and descriptions related to enzymes except:**

a. Active site – a place on an enzyme that fits the substrate.

b. Substrate – molecule(s) upon which the enzyme acts.

c. Turnover number – number of substrate molecules converted to product per enzyme molecule per second.

d. Holoenzyme – another name for a cofactor.

e. -ase – ending of most enzyme names.

Q49. **Which of the following substances are used mainly for structure and regulatory functions and are not normally used as energy sources?**

a. Lipids.

b. Proteins.

c. Carbohydrates.

Q50. **Which one of the following is a component of RNA, but not DNA?**

a. Adenine.

b. Phosphate.

c. Guanine.

d. Ribose.

e. Thymine.

Q51. **Which of the following answers consists of a pair of proteins and their correct functions?**

a. Contractile – actin and myosin.

b. Immunological – collagen of connective tissue.

c. Catalytic – enzymes.

d. Transport – haemoglobin.

Q52. **Circle T (true) or F (false) for each of the statements below.**

T   F   a. Oxygen can form three bonds since it requires three electrons to fill its outer shell.

T   F   b. Oxygen, water, NaCl and glucose are inorganic compounds.

T   F   c. There are four different kinds of amino acids found in human proteins.

T   F   d. The number of protons always equals the number of neutrons in an atom.

T   F   e. K^+ and Cl^- are both cations.

T   F   f. A strong acid has more of a tendency to contribute H^+ to a solution than a weak acid has.

T   F   g. Carbohydrates constitute about 18 to 25% of the total body weight.

T   F   h. ATP contains more energy than ADP.

T   F   i. Prostaglandins, cyclic AMP, steroids and fats are all classified as lipids.

Q53. Recognising simple chemical formula and structure. Identify each organic compound below. Write names of compounds on lines provided. 📖 *Pages 42, 44, 52.*

a. _____

b. _____

c. _____

d. _____

e. _____

Answers to questions

Q1.   a, liquid; b, gas; c, weight; d, energy; e, potential; f, kinetic; g, chemical; h, electrical; i, radiant;

Q2.   Mg, I, Cl, S, Li, Co.

Q3.   1a (6), 8b (7), 5c (53), 4d (26), 2e (20), 9f (8), 6g (19), 7h (11), 3i (17), 10j (15).

Q4.   a, electrons; b, protons; c, neutrons; d, negative; e, equal to.

Q5.   a, 19; b, 19; c, 19; d, 39.

Q6.   A molecule is produced when one or more atoms combine in a chemical reaction. An example is oxygen (O_2).
    A compound is a substance that can be broken down into two or more different elements by chemical means. An example is sodium chloride (NaCl).

Q7. H_2O and glucose.

Q8.   a, 20; b, neutrons; c, 18; d, radiation; e, half life, f, thyroid.

Q9.   a, 2; b, 8; c, valence; d, valence; e, extra; f, donor; g, positive; h, cation; i, -1; j, missing; k, accepts; l, anion; m, inert.

Q10.   a and b.

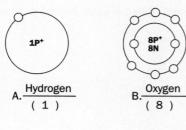

A. $\underline{\text{Hydrogen}}$
    (1)

B. $\underline{\text{Oxygen}}$
    (8)

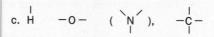

c. H   —O—   (N),   —C—

d. Atomic structure of ammonia (NH_3)

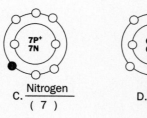

C. $\underline{\text{Nitrogen}}$
    (7)

D. $\underline{\text{Carbon}}$
    (6)

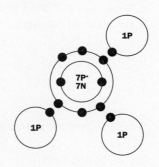

Q11. A chemical bond is a form of chemical energy which occurs when atoms of a molecule are held together by forces of attraction.

Q12. Ionic and covalent bonds.

Q13. They form weak bonds and do not bond atoms into molecules. They therefore play an important part in determining the three-dimensional shape of proteins and nucleic acids.

Q14. 3a, 2b, 1c, 2d, 1e, 1f.

Q15. 3a, 4b, 2c, 1d, 1e.

Q16. a, organic; b, organic; c, inorganic; d, organic.

Q17. a, solvent; b, large; c, large; d, mucous lining of digestive and respiratory tract, serous fluid in pleurae, pericardium of the heart and peritoneum.

Q18. 2a, 1b, 3c.

Q19. a, 4; b, 10; c, blood; d, fewer; e, 100, more. Refer also to 📖 *Page 39, Figure 2.7* to check the pH scale.

Q20. Buffers help to maintain homeostasis by converting strong acids or bases into weak acids or bases. In doing so, they maintain the pH of body fluids and blood.

Q21. An organic compound contains carbon and hydrogen, but some organic compounds may also contain oxygen, nitrogen, sulphur and phosphorus (see 📖 *Page 40*).

Q22. One to thousands of carbon atoms can react to form large molecules of many different shapes. Because of their large size and because some of them do not dissolve easily in water, these molecules are useful for building body structures.

Q23. a. Carbohydrates provide a readily available source of energy.

b. Carbohydrates can be converted into other substances. They can serve as food reserves.

Q24. Sugars, starches, glycogen and cellulose.

Q25. La, C and L for b, Ld.

Q26. a. Vitamins A, D, K and E (the order is not important).
b. Symptoms of deficiency.
c. D.
d. K.
e. A.
f. E.

Q27. Structural, contractile, transport, catalytic and regulatory.

Q28. 6a, 2b, 5c, 4d, 3e, 1f.

Q29.   SMILE, MILES, LIMES, SLIME.

Q30.   Vegan.

Q31.   Legumes, nuts, grains or seeds.

Q32.   Vitamins B_{12}, B_2 (riboflavin) and D. The minerals are: iron, zinc and calcium.

Q33.   1a, 3b, 4c, 2d

Q34.   a, sickle cell anaemia; b, denaturation; c, burns or fever.

Q35.   An enzyme is a biological catalyst and is usually a protein.

Q36.   1a, 2b, 3c.

Q37.   *Specificity* – Each enzyme only affects a particular substrate. Specificity depends on the active site of the enzyme. An enzyme only functions when its substrate can fit into the active site, comparable to a lock and key.
Efficiency – Under optimal conditions, enzymes can catalyse reactions at a greatly increased rate (see page 49 of PAP).
Control – Rate of synthesis of enzymes is controlled by gene actions. They may need cofactors or coenzymes.

Q38.   Lipase breaks down lipids. Protease breaks down proteins. Oxidase adds oxygen. Hydrolase adds water. Isomerase rearranges atoms within the molecule. Transferase transfers groups of atoms.

Q39.   a, adenine; b, ribose; c, triphosphate; d, two; e, ADP; f, phosphate.

ATP → ADP + Phosphate + Energy.

Q40.   a, cyclic AMP; b, adenylate cyclase.   **Q41.** c.   **Q42.** d.   **Q43.** b.   **Q44.** d.   **Q45.** b.   **Q46.** a.

Q47.   c.   **Q48.** d.   **Q49.** b.   **Q50.** e.   **Q51.** a.

Q52.   a, F (two bonds, since it requires two electrons); b, F (oxygen is not a compound and glucose is an organic compound); c, F (there are 20 amino acids); d, F (the number of protons equals the number of electrons); e, F (K^+ is a cation whilst Cl^- is an anion); f, T; g, F (only 2 to 3%); h, T; i, F (only prostaglandins, steroids and fats are lipids).

Q53.   a. Amino acid.
b. Monosaccharide or hexose or glucose.
c. Polysaccharide or starch or glycogen.
d. Adenosine triphosphate.
e. Fat or lipid or triglyceride (unsaturated).

Overview and key terms
The skeleton, joints and muscles

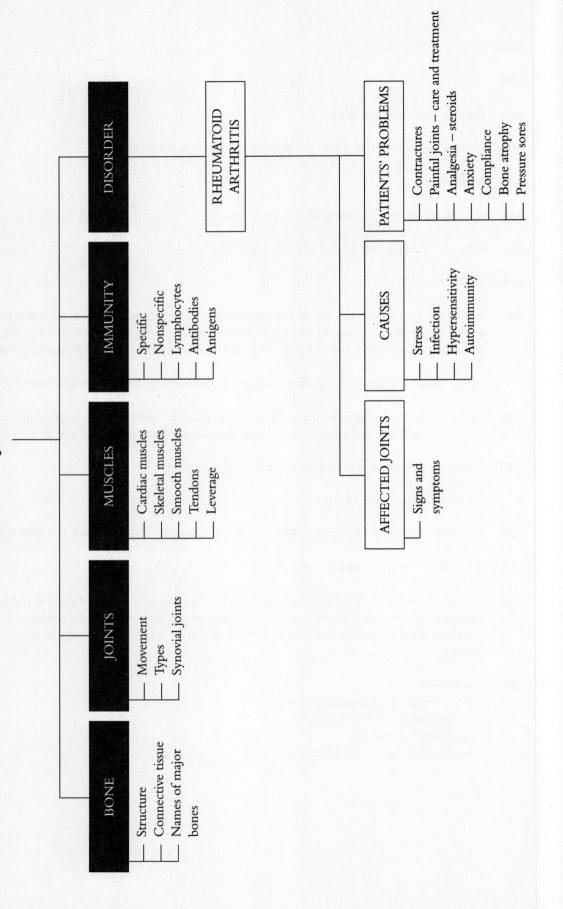

BONE
— Structure
— Connective tissue
— Names of major bones

JOINTS
— Movement
— Types
— Synovial joints

MUSCLES
— Cardiac muscles
— Skeletal muscles
— Smooth muscles
— Tendons
— Leverage

IMMUNITY
— Specific
— Nonspecific
— Lymphocytes
— Antibodies
— Antigens

DISORDER

RHEUMATOID ARTHRITIS

AFFECTED JOINTS
— Signs and symptoms

CAUSES
— Stress
— Infection
— Hypersensitivity
— Autoimmunity

PATIENTS' PROBLEMS
— Contractures
— Painful joints – care and treatment
— Analgesia – steroids
— Anxiety
— Compliance
— Bone atrophy
— Pressure sores

3. The Skeleton, Joints and Muscles

Learning outcomes

1. To learn those aspects of the normal structure and function of bones, joints, muscles and the immune system that are relevant to understanding rheumatoid arthritis.

2. To describe the disease process of rheumatoid arthritis and relate it to normal bodily structure and function.

3. To identify the patient problems that can arise in rheumatoid arthritis.

4. To relate these problems to the relevant nursing care and treatment.

Chapters 6–11

INTRODUCTION

This chapter will deal with bones, joints, muscles and associated structures that are involved in the production of movement; for example, tendons and ligaments. This chapter will link to Chapters 6–11 of PAP. In addition, topics in other chapters of PAP, such as Chapter 22 on immunity, Chapter 4 on tissues and Chapter 18 on the endocrine system will be brought in. The reason for this is that the patient scenario – a woman with rheumatoid arthritis – and this condition, require a knowledge of these structures (and their functions). This once again illustrates the point that in considering patients and their problems, one must turn to several bodily systems for a complete explanation, and, furthermore, integrate these in a way that will provide a rationale and understanding for patient care. This is the aim.

The following chapter (The Cell, Tissues and Skin) will continue with this patient scenario and look at some additional problems that are associated with cells, tissues and the skin.

At present, it is necessary to gain some understanding of bones, joints, ligaments, tendons, muscles and immunity, and the following questions will help you to do this. These questions will link to ▭ *Chapters 6–11* and also ▭ *Chapter 22*.

BONE STRUCTURE ▭ *Pages 147–52*

Q1.   What other systems of the body depend on a healthy skeletal system? Explain why, in each case.

_____

_____

_____

Q2.   The skeletal system consists of four types of connective tissue. Name these.

_____

Q3.   On Figure 3.1, label the diaphysis, epiphysis, epiphyseal plate, nutrient foramen, and medullary (marrow) cavity. Then identify the parts of a long bone listed on the Figure.

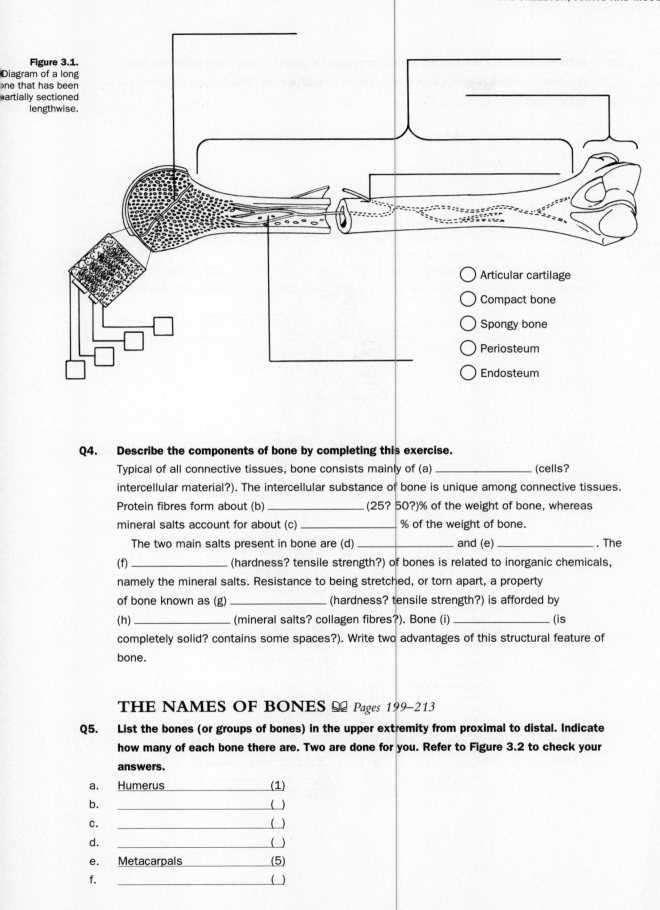

Figure 3.1.
Diagram of a long bone that has been partially sectioned lengthwise.

- ◯ Articular cartilage
- ◯ Compact bone
- ◯ Spongy bone
- ◯ Periosteum
- ◯ Endosteum

Q4.   Describe the components of bone by completing this exercise.

Typical of all connective tissues, bone consists mainly of (a) _____ (cells? intercellular material?). The intercellular substance of bone is unique among connective tissues. Protein fibres form about (b) _____ (25? 50?)% of the weight of bone, whereas mineral salts account for about (c) _____ % of the weight of bone.

The two main salts present in bone are (d) _____ and (e) _____ . The (f) _____ (hardness? tensile strength?) of bones is related to inorganic chemicals, namely the mineral salts. Resistance to being stretched, or torn apart, a property of bone known as (g) _____ (hardness? tensile strength?) is afforded by (h) _____ (mineral salts? collagen fibres?). Bone (i) _____ (is completely solid? contains some spaces?). Write two advantages of this structural feature of bone.

THE NAMES OF BONES 📖 *Pages 199–213*

Q5.   List the bones (or groups of bones) in the upper extremity from proximal to distal. Indicate how many of each bone there are. Two are done for you. Refer to Figure 3.2 to check your answers.

a.   <u>Humerus</u>   <u>(1)</u>

b.   _____   ( )

c.   _____   ( )

d.   _____   ( )

e.   <u>Metacarpals</u>   (5)

f.   _____   ( )

Q6. Refer to Figure 3.2 and list the bones (or groups of bones) in the lower extremity from proximal to distal. Indicate how many of each bone there are. One is done for you.

a. <u>Femur</u>   (1)

b. _____   ( )

c. _____   ( )

d. _____   ( )

e. _____   ( )

f. _____   ( )

g. _____   ( )

Figure 3.2.
Anterior view of the skeleton.

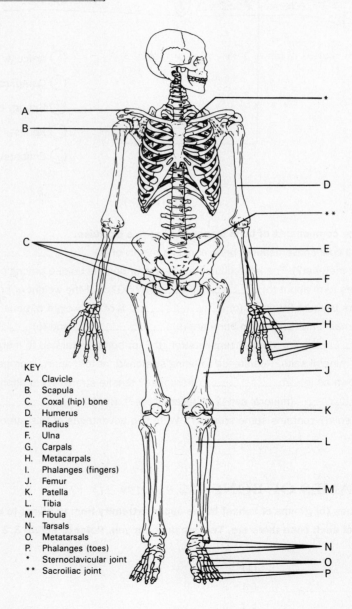

KEY
A. Clavicle
B. Scapula
C. Coxal (hip) bone
D. Humerus
E. Radius
F. Ulna
G. Carpals
H. Metacarpals
I. Phalanges (fingers)
J. Femur
K. Patella
L. Tibia
M. Fibula
N. Tarsals
O. Metatarsals
P. Phalanges (toes)
*   Sternoclavicular joint
** Sacroiliac joint

JOINTS 📖 *Pages 217–31*

Q7. **Define the term articulation (joint).**

_____

Discuss three structural factors that affect movement at joints.

_____

_____

Q8. **Name three classes of joints based on structure.**

_____

_____

Q9. **Fill in the blanks below to name three classes of joints according to the amount of movement they permit.**

a.   Synarthrosis: _____

b.   _____ : slightly moveable

c.   _____ : freely moveable

Q10. **What structural features of synovial joints make them more freely moveable than fibrous or cartilaginous joints?**

_____

_____

Q11. **On Figure 3.3, name the indicated structures.**

Figure 3.3.
Structure of a
generalized synovial
joint.

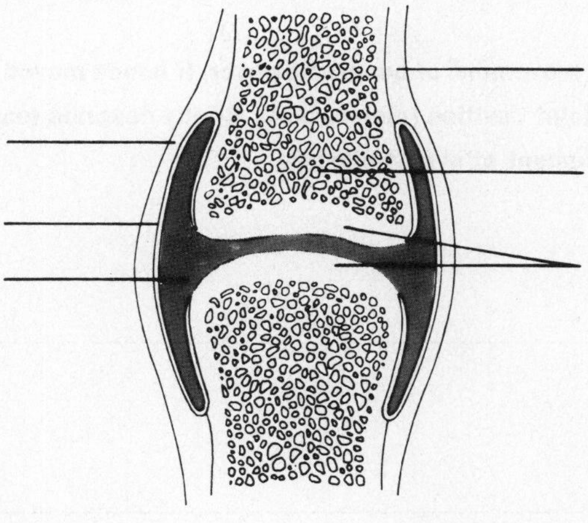

○ Articular cartilage

○ Articulating bone

○ Fibrous capsule

○ Periosteum

○ Synovial (joint) cavity

○ Synovial membrane

Q12.   Select the parts of a synovial joint (listed in the box) that fit the descriptions below.

> **1. Articular cartilage 2. Fibrous capsule 3. Ligaments 4. Synovial fluid 5. Synovial membrane**

☐ a. Hyaline cartilage that covers the ends of articulating bones, but does not bind them together.

☐ b. With the consistency of uncooked egg white or oil, it lubricates the joint and nourishes the avascular articular cartilage.

☐ c. Connective tissue membrane that lines the synovial cavity and secretes synovial fluid.

☐ d. Parallel fibres in some fibrous capsules; bind bones together.

☐ e. Together, these form the articular capsule (two answers).

Q13.   Describe the structure, function and location of the following structures that may be associated with synovial joints:

a.   Articular discs (menisci)

_____

_____

b.   Bursae

_____

_____

c.   Intracapsular ligaments

_____

_____

Q14.   The design of synovial joints permits free movement of bones. However, if bones moved too freely, they could move right out of their joint cavities (dislocation). Briefly describe four factors that account for limitation of movement at synovial joints.

a.   Articulating bones

_____

b.   Ligaments

_____

c.   Muscles

_____

d.   Soft parts

_____

Q15.   Check your understanding of types of synovial joints by choosing the type of joint that fits the description. (Answers may be used more than once.)

B. Ball and socket E. Ellipsoidal G. Gliding H. Hinge P. Pivot S. Saddle

☐   a.   Monaxial joint; only rotation possible.

☐   b.   Examples include atlas–axis joint and joint between head of radius and radial notch at proximal end of ulna.

☐   c.   Triaxial joint, allowing movement in all three planes.

☐   d.   Hip bone and shoulder joints.

☐   e.   Spool-like (convex) surface articulated with convex surface, for example elbow, ankle and joints between phalanges.

☐   f.   One type of monoaxial joint in which only flexion and extension are possible.

☐   g.   Found in joints at sternoclavicular and claviculoscapular joints.

☐   h.   Thumb joint located between metacarpal of thumb and carpal bone (trapezium).

☐   i.   Biaxial joints (two answers).

MUSCLES 📖 *Pages 238–41 & 270–4*

Q16.   Match the muscle types listed in the box with description below.

1. Cardiac 2. Skeletal 3. Smooth

☐   a.   Involuntary muscle found in blood vessels and intestine.

☐   b.   Involuntary striated muscle.

☐   c.   Striated voluntary muscle attached to bones.

☐   d.   The only type of muscle that is voluntary.

Q17.   List three functions of muscle tissue that are important for maintenance of homeostasis.

_____

_____

_____

Q18.   **Arrange the following terms (connective tissue) in correct sequence according to the amount of muscle surrounded: endomysium, epimysium, perimysium.**

(Entire muscle) → (Bundle of muscle fibres) → (Individual muscle fibre)

_____

Q19.   **Contrast the terms in the following pairs:**

a.   Tendon/aponeurosis

_____

_____

b.   Tendon/tendon sheath

_____

_____

Q20.   **Refer to Figure 3.4 and consider flexion of your own forearm as you complete this learning activity.**

In flexion, your forearm serves as a rigid rod, or (a) _____ , which moves about a fixed point, called a (b) _____ (your elbow joint, in this case). Hold a weight in your hand as you flex your forearm. The weight plus your forearm serves as the (c) _____ (effort? fulcrum? resistance?) during this movement. The effort to move this resistance is provided by contraction of a (d) _____. Note that if you held a heavy telephone book in your hand while your forearm was flexed, much more (e) _____ by your arm muscles would be required.

In Figure 3.4, identify the exact point at which the muscle causing flexion attaches to the forearm. It is the (f) _____ (proximal? distal?) end of the (g) _____ (humerus? radius? ulna?). Write an 'E' and an 'I' on the two lines next to the arrow at that point in the figure. This indicates that this is the site where the muscle exerts its effort (E) in the lever system, and it is also the insertion (I) end of the muscle.

Figure 3.4.
The lever–fulcrum principle as illustrated by flexion of the forearm.

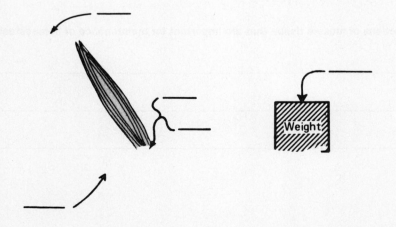

IMMUNITY 📖 *Pages 692–711*

Q21. Briefly contrast two types of resistance to disease: specific versus nonspecific.

_____

_____

Q22. Complete this exercise about cells that carry out immune responses.

Name the two categories of cells that carry out immune responses.

(a) _____ and (b) _____. Where do lymphocytes originate?

(c) _____ . Some immature lymphocytes migrate to the thymus and become

(d) _____ (B? T?) cells. Here, T cells develop immunocompetence, meaning that

these cells have the ability to (e) _____ . Some T cells become CD4$^+$ cells and

others become (f) _____ cells, based on the type of (g) _____ in their

plasma membranes. B cells mature into immune cells in (h) _____ .

Q23. Contrast two types of immunity by writing AMI before descriptions of antibody-mediated immunity and CMI before those describing cell-mediated immunity.

_____ a. Especially effective against microbes that enter cells, such as viruses and parasites.

_____ b. Especially effective against bacteria present in extracelluar fluids.

_____ c. Involves plasma cells (derived from B cells) that produce antibodies.

_____ d. Utilizes killer T cells (derived from CD8$^+$ T cells) that directly attack the antigen.

_____ e. Facilitated by helper T (CD4$^+$ T cells).

Q24. Complete this exercise on antigens.

An antigen is defined as 'any chemical substance which, when introduced into the body,

(a) _____ .' In general, antigens are (b) _____ (parts of the body? foreign substances?).

Complete the definitions of the two properties of antigens:

Immunogenicity: ability to (c) _____ specific antibodies or specific T cells.

Reactivity: ability to (d) _____ specific antibodies or specific T cells.

An antigen with both of these characteristics is called a (e) _____ .

A partial antigen is known as (f) _____ . It displays (g) _____ (immunogenicity? reactivity?) but not (h) _____ . For example, for the hapten penicillin to evoke an immune response (immunogenicity), it must form a complete antigen by combining with a (i) _____ . Persons who have this particular protein are said to be (j) _____ to penicillin.

(k) Describe the chemical nature of antigens.

_____

_____

(l) Explain why plastics used for valves or joints are not likely to initiate an allergic response and be rejected.

_____

_____

Can an entire microbe serve as an antigen? (m) _____ (yes? no?). List the parts of microbes that may be antigenic: (n) _____ .

If you are allergic to pollen in the spring or autumn or to certain foods, the pollen or foods serve as (o) _____ (antigens? antibodies?) to you. Antibodies or specific T cells form against (p) _____ (the entire? only a specific region of the?) antigen. This region is known as the (q) _____ . Most antigens have (r) _____ (only one? only two? a number of?) antigenic determinant sites.

CHECKPOINTS EXERCISE

Q25.   What is the definition of a joint?

_____

Q26.   What type of joint is the wrist?

_____

Q27.   What type of joint is the hip?

_____

Q28.   What are the three main factors that limit movement at a synovial joint?

_____

Q29.   What type of muscle is skeletal?

_____

Q30.   What is the function of B lymphocytes?

_____

Q31.   What are antibodies?

_____

Q32.   Name four antigens.

PATIENT SCENARIO

Mrs Royal is a 56-year-old married woman who has suffered from rheumatoid arthritis for a number of years. This is a condition in which the joints become inflamed, swollen and painful. It makes movement difficult, and ultimately the joints – particularly in the hand – become very distorted in appearance. For these reasons, Mrs Royal is unable to care for herself, and relies on her husband – together with support from the District Nurse – to care for her.

Her husband is now having a 'break' whilst Mrs Royal is admitted to hospital for reassessment of her condition and treatment.

RHEUMATOID ARTHRITIS

This condition is three times more common in females than in males. It appears most often between the ages of 30 and 55.

Inflammation occurs in the following joints (see Figures 3.5 and 3.6):

- The metatarsals in the feet
- The wrists
- The interphalangeal joints
- The metacarpophalangeal joints

However, the knee, ankle, hip or jaw may also be involved.

Q33.   What would you expect the appearance of these joints to be? *(Page 695).*

Q34.   Where in the joint is the synovial membrane found?

The synovial membrane is being attacked by lymphocytes (and antibodies) and to a lesser extent polymorphs *(Pages 574–6)*. This results in thickening of the membrane and it infiltrates over the articular cartilage of the joint. This, of course, will interfere with the joint and make it difficult to move. In addition, ligaments become softened and the joint becomes lax. Bone erosion may also occur. Eventually, fibrous tissue *(Page 122)* will fuse the joint and make it immoveable.

The disease is not confined to the joints, and many patients feel unwell and have a rise in body temperature, weight loss and malaise. Also, the skin becomes inelastic *(Page 130)* and rheumatoid nodules (little lumps) can appear under the skin.

Figure 3.5.
The right foot.

Plantar view

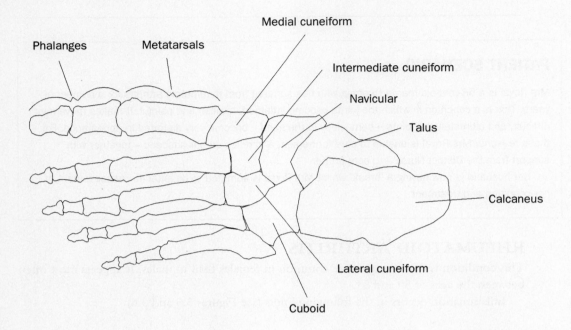

Medial view

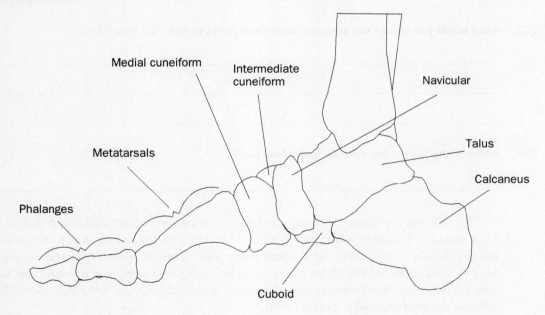

Figure 3.6.
The right hand.

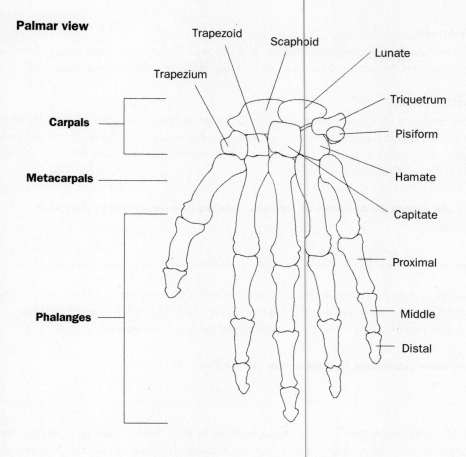

Palmar view

Trapezoid

Scaphoid

Trapezium

Lunate

Triquetrum

Pisiform

Hamate

Capitate

Carpals

Metacarpals

Phalanges

Proximal

Middle

Distal

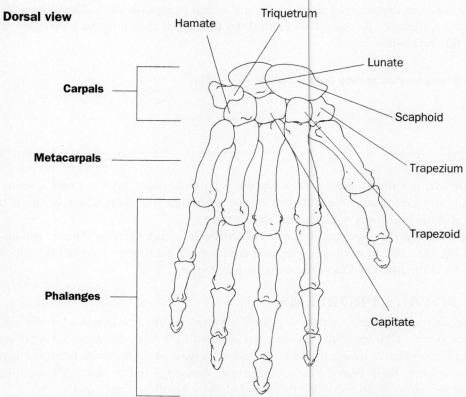

Dorsal view

Hamate

Triquetrum

Lunate

Scaphoid

Trapezium

Trapezoid

Capitate

Carpals

Metacarpals

Phalanges

The causes

The precise cause of rheumatoid arthritis is unknown. There have been many theories; they include stress, hypersensitivity, chronic or acute infection and autoimmunity.

Autoimmunity

A lot of evidence favours autoimmunity as a cause of rheumatoid arthritis. The word 'autoimmune' literally means that the immune system attacks the body ('auto' or self). Normally, the immune system can distinguish between self and non-self (i.e. foreign invaders such as bacteria and viruses).

Q35. **Bacteria and viruses are all known as antigens. How are they recognised by the body?**
📖 *Page 700*

Why, then, does the immune system attack the self? The exact details of this are not fully understood. But it is probable that the B lymphocytes *(📖 Pages 698–9)* make a mistake. They do this because body cells also have particular surface features.

Q36. **What are these cell-surface features known as?** 📖 *Page 701*

It is likely, therefore, that B lymphocytes lock on to these MHCs and try to destroy certain body cells – on the assumption that they are antigens. It is known that this happens, for example, when an organ is transplanted from one human being to another. This is the problem of organ rejection. Recipients are given drugs to suppress their immune system, and so prevent this from happening.

Q37. **How do B lymphocytes destroy body cells?** 📖 *Page 708*

Quite why this autoimmune process happens is not fully understood, nor why it should attack only certain tissues. Measurement of the antibodies (the rheumatoid factor) in a sample of blood is one way of diagnosing the condition.

One thing is certain, though: the effects of **antibody attack** 📖 *Page 708* and **phagocytosis** 📖 *Page 694* are both damaging and crippling for the patient. Pain and loss of full movement in the hands and feet can persist for many years.

MRS ROYAL'S PROBLEMS

Mrs Royal's major problem is that of painful inflamed joints. The first line of care and treatment is rest. With rest, pain becomes less acute and the body can focus on repairing damaged tissue without having to cope with the extra stress of dealing with factors such as tiredness and overwork. Nursing can, for example, encourage rest by limiting noise on a ward and perhaps tactfully restricting prolonged visits by friends and next-of-kin.

A disease like rheumatoid arthritis seems to run its course and over the years becomes less active and 'burns out'. The remainder of this chapter will help you to understand Mrs Royal's problems and the rationale for care and treatment.

Q38. **As part of her treatment, Mrs Royal may be prescribed a wrist splint; this will help to prevent flexion contractures – what are these?**

_____

_____

_____

_____

Q39. **What else can help to strengthen the wrist muscles?**

_____

_____

_____

Q40. **From your knowledge of joints, what movements should Mrs Royal's wrists be capable of?**

_____

Q41. **Mrs Royal may be prescribed aspirin (acetyl salicylic acid) tablets for pain relief. These work by inhibiting prostaglandin synthesis. What role do prostaglandins play in rheumatoid arthritis?**

_____

_____

_____

Q42.   Mrs Royal may also be prescribed steroids, which is the pharmacological name for the glucocorticoids. What are the actions of these?

_____

_____

_____

_____

Q43.   From your knowledge of steroids (📖 _Pages 545–6_) can you name four side-effects that Mrs Royal is likely to suffer from?

_____

_____

_____

Q44.   An additional problem that Mrs Royal is likely to face in taking steroids is that she shouldn't suddenly stop taking them, and if she is unwell at all, then she should consult the doctor. These two precautions are necessary, because of the way in which the release of glucocorticoids is controlled. What is the nature of this?

_____

_____

_____

Q45.   Another line of therapy for Mrs Royal may be the application of heat (sun lamp) or cold (ice packs). Can you predict the mechanism by which these may work?

_____

_____

_____

_____

Q46. What aspects of psychological reassurance may Mrs Royal require – and why?

_____

_____

_____

_____

Q47. If Mrs Royal is in a stable psychological state, then she is more likely to become compliant with her treatment, e.g. taking the correct amount of tablets at the right time. Why is this compliance important?

_____

_____

_____

_____

Q48. Whilst rest in bed is a fundamental aspect of treatment, it is not without its problems. For example, too much rest can cause contractures. Can you predict what problems may arise with bones and skin, during prolonged bedrest?

_____

_____

_____

_____

QUESTIONS FOR DISCUSSION

1. Devise a care plan for Mrs Royal that identifies problems, goals and nursing actions for each activity of daily living.

2. Compare and contrast osteoarthritis with rheumatoid arthritis.

3. Name three other autoimmune diseases and briefly discuss their features.

4. Enkephalins and endorphins are neuropeptides; name three other substances in this group and state their actions.

5. Discuss the full range of side-effects that can arise from taking steroids, and, based on these, devise an educational approach that would be appropriate for Mrs Royal.

Answers to questions

Q1.   Essentially all do. For example, muscles need intact bones for movement to occur; bones are the site of blood formation; bones provide protection for viscera of the nervous, digestive, urinary, reproductive, cardiovascular, respiratory and endocrine systems; broken bones can injure integument.

Q2.   Cartilage, bone (osseous) tissue, bone marrow and periosteum.

Q3.

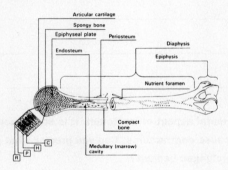

Q4.   a, intercellular material; b, 25; c, 50; d, tricalcium phosphate; e, calcium carbonate; f, hardness; g, tensile strength; h, collagen fibres; i, contains some spaces; provides channels for blood vessels and makes bones lighter in weight.

Q5.   a, humerus, (1); b, ulna (1); c, radius (1); d, carpals (8); e, metacarpals (5); f, phalanges (14).

Q6.   a, femur (1); b, patella (1); c, tibia (1); d, fibula (1), e, tarsals (7); f, metatarsals (5); g, phalanges (14).

Q7.   A point of contact between bones, cartilage and bones or between teeth and bones.

   a. Closeness with which bones fit together.
   b. Flexibility of binding tissues.
   c. Position of ligaments, muscles and tendons.

Q8.   Fibrous, cartilage, synovial.

Q9.   a, immoveable; b, amphiarthrosis; c, diarthrosis.

Q10. The space (synovial cavity) between the articulating bones and the absence of tissue between those bones (which might restrict movement) make the joints more freely moveable.

Q11.

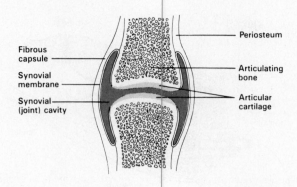

Fibrous capsule

Synovial membrane

Synovial (joint) cavity

Periosteum

Articulating bone

Articular cartilage

Q12.   1a, 4b, 5c, 3d, 2 and 5e.

Q13.   a. Pads of fibrocartilage between articular surfaces of bones maintain stability and allow bones to fit together.
b. Sacs lined by synovial membrane, filled with fluid and found between skin and bone, and between other structures, to allow movement.
c. Found within articular capsule but outside synovial cavity. Help stabilise joint.

Q14.   a. Interlocking shapes.
b. Strength and tension of ligaments.
c. Arrangement and tension of muscles.
d. Limit mobility – and so assist stability.

Q15.   Pa, Pb, Bc, Bd, He, Hf, Gg, Sh, E and Si.

Q16.   3a, 1b, 2c, 2d.

Q17.   a. Motion or movement.
b. Stabilising body positions, for example, maintaining posture and regulating organ volume, exemplified by contraction of the heart to pump out blood.
c. Generation of heat to alter body temperature.

Q18. Epimysium → perimysium → endomysium (See Figure 3.7.)

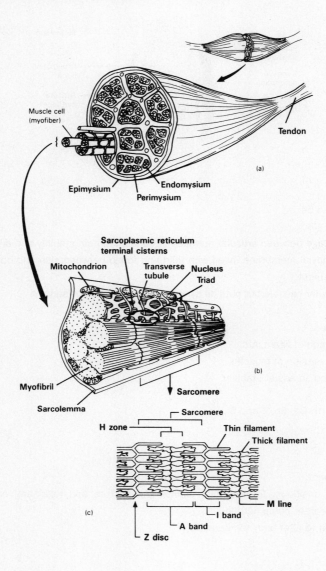

Figure 3.7. Diagram of a skeletal muscle. (a) Skeletal muscle cut to show cross section and longitudinal section with connective tissues. (b) Section of one muscle cell (myofibre). (c) Detail of sarcomere of muscle cell

Q19. a. Tendon attaches muscle to bone. Aponeurosis is a broad flat tendon that attaches to another muscle or skin.

b. Tendon sheaths enclose some tendons. They contain synovial fluid and permit tendons to slide back and forth more easily.

Q20. a, lever; b, fulcrum; c, resistance; d, muscle; e, effort; f, proximal; g, radius.

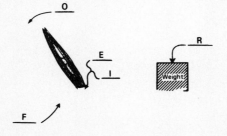

Q21.   *Non-specific* – protection against a variety of organisms; *specific* – protection against specific organisms.

Q22.   a, Lymphocytes; b, antigen presenting cells; c, from stem cells in bone marrow; d, T; e, perform immune functions against specific antigens if properly stimulated; CD8[+], antigen-receptor protein; h, bone marrow.

Q23.   CMI a, AMI b, AMI c, CMI d, AMI and CMI e.

Q24.   a, Is recognised as foreign; b, foreign substances; c, stimulate production of; d, react with (and potentially be destroyed by); e, complete antigen, or immunogen; f, hapten; g, reactivity; h, immunogenicity; i, body protein; j, allergic; k, large, complex molecules, such as proteins, nucleoproteins, lipoproteins, glycoproteins, or complex polysaccharides; l, they are made of simple, repeating subunits that are not likely to be antigenic; m, yes; n, flagella, capsules, cell walls, as well as toxins made by bacteria; o, Antigens; p, only a specific region of the; q, antigenic determinant (epitope); r, a number of.

Q25.   The point where two or more bones meet.

Q26.   Hinge joint.

Q27.   Ball and socket joint.

Q28.   Articulating bones, ligaments, muscles.

Q29.   Voluntary or striped.

Q30.   To manufacture antibodies.

Q31.   Molecules that attach to specific antigens and initiate destruction.

Q32.   Bacteria
Viruses
Foodstuffs
Chemicals
Anything foreign to the body.

Q33.   Red, painful, swollen and lacking in function. This is a characteristic response (inflammation) that the body exhibits in response to different types of damage, e.g. burns, bacterial invasion or insect bites.

Q34.   On the sides of the joints, away from the articular cartilage.

Q35.   Features on their surface – antigenic determinants – trigger antibody production.

Q36.   The major histocompatibility (MHC) antigens.

Q37.   By manufacturing antibodies which then attack the body cells (mistaking them for antigens); this produces the features of inflammation.

Q38.   A contracture is a permanent shortening of tendon and muscles that can arise because of immobility and lack of use. Patients who have had 'strokes' – if they have paralysed arms or legs – are also at risk of developing contractures in these limbs.

Flexion means to bring the bones – that make up the joint – closer together, as in bending the wrist. The joint then becomes fixed in this position, and is no longer of any functional value.

Mrs Royal's wrist is painful and so she is not inclined to use it very much and this is why a contracture may develop. A wrist splint would prevent this and would also provide support for activities such as cooking or typing.

Splints can also be used on the leg. Aids such as a long-handled comb or shoehorn can also be supplied to help Mrs Royal with her activities of daily living.

Q39. Exercises will help strengthen muscle power at the joints and in addition will stop muscles from wasting away. This is another example of the biological principle that states that if you don't use it then you lose it.

Mrs Royal's muscles will waste away because her joints are painful and she is not inclined to use them.

Patients who have had strokes or who are paralysed for other reasons, such as accidents, will also suffer from muscle wasting, unless they exercise.

The physiotherapist is the person who instigates limb movements and these regimes need to be carried on by the nurses at other times of the day. For example, a person who is paralysed and cannot move their limbs will require *passive exercises*. The limb needs to be put through its full range of movements, hence the importance of knowing the range of joint movements, as shown in, for example, 📖 *Page 223. Figure 9.3 & Page 225, Figure 9.5.*

The other reason that Mrs Royal's muscle mass may decline is that as we grow older, muscles start to *atrophy* (decrease in size).

Q40. Flexion, extension
Abduction, adduction
Circumduction
Try these movements for yourself. See 📖 *Exhibit 9.3 (Page 231) & Figures 9.3, 9.5 (Pages 222, 223, 225).*

Q41. Prostaglandins, along with other chemicals (📖 *Page 696)* contribute to producing the characteristic features of inflammation:
Pain
Redness
Heat
Swelling
Loss of function

The vasodilatation and increased capillary permeability that underlies this reaction can thus be prevented by suppressing the production of prostaglandins. Thus, in addition to pain relief, aspirin also helps quell the inflammatory process.

Aspirin also inhibits blood clotting. At least one major study has shown that this could be useful as a preventive measure in coronary thrombosis. This is a major cause of hospitalisation and mortality in middle aged men in westernised countries.

Other research suggests that a similar chemical, in red wine, will prevent blood clots from forming. The consumption of wine – particularly red – has a marked epidemiological correlation with reduction in heart attacks. For example, amongst French men, the incidence of coronary thrombosis is lower than in men in other countries. The only major difference between these groups appears to be the higher wine consumption in France.

However, aspirin has two side-effects that can limit its prolonged use. One is the erosion of the stomach lining, which can cause a **gastric ulcer**. The other is damage to the auditiory nerve (vestibulocochlear nerve; see 📖 *Page 490, Figure 16.19)* which results in a chronic ringing noise in the ears (**tinnitus**). Fortunately, there are other analgesics – without these side effects – that can be used. The so-called non steroidal anti-inflammatory drugs (NSAIDs).

Q42.   They have an anti-inflammatory action (📖 *Page 546*) and as such will, like aspirin, help to reduce the inflammation in Mrs Royal's joints. They do this by reducing mast cell numbers and phagocytosis.

However, steroids have many other actions that can give rise to side-effects. For this reason, steroids have been called a 'pharmacological blunderbuss'. They 'hit' many sites in the body, sometimes in what may seem an indiscriminate way.

Q43.   Delayed wound healing.
Mental disturbances.
Decreased resistance to infection.
Sodium and water retention – raised blood pressure.
Moon-shaped face.

Such signs and symptoms also occur in Cushing's syndrome, when the adrenal glands over-produce glucocorticoids (📖 *Page 547*). However, their occurence in patients who are taking pharmacological steroids has undoubtedly contributed to the observation that the treatment is sometimes worse than the disease.

Q44.   As the blood level of glucocorticoids rises – from adrenal gland secretion – so this suppresses the release of corticotrophin releasing hormone (CRH) from the hypothalamus, and also the release of adrenocorticotrophic hormone (ACTH) from the pituitary gland. This is an example of negative feedback control (📖 *Pages 10–11*).

ACTH stimulates the release of glucocorticoids, and without it there is no output of the these. Whilst Mrs Royal is taking steroids, her blood level is maintained, and ACTH release is suppressed. However, if she should suddenly stop taking the tablets, then her ACTH production would have to turn on immediately. But this it will not be able to do, because of the principle of, 'if you don't use it, then you lose it'. In other words, the ACTH production goes to sleep, as it were, and will take some days and possibly weeks, if she has been on the steroids for a long time, before it can come back into full production.

This can be compensated for if Mrs Royal is weaned off her steroids by, say, reducing the dosage gradually day by day. This will allow her ACTH and adrenal glands to come back into action. Stopping her steroids suddenly would mean a sudden reduction in glucocorticoid levels, and this could result in collapse and death (see Addison's disease, 📖 *Page 546*).

For the same reason, if Mrs Royal is ill, for example with flu or a chest infection, then her adrenal glands cannot step up production – as they would do in you or me. Instead, she needs to increase her steroid dose – under medical supervision.

Patients like Mrs Royal are given a card to carry with them at all times, which points out the importance of continuing to take the tablets and consulting the G.P. in case of illness. Thus, it would be an important part of Mrs Royal's education to explain to her the necessity, and reasons, for carrying this card.

Q45.   Hot water bottles, electric blankets and ice packs are traditional remedies for pain, injury and/or bruising. Indeed, they are advised in first aid e.g. take a bag of peas from the freezer and apply to a bruised limb.

It is possible that these remedies work by stimulating the release of endorphins (endogenous morphines) and **enkephalins**, which then function to inhibit painful impulses (see 📖 *Page 430 & Exhibit 14.4* for more details on enkephalins and endorphins).

It is suspected that pain-relieving methods, such as acupuncture and transcutaneous electrical nerve stimulation work in a similar way, that is, by stimulating nerves under the skin which then transmit nervous impulses to the spinal cord, and these lead to the release of the endorphins, etc. The painful impulses, from Mrs Royal's hands, are blocked at the level of the spinal cord and thus never reach conscious perception in the brain.

Q46.   Rest is the first principle of all treatment – and vital for patients like Mrs Royal, who are in pain. Adequate rest is both a physical and a mental state – and putting someone into bed does not necessarily guarantee the latter. Mrs Royal may worry about her home, her husband or job, and it is only through developing a relationship with her, and coming to know the details of her life, that a plan can be formulated to deal with these individual issues.

If Mrs Royal is mentally relaxed and comfortable about these matters, then this can influence her physical state. For example, it is well recognised – and proven by research – that reducing anxiety can also help decrease the amount of pain that a patient feels. It is possible that this works through the release of endorphins and enkephalins. The action of the mind on the body is called *psychosomatic* (psyche = mind, soma = body), although this term is usually reserved for its involvement in physical diseases that are supposedly caused by the mind, e.g. the role of mental stress in coronary artery disease or skin disease.

Q47. Compliance is important, because only if she strictly adheres to treatment regimes, can decisions be made about their effectiveness. On the basis of this, a particular line of treatment – or tablet – may be stopped or changed. The importance of complying with steroid treatment has already been discussed (Q44.).

Good information and communication can also help set realistic goals and expectations for the success of Mrs Royal's hospitalisation. If her sights are set at the correct level – and not over-optimistic or pessimistic – then false expectations can be avoided. From Mrs Royal's point of view, false expectations can only lead to frustration, stress and anger, when the high hopes do not materialise. This is probably particularly important in relation to surgical outcomes. Surgery is sometimes tried on diseased joints e.g. removing the diseased synovial membrane (synovectomy).

Q48. We have already seen in this chapter, and will see again in Chapters 12 and 13, examples of the biological principle of – don't use it and you lose it! Mrs Royal's bones will start to waste away (**atrophy**) if she remains confined to bed. In order to remain healthy, bones require to be physically stressed by movements, such as standing and walking. Without this, they thin out and become less dense as a result of losing some of their calcium. Thus, they are then more liable to fracture. This process can take some weeks and months, so a patient who is in bed for a few days or a week is not at risk.

The problem of bone atrophy and immobility has been indirectly recognised for many years as leading to the problem of kidney stones in patients who have suffered damage to the spinal cord and are paralysed. Because of immobility, the bones atrophy and the calcium that is released is then excreted via the kidneys. This excess calcium then becomes deposited in the urinary tract and forms stones.

Further evidence for this mechanism came as a result of the astronaut and space research programme in the 1960s. Prior to – and following – a journey into space, the astronauts would be medically examined and undergo blood tests. These were then repeated on return to Earth.

As a result, the blood calcium level was found to be higher on return to Earth. This was due to the cramped conditions, zero gravity and consequent lack of mobility on board the space ship. The astronaut's bones were thinning out and releasing calcium into the bloodstream.

One of the greatest dangers of bedrest – and the commonest – are pressure sores. As the name suggests, these can also occur as a result of pressure from chairs and trolleys. The skin will soon break down under pressure – perhaps in a matter of hours – and start to form an ulcer. The following chapter (The Cell, Tissues and Skin) looks at the causes, prevention and treatment of pressure sores.

From what has been said so far, it can be seen that there is often a fine line between the curative and pathological (disease) effects of rest. Figure 3.8 is a summary of the problems of bedrest.

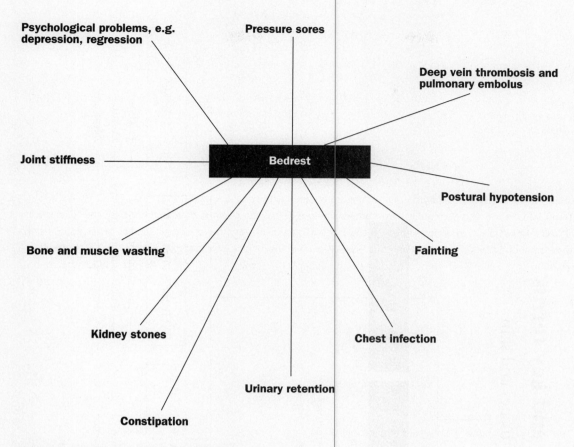

Figure 3.8. A summary of the problems of bedrest.

Overview and key terms

The cell, tissues and skin

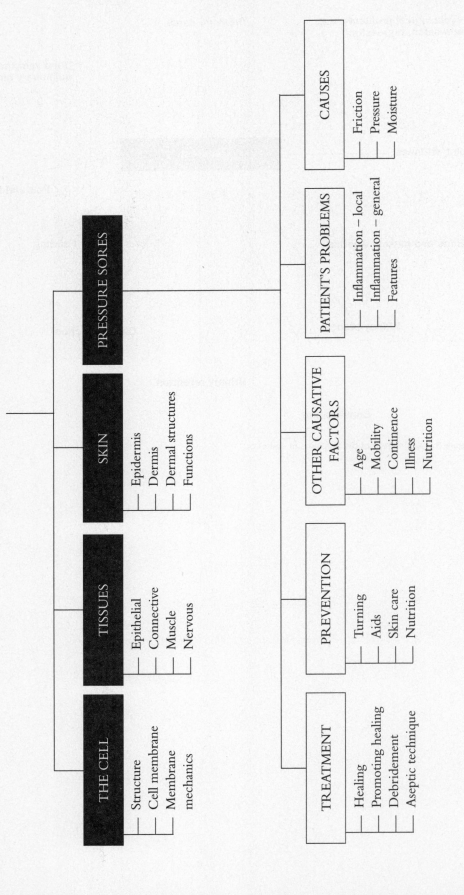

4. The Cell, Tissues and Skin

(The Integumentary System)

Learning outcomes

1. To learn those aspects of cells, tissues and the skin that are associated with pressure sores.

2. To define a 'pressure sore' and explain its causes and developmental stages.

3. To describe the local and general features of inflammation.

4. To explain the predisposing factors in the formation of pressure sores.

5. To discuss the principles of prevention in relation to pressure sores.

6. To discuss the principles of pressure sore treatment.

Chapters 3, 4, 5

INTRODUCTION

This chapter will deal with the cell, tissues and the skin. It will also continue with the a Patient Scenario about Mrs Royal, a 56-year-old woman who suffers from rheumatoid arthritis. Mrs Royal was prone to contractures and muscle weakness. This was partly because of her condition, but also as a result of bedrest. Although bedrest is a form of treatment, it is fraught with hazards, and these problems can afflict a great many other patients who may, for whatever reason, be confined to bed.

The prime purpose of this chapter is to consider the subject of pressure sores – perhaps the major hazard of bedrest – and look at exactly what they are, how they occur and how they can be prevented or treated. The first step in doing this is for you to tackle the following questions that are based on cells, tissues and the skin. Then follows the Scenario, some information about pressure sores and questions that will help you to extend that knowledge.

THE CELL *Pages 57–69*

Q1.   Label all of the parts of Figure 4.1, using the labels below.

Figure 4.1.
Generalised
animal cell.

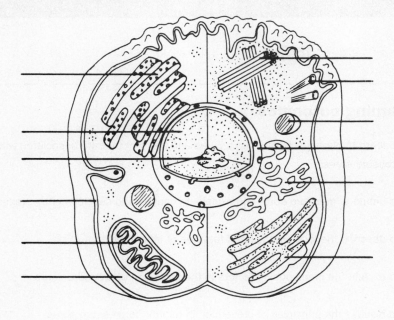

Granular (rough) endoplasmic reticulum	Centriole
Chromatin	Microtubule
Nucleolus	Lysosome
Plasma (cell) membrane	Nuclear membrane
Mitochondrion	Agranular (smooth) endoplasmic reticulum
Cytosol	Golgi complex

Q2.   Refer to *Page 59, Figure 3.2*, to complete the following exercise about the fluid mosaic model of the plasma membrane. Label the parts (a – e) on Figure 4.2, here. Now use the lines provided next to the name of each membrane part to write one or more functions for each part.

a. Phospholipid polar 'head' _____

b. Phospholipid nonpolar 'tail' _____

c. Integral protein _____

d. Glycoprotein _____

e. Cholesterol _____

Figure 4.2.
asma membrane,
ording to the fluid
mosaic model.

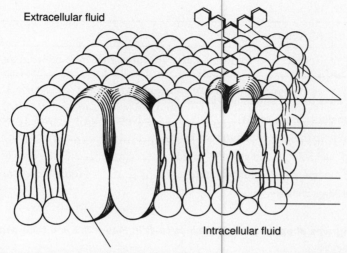

Extracellular fluid

Intracellular fluid

Q3. **Complete the following table about the mechanisms of movement of materials across membranes.**

Name of Process	What moves (particles or water)?	Direction, (e.g. high to low concentration)?	Membrane necessary (yes or no)?	Carrier necessary (yes or no)?	Active or passive?
a. Simple diffusion					
b.	Water	From high to low concentration of water across semi-permeable membrane			
c.		From high pressure area to low pressure area			
d. Facilitated diffusion					
e. Primary active transport		From low to high concentration of solute			
f. Phagocytosis			Yes		
g.	Water	From outside cell to inside cell			
h. Exocytosis					Active

TISSUES 📖 *Pages 97–120*

Q4.   Complete the table about the four main classes of tissues.

Tissue	General functions
Epithelial tissue	a.
Connective tissue	b.
c.	Movement
d.	Initiates and transmits nerve impulses that help coordinate body activities

Q5.   Describe the structure of epithelium in this exercise.

Epithelium consists mostly of (a) _____ (closely packed cells? intercellular material with few cells?). Epithelium is penetrated by (b) _____ (many? no?) blood vessels. A term meaning 'lacking in blood vessels' is (c) _____. Epithelium (d) _____ (has? lacks?) a nerve supply. Epithelium (e) _____ (does? does not?) have the capacity to undergo mitosis.

Q6.   Study the diagrams of epithelial tissue types (a–f) in Figure 3.3 and then write the name of each tissue.

Figure 4.3. Diagrams of different types of epithelial tissue.

a. _____

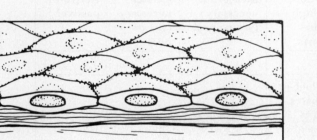

b. _____

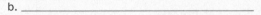
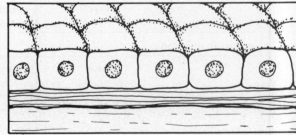

c. _____

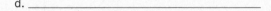
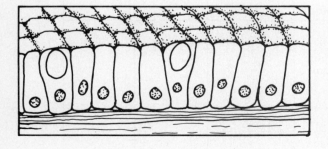

d. _____

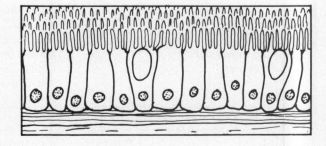

e. _____   f. _____

Q7.   **Check your understanding of the most common types of epithelium listed in the box by matching them with the phrases that describe them.**

> 1. Pseudostratified columnar 2. Simple squamous 3. Simple columnar, ciliated 4. Stratified squamous 5. Simple columnar, unciliated 6. Stratified transitional 7. Simple cuboidal

☐   a.   Lines the inner surface of the stomach and intestine.

☐   b.   Lines the urinary tract, as in the bladder, permitting distension.

☐   c.   Lines mouth; present on outer surface of skin.

☐   d.   Single layer of cube-shaped cells; found in kidney tubules and ducts of some glands.

☐   e.   Lines air sacs of lungs where thin cells are required for diffusion of gases into blood.

☐   f.   Not a true stratified epithelium; all cells on basement membrane, but some do not reach surface of tissue.

☐   g.   Endothelium and mesothelium contain this.

Q8.   **Keratin is a (carbohydrate? protein?). What is its function?**

_____

_____

Q9.   **List three locations of nonkeratinized stratified squamous epithelium.**

_____

_____

THE SKIN 📖 *Pages 127–37*

Q10. **Answer these questions about the two parts of skin. Label them (bracketed regions) on Figure 4.4.**

The outer layer is named the (a) _____. It is composed of (b) _____ (connective tissue? epithelium?). The inner portion of skin, called the (c) _____, is made of (d) _____ (connective tissue? epithelium?). The dermis is (e) _____ (thicker? thinner?) than the epidermis.

Q11. **Most sensory receptors, nerves, blood vessels and glands are embedded in the (epidermis? dermis?). Label all the lines on the right side of Figure 4.4, using the following:**

Arrector pili (hair) muscle

Blood vessel

Hair follicle

Sebaceous (oil) gland

Sudoriferous (sweat) gland

Touch (Meissner's) receptor

Pressure (lamellated or Pacinian) corpuscle

Nerve

Figure 4.4.
Structure of the skin.

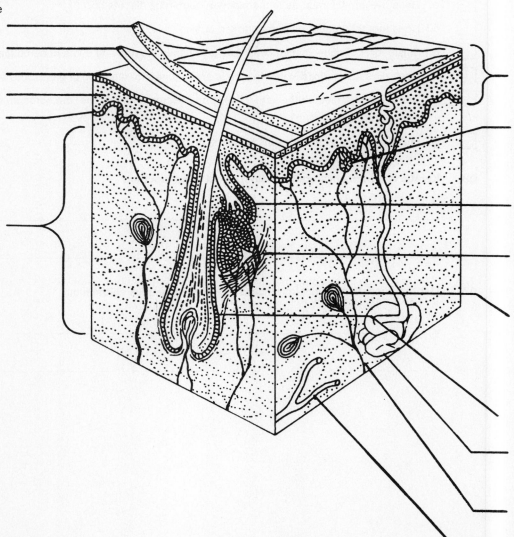

Q12.   The tissue underlying skin is called subcutaneous, meaning (a) _____ . This layer is also called (b) _____ . It consists of two types of tissue, (c) _____ and (d) _____ . What functions does subcutaneous tissue serve?

_____

Q13.   Skin may be one of the most underestimated organs in the body. What functions does your skin perform while it is 'just lying there' covering your body? List seven functions.

_____

_____

_____

Q14.   Label each of the five layers on the left side of Figure 4.4

Q15.   In which areas of the body are Sebaceous Glands largest?

_____

Q16.   Describe the composition of perspiration (sweat) and state its functions.

_____

_____

Q17.   Check your understanding of skin glands by stating whether the following descriptions refer to sebaceous, sudoriferous, or ceruminous glands.

a.   Sweat glands _____ .

b.   Glands leading directly to a hair follicle; secrete sebum, which keeps hair and skin from drying out _____ .

c.   Line the outer ear canal; secrete earwax _____ .

CHECKPOINTS EXERCISE

Q18. During cell division, chromatin becomes visible and is known as what?

_____

Q19. What are the functions of chromosomes and their constituent parts, the genes?

_____

Q20. What type of tissue makes up the skin?

_____

Q21. In what parts of the body would you expect to find heavily keratinised epithelium?

_____

Q22. The epidermis is unusual in that it is a part of the body that does not contain any what?

_____

Q23. What is the effect on the skin of excessive washing and sebum removal?

_____

PATIENT SCENARIO

Mrs Royal had been admitted to hospital both to give her husband a rest and to have her condition re-assessed. Mrs Royal suffers from rheumatoid arthritis, a painful and crippling condition of the hands and other joints. Because of this condition, Mrs Royal has problems with mobility and relies on others to help move her into and out of bed. She also requires assistance to move into different positions in bed. For these reasons, Mrs Royal is apt to remain immobile for lengthy periods of time. As a result, she is now developing a pressure sore.

The remainder of this chapter will deal with pressure sores. It will examine what they are, why they occur and how they can be prevented and treated. This discussion will once again be related to normal bodily structure and function. Also, topics in other chapters, will be brought in, to help explain the rationale for the care of pressure sores. For example, on the **inflammatory process** and **wound healing**.

Figure 4.5.
Shearing forces and
pressure points in a
semi-recumbent
patient.

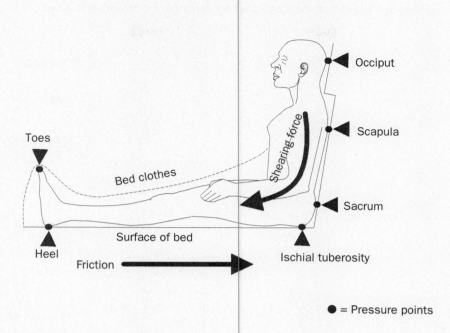

= Pressure points

PRESSURE SORES

These arise on the skin surface because of the effects of pressure – particularly over bony prominences. They used to be called 'bedsores', which indicated their chief causative factor. But it is now recognized that sustained pressure from a chair, trolley or operating table can equally well cause the damage.

A pressure sore represents damage to the skin cells, resulting either from direct pressure – which squeezes blood away from the skin surface – or from shearing forces. The latter occur when the skin is stretched against a firm surface; imagine a patient's sacral region shearing against the bed surface when they sit in an upright position. This damage will initially result in a skin abrasion, but if it is prolonged and unrelieved, a deep **ulcer crater** can develop. Figure 4.5 shows the main pressure points and shearing forces in a patient who is sitting in bed. The majority of pressure sores occur on the sacrum and heels.

Classification of pressure sore types

There are various ways in which authors and researchers have attempted to classify pressure sores. The most common is according to visual severity:

(1) The skin is permanently discoloured – perhaps reddened or blistered, but the skin is not broken.
(2) The epidermis is broken.
(3) There is destruction of the skin but not the underlying tissues.
(4) Both skin and underlying tissues are damaged, and a cavity is formed.

Q24. What tissues underlie the dermis? *Page 130*

Figure 4.6 shows that the major sites for sores are the sacrum and heels.

Figure 4.6.
A survey of pressure sore positions (J. A. David (1983). An investigation of the current methods used in nursing for the care of patients with established pressure sores. Nursing practice research unit. Northwich Park Hospital and Clinical Research Centre.)

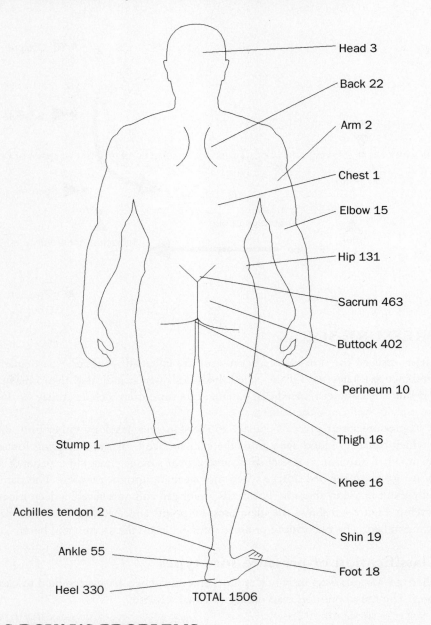

Head 3

Back 22

Arm 2

Chest 1

Elbow 15

Hip 131

Sacrum 463

Buttock 402

Perineum 10

Thigh 16

Knee 16

Shin 19

Foot 18

Stump 1

Achilles tendon 2

Ankle 55

Heel 330

TOTAL 1506

MRS ROYAL'S PROBLEMS

Q25. Which structures in the dermis, if compressed, are likely to lead to pressure sore formation?

_____

_____

_____

_____

Q26. When the skin is damaged by pressure or by burns, chemicals or microbial invasion, then it reacts in a characteristic way. What is this known as, and what are its features? 📖 *Page 695*

_____

_____

_____

Q27. Describe the underlying physiological changes that give rise to the features of inflammation.

_____

_____

_____

_____

Q28. These changes are all localised, but Mrs Royal is also likely to develop a rise in body temperature. Why is this? 📖 *Page 856*

_____

_____

_____

_____

Q29. What will you be able to observe about Mrs Royal when her temperature starts to fall? What nursing measures can support this?

_____

_____

_____

_____

Q30. **How is Mrs Royal likely to feel when her body temperature is raised?**

_____

_____

_____

_____

FACTORS IN THE FORMATION OF PRESSURE SORES

We have already noted pressure and shearing forces as the principal direct causes of sores. But is there anything else that can (perhaps indirectly) predispose Mrs Royal to developing pressure sores?

Surveys of the incidence of pressure sores in hospitals have been carried out. From these it is seen that the incidence of sores can be variable – from 2% to 8% of all patients. The distribution of sores is highest amongst patients with the following characteristics:

Age

There is an increase in the prevalence of pressure sores as age increases. Skin becomes less elastic as we grow older.

Mobility

The incidence of sores increases as patient mobility decreases. The incidence is particularly high in those patients who are paralysed and unable to move. In this respect, Mrs Royal is particularly at risk. Also, patients who are confused or unconscious are also likely to be mostly immobile.

Continence

Incontinent patients are more likely to develop sores. Urine and faeces undoubtedly damage the skin and thus predispose it to breakdown.

Concurrent illness

Certain groups of patients seem to be predisposed to pressure sores. For example, **orthopaedic patients** – perhaps with broken limbs – do not move very much, or can find it difficult. Patients with diseases of the blood vessels also have an increased incidence – perhaps because the skin does not receive an adequate supply of O_2 and nutrients. Mrs Royal's arteries may not be in the best of condition both because of her illness and because of her age.

Patients suffering from **neurological disorders** are often unconscious/semi-conscious and/or paralysed – thus they are not inclined to move around and ease the pressure on their skin.

Nutrition

This does not seem to affect sore development directly, but it does contribute to general health and so may have an effect. It certainly has an effect on pressure sore healing, because of the necessity for **protein** and **calories**, in order to build new skin, as well as **vitamin C**, which has long been associated with wound healing.

All of these factors have been combined into pressure-sore risk assessment scales, such as the **Norton scale** (Table 4.1). There is an almost linear relationship between the score that can be obtained, and the risk of developing a sore. Patients with a score of 14 or less are at risk. Those scoring less than 12 are particularly at risk. Thus, the nurse can use this scale to assess patients and so target preventive measures on those most at risk.

Table 4.1. The Norton scale.

Physical condition	Mental state	Activity	Mobility	Incontinence
Good 4	Alert 4	Ambulant 4	Full 4	None 4
Fair 3	Apathetic 3	Walks with	Slightly	Occasional 3
Poor 2	Confused 2	help 3	limited 3	Usually
Very bad 1	Stuporous 1	Chairbound 2	Very	urinary 2
		Bedfast 1	limited 2	Double 1
			Immobile 1	

Q31. **Mrs Royal is in reasonably good condition, having been looked after by her husband; however, what would you put her Norton score at?**

_____

Whilst these assessments are subjective – a different nurse may reach a different score – they are useful in helping to concentrate efforts on what is a major problem in today's Health Service. Figure 4.7 (next page) provides a summary of factors involved in pressure sore development.

Q32. **Based on what you know of the causes of pressure sores, what is the most important aspect of pressure sore prevention for Mrs Royal?**

_____

_____

_____

_____

Q33. **What else can be done to help prevent the development of pressure sores in Mrs Royal?**

_____

_____

_____

_____

_____

Figure 4.7.
A summary of
factors involved in
pressure sore
development.

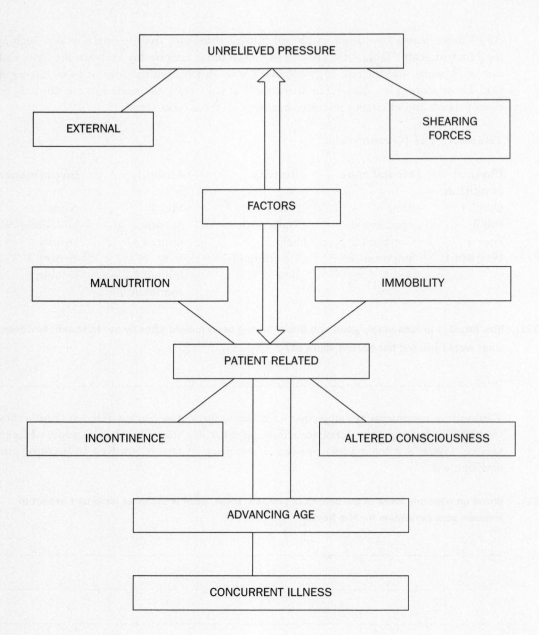

Q34.   **Should Mrs Royal start to develop a sore, then the skin will start to redden and turn a dark plum colour. What is this due to?** 📖 *Pages 695–6*

_____

_____

_____

Q35. Once Mrs Royal's pressure sore starts to heal, then it will go through various phases (📖 *Pages 136–7*). Briefly describe these.

_____

_____

_____

_____

_____

Q36. What part of Mrs Royal's treatment is likely to have an effect on the healing of her pressure sore?

_____

_____

_____

Q37. What factors will help promote the healing of a pressure sore?

_____

_____

_____

_____

QUESTIONS FOR DISCUSSION

1. Are there any situations in hospital in which patients are more at risk of developing pressure sores? How can this risk be minimised?

2. Are there any other factors which could be added to the Norton scale to improve its accuracy? Does research into pressure-sore risk-assessment scales indicate that any one scale is the best?

3. What research evidence is there that cushions, pads and sheepskins are effective in relieving pressure? Is any one type better than the other?

4. Compare and contrast the following dressing materials in relation to their usefulness in treating a sacral pressure sore:

Hydrocolloids
Polyurethane foam
Alginates
Non-adherent dressings

5. With reference to their actions, discuss what evidence there is that some lotions may be better than others in treating pressure sores.

Answers to questions

Q1.

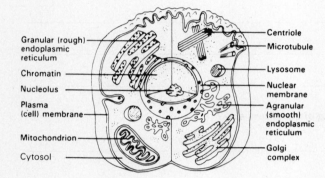

Q2.

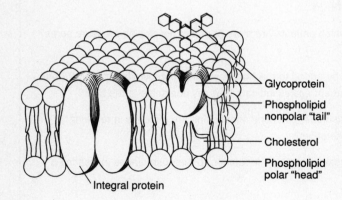

Q3.

Name of process	What moves (particles or water)?	Direction (e.g. high to low concentration)?	Membrane necessary (yes or no)?	Carrier necessary (yes or no)?	Active or passive?
a. Simple diffusion	Particles or water	From high to low concentration of solute	No	No	Passive
b. Osmosis	Water	From high to low concentration of water across semi-permeable membrane	Yes	No	Passive
c. Filtration	Particles or water	From high pressure area to low pressure area	Yes (or other barrier, such as filter paper)	No	Passive
d. Facilitated diffusion	Particles such as glucose	From high to low concentration of solute	Yes	Yes	Passive
e. Primary active transport	Solutes such as glucose or ions (Na+, K+)	From low to high concentration of solute	Yes	Yes	Active
f. Phagocytosis	Large particles	From outside of cell to inside of cell	Yes	No	Active
g. Pinocytosis	Water	From outside of cell to inside of cell	Yes	No	Active
h. Exocytosis	Large molecules or particles	From inside of cell to outside of cell	Yes	No	Active

Q4. a. Covers and lines the body.

b. Binds, supports and protects the body. Blood acts as a transport system.

c. Muscle.

d. Nervous tissue.

Q5. a, Closely packed cells; b, No; c, avascular; d, has; e, does.

Q6. a. Simple squamous epithelium.

b. Simple cuboidal epithelium.

c. Simple columnar epithelium (unciliated).

d. Simple columnar epithelium (ciliated).

e. Stratified squamous epithelium.

f. Pseudostratified columnar epithelium, ciliated.

Q7. 5a, 6b, 4c, 7d, 2e, 1f, 2g.

Q8. Protein; waterproofs, resists friction, and repels bacteria.

Q9. Examples of locations: wet surfaces such as lining of the mouth, tongue, oesophagus, and parts of epiglottis and vagina.

Q10. a, Epidermis; b, epithelium;
c, dermis; d, connective tissue;
e, thicker.

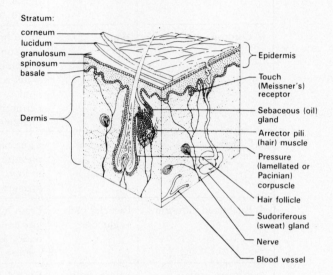

Stratum:
corneum
lucidum
granulosum
spinosum
basale

Dermis

Epidermis

Touch (Meissner's) receptor

Sebaceous (oil) gland

Arrector pili (hair) muscle

Pressure (lamellated or Pacinian) corpuscle

Hair follicle

Sudoriferous (sweat) gland

Nerve

Blood vessel

Q11. Dermis. See figure above.

Q12. a, Under the skin; b, superficial fascia or hypodermis; c, areolar; d, adipose. Anchors skin to underlying tissues and organs.

Q13. 1. Regulates body temperature.
2. Protects.
3. Detects sensations.
4. Excretion.
5. Immunity.
6. Blood reservoirs.
7. Synthesis of vitamin D

Q14. See figure above.

Q15. Breast, face, neck and upper chest.

Q16. Composed of water, NaCl, urea, uric acid, ammonia, sugar, lactic and ascorbic acid. It helps to regulate body temperature.

Q17. a. Sudoriferous.
b. Sebaceous.
c. Ceruminous.

Q18. Chromosomes.

Q19. The genes direct the synthesis of proteins inside the cell.

Q20. Stratified squamous epithelium.

Q21. On the soles of the feet or toes as 'hard skin'. Possibly on the hands, in manual workers.

Q22. Blood vessels.

Q23. It will become dry and possibly reddened, and start to crack. Cream can help prevent this by replacing the washed out sebum.

Q24. A variable amount of fat and muscle.

Q25. The capillaries. Pressure within them is quite low (20–40mmHg; (📖 *Page 631)* and sustained pressure will oppose this and disrupt blood flow. Without blood bringing O_2 and nutrients and removing CO_2 and waste products, the skin cells will start to die. Healthy people avoid this by regular movement – think of sitting on a hard chair for a long period of time.

The other factor that will disrupt blood supply to the skin is friction (shearing forces). These will tear delicate capillaries, and this will release blood into the tissues. Once blood loses its O_2 it will turn the skin a purple, plum colour. The shearing force can also physically strip away the skin, in the same way, but not quite so quickly, as a graze will occur as a result of a fall.

Shearing forces seem to be more effective on skin that is damp – from perspiration or urine. Hence, incontinent patients are at an increased risk of developing pressure sores.

Q26. This is the inflammatory reaction. The affected area is red, swollen, warm, and painful, and there is loss of function. This is a homeostatic response, in that it is the body's way of trying to dispose of dead tissue or microbes and promote tissue repair.

Q27. Firstly there is **vasodilatation** (vaso=vessel; dilatation=widening). This leads to an increased blood flow to the tissues, and thus the skin becomes a red colour (**hyperaemia**). This would be the first sign of a pressure sore developing, and as such would be an important nursing observation. There are several substances that contribute to vasodilatation, including histamine and prostaglandins *(📖 Page 692).*

In addition to dilatation, the capillaries also become increasingly permeable. As a result, cells and large molecules such as figrinogen escape through the capillary wall into the tissues. The release of fibrinogen promotes clotting *(📖 Page 530)* and this traps microbes, etc. at the site. Antibodies *(📖 Page 702)* will attack the microbes, and white blood cells will act as phagocytes (Phagus = to eat) and engulf and destroy the microbes. The increased capillary permeability also allows water to escape into the tissues, and this results in swelling.

The result of this inflammatory process is the production of **pus**. This is composed of water, dead skin cells and microbes. This can be seen on a small scale at the site of infected pimples and boils.

Q28. A rise in body temperature (fever or pyrexia) is a fundamental sign of inflammation. Bacteria release chemicals called toxins, which travel in the bloodstream. In the hypothalamus *(📖 Page 855)* is found the centre controlling the body temperature. It is here that the toxins interfere.

The 'thermostat' is re-set by the toxins, to a higher figure – say 39°C. The control centre then starts to raise body temperature to this new level. Hence, the patient feels cold and starts to shiver (the muscles are producing heat by undergoing involuntary movements).

Hormonal changes from adrenaline and thyroxine *(📖 Pages 538 and 548)* start to speed up metabolism and thus heat production. Mrs Royal will feel the necessity to warm up in bed with extra blankets, etc.

When a patient complains of feeling cold, then their body temperature is rising. A raised body temperature may 'break' spontaneously, or we can take a drug such as aspirin, which will help lower the body temperature by interfering with prostaglandin production. This is involved in resetting the hypothalamic thermostat.

Q29. There are three changes that will be observable (apart from a visible thermometer reading):

(1) Vasodilatation will bring blood and heat to the skin, making it appear pink or red.
(2) Perspiration will extract heat from the skin, in evaporation.
(3) Behavioural changes. Mrs Royal may shed her dressing gown and/or blankets.

Perspiration can be assisted by **tepid sponging**. This means using flannels dipped in tepid water and applied to the body. This, together with a fan, will encourage heat loss from the body. It is important to use tepid water because the use of ice water would produce vasoconstriction – the body's response to cold – and thus drive blood (and heat) into the core of the body. This would delay heat loss from the body. When Mrs Royal's temperature reaches 37°C then the hypothalamus will switch off the above mechanisms. This type of control is another example of negative feedback (📖 *Page 10 and Figure 5.7, Page 138*).

All of this begs the question – What is the purpose of a rise in body temperature? Firstly, it seems to intensify the effect of **interferon** on the destruction of viruses. Also, antibody and T cell production increase (📖 *Pages 705–8*). In addition, bacterial growth is inhibited by high temperatures.

Also, blood flow increases and thus the delivery of white blood cells (phagocytes) will improve. Finally, high temperatures increase the rate of chemical reactions, and tissue repair mechanisms may thus be increased.

Q30. Malaise is a characteristic feature of all illnesses that involve an infection and a rise in body temperature. Think about how you feel if you contract influenza. Perhaps this is our body's own way of ensuring rest, and thus channelling all its resources into the body defences (immune system) and repair process. Accompanying these feelings of listlessness, is often a very much reduced and poor appetite. Patients, like Mrs Royal, will often need a lot of enticement and coaxing in order to ensure that sufficient calories and proteins are ingested. These are important if her sore is to heal.

Unfortunately, the disadvantage with malaise is that it makes the patient reluctant to move – and this will in turn perhaps lead to other pressure sores; and the complications of bedrest. However, treatment with drugs such as aspirin will not only reduce the temperature but also make Mrs Royal feel less lethargic and more like moving.

Figure 4.8 provides a summary of the features of inflammation.

Q31. 13 to 16. Thus she is on the border of being at risk.

Q32. Regular movement will prevent any effects of unrelieved pressure. This needs to be done regularly during both the day and the night. If Mrs Royal is unable to move herself, then it is an important nursing function to carry this out for her. It has been said that a nurse can put anything on a pressure area – except the patient.

Mrs Royal will need help – and pain relief – in order to turn successfully from side to side in bed. Also, it is important for her to get up and out of bed.

Figure 4.8. A summary of the features of inflammation.

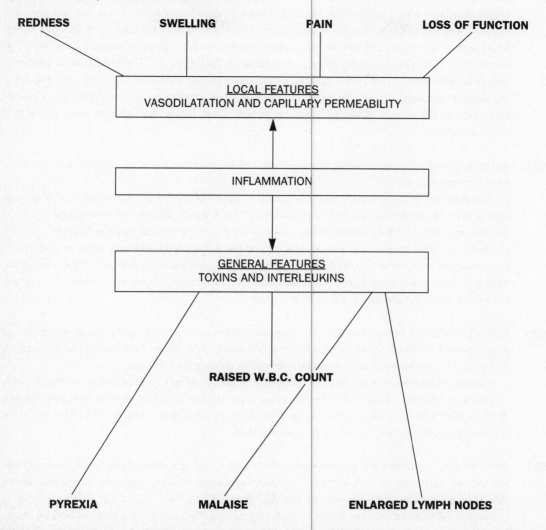

Q33. A soft mattress or a cushion is a vital element in relieving the effects of pressure on the skin. The so-called ripple mattress consists of air cells that alternately inflate and deflate, and this helps to redistribute the effects of pressure on someone, like Mrs Royal, who finds it difficult to move.

Sheepskins are also used. It is claimed that they reduce the accumulation of moisture on the skin – a major factor in sore formation. For this reason the skin should be kept clean and dry. The use of a barrier cream – which applies a waterproof layer to the skin – may be useful if Mrs Royal becomes incontinent.

Traditionally, nurses have massaged the skin with soap and water, in the hope of improving the circulation. However, there is evidence that this may do more harm than good, by disrupting the small capillaries in the skin and thus contributing to sore formation. Excessive washing of the skin will remove the oily secretion of the sebaceous glands, and this is likely to make the skin crack and break more easily.

Nutritional factors are important in maintaining a healthy skin. Protein is necessary for skin to regenerate and repair, because it is the major structural component. Vitamins A, B₆ and C are also necessary for healthy skin. Also, Mrs Royal is taking steroids (glucocorticoids) *(Page 545)* to reduce the inflammation of her arthritis. These will stimulate the breakdown of protein and new skin. This would lead to delayed healing, should a sore develop.

Q34. It is blood beneath the skin. Red blood cells escape from damaged capillaries and then, losing their oxygen, they turn a dark colour (📖 *Page 570*) deoxygenated haemoglobin). Over the next few days the red cells and haemoglobin are broken down, and removed from the site by phagocytes (white blood cells). The progress of this can be followed by observing the colour changes in the skin. The haemoglobin is broken down into bilirubin and biliverdin (📖 *Page 573*) and the skin turns from a dark to a yellow color. (The same pigments turn the skin yellow in jaundice.) Over the next few days, the yellow fades away. This is the same process that is seen in the resolution of damage (a bruise) elsewhere on the skin. If, however, pressure remains, then further damage may keep the skin a red/plum colour.

Q35. (i) *The inflammatory phase* – during which a blood clot forms in the wound to unite the wound edges. Vasodilatation also occurs.

(ii) *The migratory phase* – the clot forms a scab and epithelial cells migrate beneath it to bridge the wound. Scar tissue forms and blood vessels regrow. Thus it should appear pink and healthy.

(iii) *The proliferative phase* – epithelial cells, scar tissue and blood vessels continue to grow.

(iv) *The maturation phase* – the scab breaks off and the epidermis is renewed. Blood vessels return to normal, and thus the wound turns from a pink to a more pale colour. A pink appearance during the healing process is a healthy sign, because it means that blood (with oxygen and nutrients) is reaching the wound. Thus, the conditions for repair are present.

Q36. The fact that she is taking steroids (corticosteroids) will lead to a delay, and possibly disruption, of wound healing. Steroids utilise protein for heat and energy (📖 *Pages 545–6*). This is unusual, as protein is normally reserved as a structural material for building body tissues.

However, when steroid levels are high – through medication or as a general feature of stress, such as illness or accident – then protein can be converted to glucose. The latter is then available as extra 'fuel' for body cells, at what may be a time of crisis for the body. But in Mrs Royal's case, this state is maintained permanently, by her taking steroid tablets.

Q37. Adequate rest is probably the cornerstone of all treatment, and is a prerequisite for all forms of healing and recovery; vitamin C, from fresh fruit and vegetables, is also necessary for wound healing (📖 *Page 852*), as are minerals such as zinc (📖 *Page 849*).

Surgical intervention can also assist in promoting healing. For example, the removal of dead tissue (**debridement**) with a scalpel, under anaesthetic, is necessary when a lot of dead tissue is present in a wound. This can be followed by the use of sterile dressing materials (**aseptic technique**). In addition, the wound can be swabbed with antiseptics, such as saline, when the dressing is renewed. If there is any infection in the wound, then Mrs Royal can be given **antibiotics** (e.g. penicillin) to help kill these off. Figure 4.9 provides a summary of the principles of pressure sore prevention and treatment.

Figure 4.9. Pressure sores: A summary of prevention and treatment

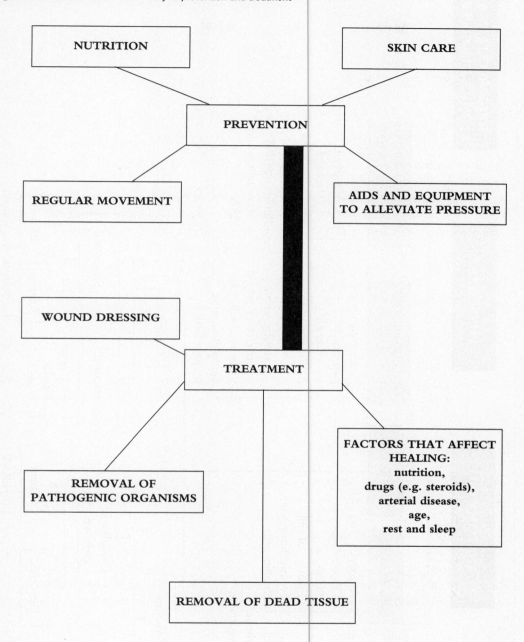

Overview and key terms

Nervous tissue

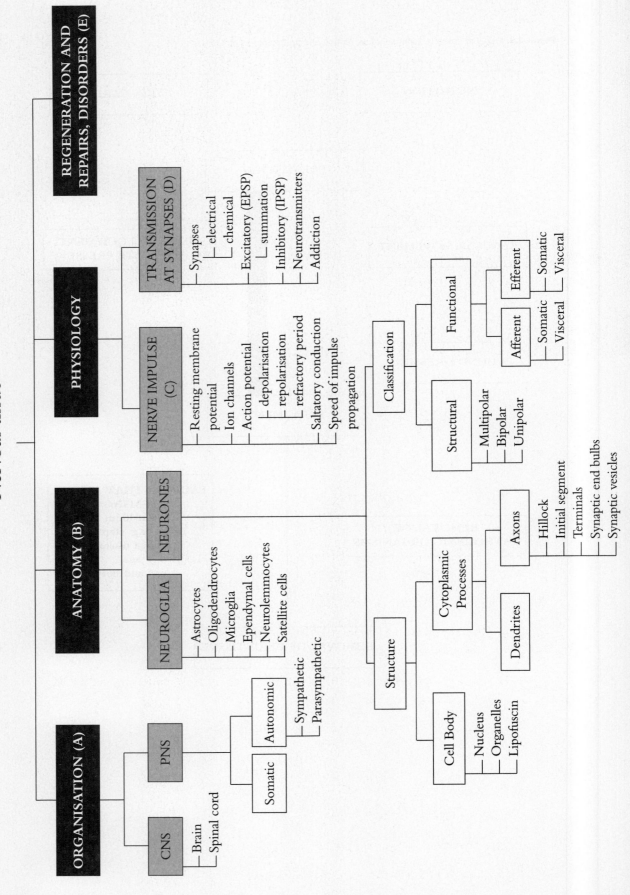

5. Nervous Tissue

Learning outcomes

1. To identify the three basic functions of the nervous system in maintaining homeostasis.

2. To classify the organs of the nervous system into central and peripheral divisions.

3. To describe the structure and functions of neuroglia, neurones, grey and white matter.

4. To describe the cellular properties that permit communication among neurones and muscle fibres.

5. To outline the factors that contribute to generation of a resting membrane potential.

6. To compare the basic types of ion channels and explain how they relate to action potentials and graded potentials.

7. To outline the sequence of events involved in generation of nerve impulses and also those of synaptic transmission.

8. To distinguish between spatial and temporal summation.

9. To give examples and functions of excitatory and inhibitory neurotransmitters.

10. To list four ways that synaptic transmission may be enhanced or blocked.

11. To outline the various types of neuronal circuits in the nervous system.

12. To describe damage and repair in peripheral neurones.

13. To outline the symptoms and causes of epilepsy.

Chapter 12

INTRODUCTION

The body is controlled by two main regulating systems, the *nervous* and *endocrine* systems. The nervous system is dependent on chemicals known as *neurotransmitters* for its functions, whilst the endocrine system is dependent on hormones. The endocrine system will be discussed in Chapter 11.

The nervous system will be dealt with in six chapters, as it is such a complex and vast topic. This chapter will relate to nervous tissue, Chapter 6 will focus on the spinal cord and spinal nerves, Chapter 7 will relate to the brain and cranial nerves, Chapter 8 will be an introduction to sensory, motor and intergrative systems, Chapter 9 will focus on the special senses and Chapter 10 concludes with the autonomic nervous system.

Understanding the nervous system should help any nurse to provide better care for individuals with physical or mental problems, especially when they are unable to cope with the daily activities of living, such as patients with cerebrovascular accident (stroke), Parkinson's disease, multiple sclerosis, and schizophrenia.

This study will be an attempt to introduce you to the various parts of the nervous system so that you are able to develop a better understanding of this complex and interesting system.

NERVOUS SYSTEM DIVISIONS 📖 *Page 347*

There are two principal divisions of the nervous sytem.

Q1. **Name the two principal divisions of the nervous system.**

_____

Q2. **Name the two main groups of nerves that form the peripheral nervous system, and indicate from where they arise.**

_____

_____

Q3 **List three principal functions of the nervous system.**

_____

Nervous tissue consists of two types of cells, **neurones** and **neuroglia**. Neuroglia are cells that act as support and protect the neurones. Neurones are nerve cells and as such they transmit nerve impulses, which are essential for the function of the nervous system. The functions are dependent on an intricate balance between **potassium** and **sodium ions** found in and around the nerve cells. Nerves can interact with nerves and this is referred to as **synapse**, and nerve can also interact with muscles (referred to as **neuromuscular junction**) or gland .

Q4. Check your understanding of the organisation of the nervous system by selecting the term(s) that best fit the descriptions below.

1. Afferent 2. Efferent 3. Autonomic nervous system 4. Central nervous system 5. Peripheral nervous system 6. Somatic nervous system

☐   a. Brain and spinal cord.

☐   b. Sensory nerves.

☐   c. Carries information from the central nervous system to skeletal muscles.

☐   d. Consists of sympathetic and parasympathetic divisions.

For question 5, 📖 *Pages 348–9*

When you have answered question 5, you should understand the differences between the neuroglia and neurones.

Q5. Write 'neurones' or 'neuroglia' after descriptions of these cells.

a. Conduct impulses from one part of the nervous system to another: _____ .

b. Provide support and protection for the nervous system : _____ .

c. Bind nervous tissue to blood vessels, form myelin and serve phagocytic functions: _____ .

d. Smaller in size, but more abundant in number : _____ .

Q6. Fill in the table below, which relates to neuroglia.

TYPE	DESCRIPTION	FUNCTIONS
	Star-shaped cells	
Oligodendrocytes		
		Phagocytic
		Line ventricles of brain and central canal of spinal cord

Myelin 📖 *Pages 349–54*

Myelin is an important component of some nerves. The exercise below will assist you in understanding the role of myelin.

Q7. Myelin consists of (a) _____ and (b) _____ . Axons that are covered with myelin sheath are said to be (c) _____ and those without are referred to as being (d) _____ .

     The neuroglia that produce myelin sheaths in the peripheral nervous system are called neurolemmocytes or (e) _____ cells. The neuroglia that produce myelin sheaths in the central nervous sytem are known as (f) _____ .

Q8.   Figure 5.1 shows a neurone. Label all the parts indicated (1–10).

Figure 5.1.
Structure of a typical
neurone as
exemplified by an
efferent (motor)
neurone.

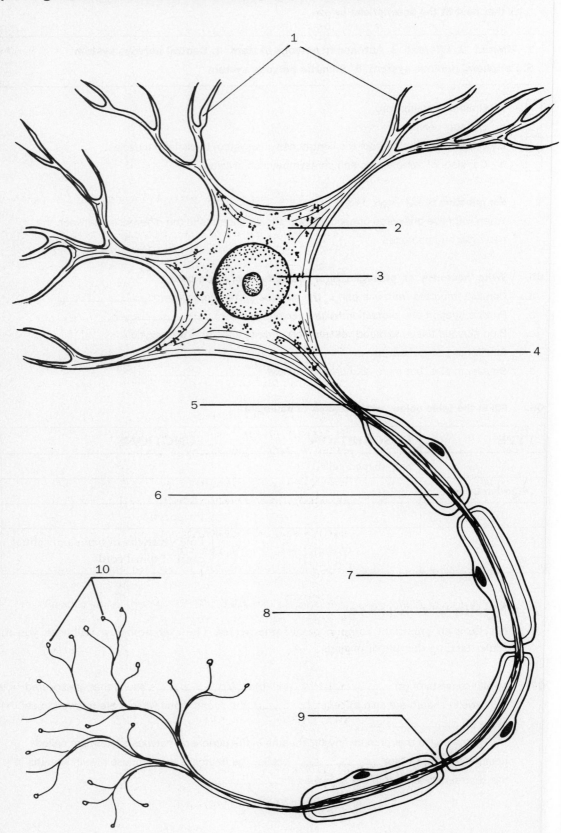

Q9. **Match the parts of the neurone listed in the box with the descriptions below.**

---

1. Axon 2. Cell body 3. Dendrite 4. Lipofuscin 5. Mitochondrion 6. Neurofibril 7. Chromatophilic substance (Nissl bodies)

☐ a. Contains nucleus; cannot regenerate, since it lacks mitotic apparatus.

☐ b. Yellowish brown pigment that increases with age; appears to be byproduct of lysosomes.

☐ c. Provides energy for neurones.

☐ d. Long, thin filament that provides support and shape for the cell.

☐ e. Orderly arrangement of endoplasmic reticulum; site of protein synthesis.

☐ f. Conducts impulses towards cell body.

☐ g. Conducts impulses away from cell body; has synaptic end bulbs that secrete neurotransmitter.

Q10. **Identify the statements that describe a neurone and those that describe a nerve.**

a. A single nerve cell; consists of a cell body with axon and dendrites:_____ .

b. Bundle of axons and dendrites of many neurones, both afferent and efferent, somatic and autonomic; contains no cell bodies:_____ .

c. Located entirely outside the central nervous system (CNS) and inside the peripheral nervous system (PNS); macroscopic in diameter:_____ .

Axonal transport 📖 *Pages 353–4.*

There are two types of transport system that carry materials from the cell body to the axon terminals and back.

Q11. **Name the two types of axonal transport and briefly contrast their functions.**

_____

_____

_____

Q12. **Which type of axonal transport is involved in the spread of herpes and rabies viruses?**

_____

Neurones are classified according to their structures and functions. Questions 13 and 14 should help you to understand the classification of neurones.

Q13.   Fill in the blank, outlining the appropriate structure, the type of neurone or description.

Structure	Types of neurones	Description
Have several dendrites	a.	Most neurones in brain and spinal cord
b.	Bipolar	c.
Have just one process extending from cell body	d.	Are always sensory

Q14.   Identify the type of nerve fibre that transmits each of the kinds of nerve impulses listed below.

> **1. General somatic afferent 2. General somatic efferent 3. General visceral afferent**
> **4. General visceral efferent**

☐   a. All autonomic nervous system (ANS) fibres are of this type.

☐   b. Pain from a thorn in your skin is sensed via fibres of this type.

☐   c. Pain from a spasm of smooth muscle in the gallbladder is sensed by means of fibres of this type.

☐   d. With your eyes closed, you can tell the position of your skeletal muscles and joints due to nerve impulses that pass along this type of fibre.

☐   e. In order to increase your heart rate, impulses pass from your brain to your heart via this type of nerve fibre.

☐   f. These nerve fibres carry impulses from the CNS to muscles in your fingers used in writing.

Q15.   Briefly explain how myelination relates to:

a.   The colour of white matter.

_____

b.   The colour of grey matter.

_____

c.   The speed of nerve impulse transmission.

_____

Q16. Complete the table about structures in the nervous system.

Structure	Colour (grey or white)	Composition (cell bodies or nerve fibres)	Location (CNS or PNS)
Nerve	White	a.	b.
Tract	c.	d.	CNS
Nucleus	Grey	e.	f.

NEUROPHYSIOLOGY 📖 *Pages 356–64*

Now that you have been exposed to the structure of the neurones, it is appropriate to look at their functions. For example, how do neurones transmit impulses? You will meet the terms: resting membrane potential, depolarisation, repolarisation and sodium and potassium ions.

Q17. Study Figure 5.2 and then complete the following exercises.

Label the major cation in each site (indicated by the large circles). Also label the major anion inside the neurone. (Values for all of these ions are indicated in 📖 *Page 909, Figure 27.4.*)

The arrows indicate the types of transport process for each ion (differences in thickness of arrows indicate relative rates of the processes). Identify the two transport processes. Then complete the exercise that follows.

Figure 5.2.
Diagram of a nerve cell.

○ Diffusion
○ Active transport pump

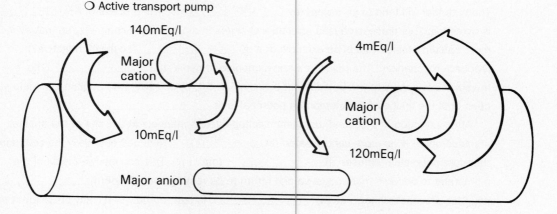

The ion that is 14 times more concentrated outside the nerve cell is (a) _____ whilst the ion that is most concentrated inside the nerve cell is (b) _____ .
The major anion inside the nerve cell is (c) _____ . Close to the neurone plasma membrane, there is a small build-up of (d) _____ (negative? positive?) charges.
Since a difference in electrical charge exists between the inside and the outside of the neurone, the resting plasma membrane is said to be (e) _____ . This difference in charge (between the inside and the outside of the membrane) is said to be the resting membrane (f) _____ . This is a form of potential energy, which is measured in (g) _____ . In a resting membrane, this value is approximately (h) _____ mV.

Q18. **Complete this exercise about roles of ion channels in development of membrane potentials.**

There are two kinds of ion channels: (a) _____ channels that are always open and (b) _____ channels that require a stimulus to activate opening or closure. The plasma cell of a membrane is more permeable to (c) _____ ions, since there are more leakage channels for these ions.

Q19. **Complete this exercise about gated channels. In a–c, choose your answer from the following: voltage/chemically/mechanically/light gated channels.**

a. Channels in receptors for hearing in the ear : _____ .

b. Channels responsive to the neurotransmitter acetylcholine : _____ .

c. Channels in neurones responsive to vibrations: _____ .

d. The presence of chemically, mechanically, or light gated channels in membranes permits _____ potentials, which vary according to the number and duration of channel openings.

e. Voltage gated channels for sodium and potassium are involved in development of an _____ potential (or impulse).

Q20. **Check your understanding of how a nerve impulse occurs, by completing the exercise below.**

A stimulus causes the nerve cell membrane to become (a) _____ (more? less?) permeable to sodium ions. Na^+ ions can then enter the cell as voltage gated sodium (b) _____ become activated and open.

At rest, the membrane has a potential of (c) _____ mV. As sodium ions enter the cell, the inside of the membrane becomes more (d) _____ (positive? negative?). The potential will tend to go toward (e) _____ mV. The process of (f) _____ is occurring. This process causes structural changes in more sodium channels, so that even more sodium enters. This is an example of a (g) _____ (positive? negative?) feedback mechanism. The result is a nerve impulse or nerve (h) _____ . The membrane is completely depolarised at exactly (i) (-50, 0, or +30?) mV. Sodium channels stay open until the inside of the membrane potential is (j) _____ at +30 mV.

After a fraction of a second, potassium voltage gated channels at the site of the original stimulus open. K^+ is more concentrated (k) _____ (inside? outside?) the cell, and therefore potassium diffuses (l) _____ (out? in?). This causes the inside of the membrane to become more negative and return to its resting potential of (m) _____ mV. This process is known as (n) _____ . In fact, outflow of K^+ may be so great that (o) _____ occurs, in which the membrane potential becomes closer to (p) _____ (-50? -90?) mV.

During depolarisation, the nerve cannot be stimulated at all. This period is known as the (q) _____ refractory period. (r) _____ (large? small?) diameter axons have a longer absolute refractory period, which is about (s) _____ (0.4? 4? 40?) msec. In other words, slower impulses are likely to occur along (t) _____ (large? small?) diameter neurones. Only a stronger than normal stimulus will result in an action potential during the (u) _____ refractory period, which corresponds roughly with (v) _____ (repolarisation? or depolarisation?).

The nerve impulse is essentially a wave of negativity along the (w) _____ (inside? outside?) of the nerve cell membrane. The impulse is propagated (or (x) _____) along the nerve cell membrane, as adjacent areas are depolarised, causing more channels to be activated and more (y) _____ to enter.

Q21. **Now that you have completed question 20, check that you understand nerve action potential by referring to Figure 5.3. Identify the correct letter label on the diagram and place it against the appropriate description.**

Figure 5.3.
Diagram of an
action potential.

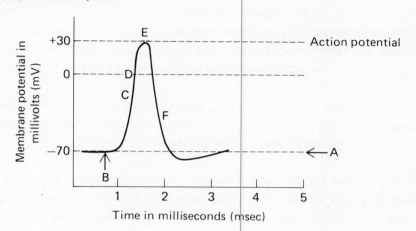

a. The stimulus is applied at this point.
b. Resting membrane potential is at this level.
c. The membrane becomes so permeable to K⁺ that K⁺ diffuses rapidly out of the cell.
d. The membrane is becoming more positive inside as Na⁺ enters; its potential is –30 mV. The process of depolarisation is occurring.
e. The membrane is completely depolarised at this point.
f. The membrane is repolarising at this point.
g. Reversed polarisation occurs; enough Na⁺ has entered so that this part of the cell is more positive inside than outside.

Q22. **Define these two terms:**

a. Threshold stimulus.

_____

_____

_____

b. All-or-none principle.

_____

_____

_____

Understanding saltatory conduction and speed of impulses according to fibre thickness and temperature 📖 *Pages 362–4*

When you have read this section in your text and completed question 23 you should be able to understand how myelination of nerves can affect their conducting properties.

Q23. **Complete the exercise, which describes how myelination, fibre thickness and temperature affect the speed of impulse propagation.**

Saltatory conduction occurs along (a) _____ nerve fibres. Saltatory transmission is (b) _____ (faster? slower?) and takes (c) _____ (more? less?) energy than continuous conduction. Type A fibres have (d) _____ diameter and are covered with myelin, and therefore they are (e) _____ fibres. The A fibres conduct impulses (f) _____ (rapidly? slowly?). Give two examples of A fibres: _____ _____ .

Type C fibres have (g) _____ diameter and they do not contain myelin, and therefore they are called (h) _____ fibres. These fibres conduct impulses (i) _____ (rapidly? slowly?). Give two examples of C fibres: _____ _____ .

Since it is known that (j) —————————— (warm? cool?) nerve fibres conduct impulses faster, in a situation where the opposite effect is desired (e.g. to reduce pain stimulus), a (k) —————————— compress such as ice may be applied to the affected area.

Q24. **Contrast the action potentials of nerve and muscle by completing the table below.**

Tissue	Resting membrane potential	Duration of nerve impulse
Neurone	a.	b.
Muscle	c.	d.

ELECTRICAL AND CHEMICAL SYNAPSES 📖 *Pages 364–8*

A synapse allows communication between nerves or muscles. Synapses are essential for the proper functioning of the nervous system, as they allow information to be integrated and filtered. Synapses are also dependent on the various chemicals known as neurotransmitters and, if they do not respond because of structural damage or other problems, this can give rise to psychiatric disorders. It is not therefore surprising that in many psychiatric disorders medications that are prescribed act at the synaptic level.

Q25. **Figure 5.4 shows a schematic representation of a synapse between two neurones.**
a.   Label all the parts (1–7).
b.   If the dots represent a type of neurotransmitter that causes chloride channels to be opened, explain the likely consequence upon the postsynaptic neurone.

Figure 5.4.
Diagram of a
synapse.

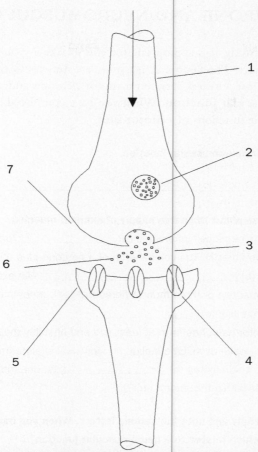

Q26. **Complete the exercise below, which deals with transmission at synapses.**

The minute space between two neurones is known as a (a) _____ . The point at
which a neurone comes close to contacting a muscle is known as a (b) _____ .

There are two types of synapse, chemical and (c) _____, which is designed to
allow spread of an ionic current from one neurone to the next. These synapses consist of
(d) _____ junctions made of hundreds of tubular proteins called (e) _____.
Gap junctions are common in (f) _____ and cardiac muscle where a group of muscle
fibres work in synchrony.

When a nerve impulse arrives at the synaptic end bulb of the (g) _____ neurone,
the depolarising phase causes (h) _____ channels to open, and (i) _____
flows inside the cell. This causes exocytosis of synaptic (j) _____ and therefore
(k) _____ is released into the (l) _____ _____ and makes
its way towards the (m) _____ membrane.

If the neurotransmitter causes depolarisation of the postsynaptic membrane, this is known
as an (n) _____ response and hence an (o) _____ _____
potential.

On the other hand, an inhibitory postsynaptic potential occurs when the neurotransmitter
causes (p) _____ . Two ions may be responsible for IPSP; one because its influx in
the postsynaptic membrane causes the inside of the membrane to become more
(q) _____ ; the other ion, (r) _____ because its outflow through gated
channels also causes the inner membrane to become more (s) _____ .

MOTOR NEURONE AND NEUROMUSCULAR JUNCTION

📖 *Pages 239–40*

At this stage in your study, it is appropriate for you to take a look at how neurones cause a muscle fibre to contract. The neurones that stimulate muscles to contract are called **motor neurones**. The synapse formed between a motor neurone and a skeletal muscle fibre is called the **neuromuscular junction**. When you have completed questions 27 and 28, you should understand the functions of a **motor unit**.

Q27.   Give another name for neuromuscular junction.

_____

Q28.   Complete this exercise about the nerve supply of skeletal muscles.

In most cases, a single nerve cell innervates (a) _____ (one muscle fibre? an average of 150 muscle fibres?). The combination of a neurone plus the muscle fibres it innervates is called a (b) _____ _____ . An example of a motor unit that is likely to consist of just two or three muscle fibres precisely innervated by one neurone is the laryngeal muscles controlling (c) _____ .

In other words, motor neurones form at least two and possibly thousands of branches called (d) _____ , each of which supplies an individual skeletal muscle fibre. When the motor neurone 'fires', it stimulates (e) _____ (just one muscle fibre supplied by one axon? all muscle fibres within that motor unit?).

Q29.   Study Figure 5.5 carefully and note the various letters. When you have done this, complete the exercise below, which relates to a neuromuscular junction.

The diagram shows the portion of a motor unit at which a branch of one neurone stimulates a single muscle fibre. An impulse travels along an axon, at (a) _____ (letter?) toward one muscle fibre: (b) _____ (letter?). The axon is enlarged at its end into a bulb-shaped synaptic (c) _____ (at letter B).

The nerve impulse causes synaptic vesicles (d) _____ (letter?) to fuse with the plasma membrane of the axon. Next, the vesicles release the neurotransmitter (e) _____ (letter?) named (f) _____ into the synaptic cleft (g) _____ (letter?).

The region of the muscle fibre membrane (sarcolemma) close to the axon terminals is called a (h) _____ . This site contains specific (i) _____ (letter G) that recognise and bind to acetylcholine (ACh). A typical motor end plate contains about (j) _____ million ACh receptors.

The effect of ACh is to cause Na$^+$ channels in the sarcolemma to (k) _____ , so that Na$^+$ enters the muscle fibre. As a result, an action potential is initiated, leading to (l) _____ of the muscle fibre. The diagnostic technique of recording such electrical activity in muscle cells is called (m) _____ .

The combination of the axon terminals and the motor end plate is known as a (n) _____ _____ . At only one site along a muscle fibre does a nerve approach a muscle cell to innervate it. In other words, there is/are usually (o) _____ (only one? many?) neuromuscular junctions, labelled (p) _____ (letter?) on the figure, for each muscle fibre.

Figure 5.5.
Diagram of a neuro-
muscular junction.

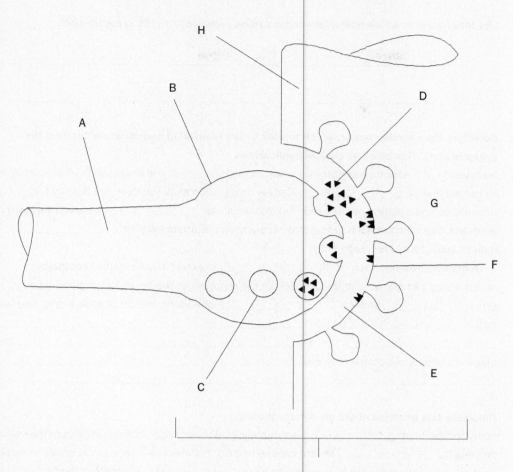

More about postsynaptic potentials

Q30. **Complete the following exercise about postsynaptic potentials.**

Usually a single EPSP within a single neurone (a) _____ (is? is not?) sufficient to
cause a threshold potential and initiate a nerve impulse. Instead, a single EPSP can cause
(b) _____ (partial? total?) depolarisation. If neurotransmitters are released from a
number of presynaptic end bulbs at one time, their combined effect may produce threshold
EPSP of about (c) _____ mV. This phenomenon is known as (d) _____
summation. Temporal summation is that due to accumulation of transmitters from
(e) _____ (one? many?) presynaptic end bulbs over a period of time.

Removal of neurotransmitter

Any excess of neurotransmitter in the synaptic cleft needs to be removed, otherwise it
could interfere with the normal function of the postsynaptic neurone. Questions 31 and
32 should help you to understand how a neurotransmitter can be removed from the
synaptic cleft.

Q31. **List three ways in which neurotransmitter can be removed from the synaptic cleft.**

_____

_____

Q32. **Complete the exercise below, which relates to the removal of neurotransmitter from the synaptic cleft. This also has clinical applications.**

Inactivation of a neurotransmitter may occur by means such as the degradation of acetylcholine by the enzyme (a) _____ . Certain drugs (such as physostigmine) destroy this enzyme, so postsynaptic neurones or muscles would (b) _____ (remain? be less?) activated. The effect of such a drug may be useful in the treatment of (c) _____ (see Chapter 10 of PAP, page 265).

A neurotransmitter such as (d) _____ may be recycled by the presynaptic neurone that had released it. Cocaine blocks the reuptake of two neurotransmitters, namely, (e) _____ and (f) _____ . The short-term effects of such a drug may lead to _____

_____ . The long-term effects of cocaine may lead to _____

_____ .

Q33. **Complete this exercise about neurotransmitters.**

Acetylcholine is (a) _____ toward skeletal muscle, but ACh released from the vagus nerve is (b) _____ toward cardiac muscle. So when the vagus nerve sends impulses to your heart, your pulse (heart rate) becomes (c) _____ (faster? slower?).

GABA and glycine are both (d) _____ (excitatory? inhibitory?) neurotransmitters. They act by opening (e) channels, leading to IPSPs. The most common inhibitory transmitter in the brain is (f) _____ , whereas (g) _____ is more commonly released by neurones in the spinal cord. Strychnine is a chemical that blocks (h) _____ receptors so that muscles are not properly inhibited (relaxed). Strychnine is likely to lead to death, because the muscles of the (i) _____ cannot relax, so that air that is high in carbon dioxide cannot be exhaled.

Question 34 will introduce you to changes in synaptic transmission as a result of changes in the chemical and physical environment of the neurone.

Q34. **This question is about a clinical challenge. Complete the exercise.**

Alkalosis tends to (a) _____ the neurones of the central nervous system, leading to tingling, spasms and possibly convulsions. Acidosis tends to (b) _____ the central nervous sytem, leading to (c) _____ .

Q35. **Check your understanding of chemicals that affect transmission at synapses and neuromuscular or neuroglandular junctions by completing this activity. Write 'E' if the effector is excitatory or 'I' if the effector is inhibitory. Then match the chemicals below (1–5) with the appropriate statement.**

1. Hypnotics, tranquillisers, anaesthetics 2. Caffeine, benzedrine, nicotine 3. Botulism toxin, inhibiting contraction 4. Curare, a muscle relaxant 5. Nerve gas, physostigmine

☐ a. A chemical that inhibits release of ACh: _____ .

☐ b. A chemical that competes for the ACh receptor sites on muscle cells: _____ .

☐ c. A chemical that inactivates acetylcholinesterase : _____ .

☐ d. A chemical that increases the threshold (for example, from –60 to –40) of a neurone: _____ .

☐ e. A chemical that decreases the threshold: _____ .

Neuronal circuits 📖 Pages 369–70

Nerves are organised into complicated patterns called **neuronal pools**. Neuronal pools are arranged into patterns called **circuits**. Question 36 should help you to understand such circuits.

Q36. **Match the types of circuit in the box with related descriptions. Answers may be used more than once.**

1. Converging 2. Diverging 3. Reverberating 4. Parallel after-discharge

☐ a. Impulse from a single presynaptic neurone causes stimulation of increasing numbers of cells along the circuit.

☐ b. An example is a single motor neurone in the brain that stimulates many motor neurones in the spinal cord, therefore activating many muscle fibres.

☐ c. Branches from a second and third neurone in a pathway may send impulses back to the first, so the signal may last for hours, as in co-ordinated muscle activities.

☐ d. One postsynaptic neurone receives impulses from several fibres.

☐ e. A single presynaptic neurone stimulates intermediate neurones, which synapse with a common postsynaptic neuron, allowing this neurone to send out a stream of impulses, as in precise mathematical calculations.

REGENERATION AND REPAIR OF NERVOUS TISSUE
📖 Pages 370–1

It is important to recognise that mammalian neurones have very limited power of regeneration. Therefore, if neurones are damaged, their functions may be lost forever. In many nervous system disorders, where there is degeneration of neurones, a cure is not possible. This is indeed a very big problem in terms of health care delivery, for the number of individuals who are affected with Parkinson's disease or Alzheimer's disease is likely to increase as the elderly population increases (due to the fact that they are living much longer). Such disorders are also associated with dementia.

When you have answered Questions 37–39, you should have a better understanding of nerve regeneration and repair.

Q37   **Which one of the following can regenerate if destroyed? Give the rationale for your answer.**

a.   Neurone cell body.

b.   CNS nerve fibre.

c.   PNS nerve fibre.

_____

Q38.   **Answer these questions about nerve regeneration.**

In order for a damaged neurone to be repaired, it must have an intact cell body and also a

(a) _____ . Axons in the CNS cannot regenerate, because they lack a

(b) _____ . When a nerve fibre (axon or dendrite) is injured, the changes that follow

in the cell body are called (c) _____ . Those that occur in the portion of the fibre

distal to the injury are known as (d) _____ _____ .

Q39.   **Explain how peripheral nerves regenerate by describing each of these events.**

a.   Chromatolysis.

_____

_____

b.   Wallerian degeneration.

_____

_____

c.   Retrograde degeneration.

_____

_____

You have now concluded the first part of your study of the nervous system. Well done! You may wish to check your progress by attempting the Checkpoints Exercise.

CHECKPOINTS EXERCISE

Q40.   **Arrange the following structures that are involved in transmission across a synapse, in sequence from first structure to last.**

a.   Presynaptic end bulb.

b.   Postsynaptic neurone.

c.   Synaptic cleft.

_____

Q41. **Choose the one false statement.**

a. The membrane of a resting neurone has a membrane potential of − 70mV.

b. In a resting membrane, permeability to K$^+$ ions is about 100 times less than permeability to Na$^+$ ions.

c. C fibres are thin, unmyelinated fibres with a relatively slow rate of nerve transmission.

d. C fibres are more likely to innervate the heart and bladder than structures (such as skeletal muscles) that must make instantaneous responses.

Q42. **Which one of the following is an incorrect description?**

a. Neurolemmocyte: myelination of neurones in the PNS.

b. Oligodendrocytes: myelination of neurones in the CNS.

c. Astrocytes: form an epithelial lining of ventricles of the brain.

d. Microglia: phagocytic.

Q43. **Which one of the following is the location for synaptic end bulbs?**

a. At the ends of axon terminals.

b. On axon hillocks.

c. On neurone cell bodies.

d. At the ends of dendrites.

e. At the ends of both axons and dendrites.

Q44. **Which one of the following is synonymous with afferent?**

a. Autonomic.

b. Somatic.

c. Peripheral.

d. Motor.

e. Sensory.

Q45. **Which one of the following is likely to occur, if an excitatory transmitter substance changes the membrane potential from –70 to –65 mV?**

a. Impulse conduction.

b. Partial depolarisation.

c. Inhibition.

d. Hyperpolarisation.

Q46.   Circle 'T' (true) or 'F' (false) for each of the following statements.

T   F   a. The concentration of potassium ions is considerably greater inside a resting cell
                      than outside it.

T   F   b. Since CNS fibres contain no neurolemma, and the neurolemma produces myelin,
                      CNS fibres are all unmyelinated.

T   F   c. Generally, release of excitatory transmitter by a single presynaptic end bulb is
                      sufficient to develop an action potential in the postsynaptic neurone.

T   F   d. Epilepsy is a condition that involves abnormal electrical discharges within neurones
                      of the brain.

T   F   e. In the converging circuit, a single presynaptic neurone influences several
                      postsynaptic neurones (or muscle or gland cells) at the same time.

T   F   f. Action potentials are measured in milliseconds, which are thousandths of a second.

T   F   g. Nerve fibres with a short absolute refractory period can respond to more rapid
                      stimuli than nerve fibres with a long absolute refractory period.

T   F   h. Most neurones in the central nervous system are classified as unipolar.

T   F   i. A stimulus that is adequate will temporarily increase permeability of the nerve
                      membrane to Na$^+$.

T   F   j. The brain and spinal nerves are parts of the peripheral nervous system.

Answers to questions

Q1. The central and peripheral nervous system.

Q2. Cranial nerves that arise from the brain and spinal nerves that arise from the spinal cord.

Q3. Sensory, integrative and motor. 📖 *Page 347.*

Q4. 4a, 1b, 2c, 6d.

Q5. a, neurones; b, neuroglia; c, neuroglia; d, neuroglia.

Q6. See 📖 *Pages 348–52*, and especially Exhibit 12.1, page 349.

Q7. a, Lipid; b, protein (you might have got them the other way round); c, myelinated; d, unmyelinated; e, Schwann; f, oligodendrocytes.

Q8. 1, Dendrites; 2, Cell body; 3, Nucleus; 4, Axon hillock; 5, Axon; 6, Myelin sheath; 7, Nucleus of Schwann cell; 8, Myelin; 9, Node of Ranvier; 10, Synaptic end bulbs or terminals.

Q9. 2a, 4b, 5c, 6d, 7e, 3f, 1g.

Q10. a, Neurone; b, nerve; c, nerve.

Q11. Slow axonal transport and fast axonal transport. Slow axonal transport moves material about 1 to 5 mm per day, whilst fast axonal transport moves material from 200 to 400 mm per day.

Q12. Fast axonal transport.

Q13. a, Multipolar neurones. b, Have one dendrite and one axon. c, In the retina of the eye, the inner ear and the olfactory area of the brain. d, Unipolar.

Q14. 4a, 1b, 3c, 1d, 4e, 2f.

Q15. a. Consists of myelinated fibres. Myelin is white.
b. Consists of unmyelinated fibres, cell bodies and neuroglia.
c. Speeds conduction by saltatory effect.

Q16. a, Nerve fibres; b, PNS; c, White; d, Nerve fibres; e, Cell bodies; f, CNS.

Q17.

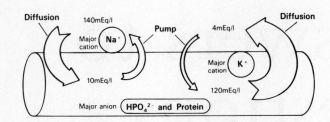

a, sodium; b, potassium; c, organic phosphates and amino acids in proteins; d, negative; e, polarised; f, potential; g, millivolts; h, −70.

Q18.   a, Leakage; b, gated; c, potassium.

Q19.   a, mechanically; b, chemically; c, mechanically; d, graded; e, action.

Q20.   a, more; b, channels; c, −70; d, positive; e, −60; f, depolarisation; g, positive; h, action potential; i, 0; j, reversed; k, inside; l, out; m, −70; n, repolarisation; o, hyperpolarisation; p, −90; q, absolute; r, small; s, 4; t, small; u, relative; v, repolarisation; w, outside; x, transmitted; y, Na^+.

Q21.   Ba, Ab, Fc, Cd, De, Ff, Eg.

Q22.   a. If a membrane is depolarised (about −55 mV) to a critical level when a stimulus is applied, this is known as the threshold stimulus.

b. If depolarisation reaches a threshold level of −55 mV, an action potential will occur, and it has a constant and maximum strength, however great the stimulus. Obviously this depends on the state of the nerve or muscle.

Q23.   a, myelinated; b, faster, since nodes of Ranvier have a high density of voltage gated Na^+ channels; c, less; d, largest; e, myelinated; f, rapidly.

Sensory nerves such as those for touch, position of joints and temperature, and nerves to skeletal muscles.

g, Smallest; h, unmyelinated; i, slowly; Examples are nerves that carry impulses to and from the viscera.

j, warm; k, cold.

Q24.   a, Higher (−70 mV); b, Shorter (0.5–2 ms); c, Lower (−90 mV); d, Longer (1.0–5.0 ms for skeletal muscle, 10–300 ms for cardiac and smooth muscle).

Q25.   a. 1, Presynaptic neurone; 2, vesicle; 3, synaptic bouton or end bulb or terminal; 4, synaptic cleft; 5, postsynaptic neurone; 6, neurotransmitter; 7, neurotransmitter receptor.

b. The inside of the membrane will become more negative, thus causing hyperpolarisation. In other words, this will be an inhibitory response.

Q26.   a, Synapse; b, neuromuscular junction; c, electrical; d, gap; e, connexons; f, smooth; g, presynaptic; h, calcium; i, calcium; j, vesicles; k, neurotransmitter; l, synaptic cleft; m, postsynaptic; n. excitatory; o, excitatory postsynaptic; p, hyperpolarisation; q, negative; r, K^+; s, negative.

Q27.   Myoneural junction.

Q28. a, An average of 150 muscle fibres; b, motor unit; c, speech; d, axons; e, all muscle fibres within that motor unit.

Q29. a, A; b, H; c, terminal; d, C; e, D; f, acetylcholine; g, E; h, motor end plate; i, receptors; j, 30–40; k, open; l, contraction; m, electromyography; n, neuromuscular junction; o, only one; p, I.

Q30. a, is not; b, partial; c, –55; d, spatial; e, one.

Q31. Diffusion, enzymatic degradation and uptake into the cells (mainly presynaptic terminal). For more elaboration, please refer to 📖 *Page 366.*

Q32. a, Acetylcholinesterase; b, remain; c, myaesthenia gravis (such drugs may help activate muscles of persons with myasthenia gravis, since many of their neurotransmitter receptors are destroyed, and the extra activation of ACh can enhance the response of remaining receptors. On the other hand, use of some powerful anticholinesterase drugs, such as nerve gases causes profound and lethel effects; d, noradrenaline; e, noradrenaline; f, dopamine.
Short-term effects: increased heart rate, blood pressure, blood sugar and body temperature, along with euphoria.
Long-term effects: depletion of dopamine, with harmful effects on heart and/or other organs.

Q33. a, Excitatory; b, inhibitory; c, slower; d, inhibitory; e, chloride; f, GABA; g, glycine; h, glycine; i, diaphragm.

Q34. a, Stimulate; b, depress; c, decrease level of consciousness.

Q35. Ia (3), Ib (4), Ec (5), Id (1), Ee (2).

Q36. 2a, 3b, 3c, 1d, 4e.

Q37. a. No. About six months after birth, the mitotic mechanism is lost.
b. No. CNS nerve fibres lack the neurolemma necessary for regeneration, and scar tissue builds up by proliferation of astroglia.
c. Yes. PNS fibres do have neurolemma.

Q38. a, Neurolemma; b, neurolemma; c, chromatolysis; d, Wallerian degeneration.

Q39. All three are explained under Disorders: Homeostatic Imbalances in 📖 *Page 372.*

Q40. a, c, b.

Q41. b.

Q42. c.

Q43. a.

Q44. e.

Q45. b.

Q46. Ta, Fb, Fc, Fd, Fe, Tf, Tg, Fh, Ti, Fj.

Overview and key terms
The spinal cord and the spinal nerves

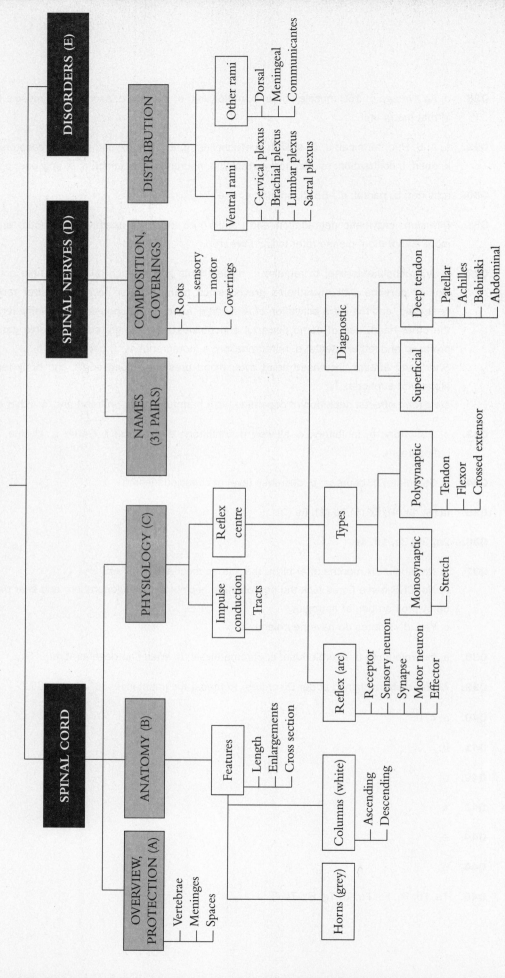

6. Spinal Cord and Spinal Nerves

Learning outcomes

1. To describe the structure and functions of the spinal cord.

2. To descibe the functions of the principal sensory and motor tracts of the spinal cord.

3. To outline the components of the reflex arc and its relationship to homeostasis.

4. To describe the composition and coverings of a spinal nerve.

5. To define and describe the composition and distribution of nerves of the cervical, brachial, lumbar and sacral plexuses.

6. To outline the effects of spinal cord injury.

7. To explain the causes and symptoms of neuritis, sciatica, shingles and poliomyelitis.

Chapter 13

INTRODUCTION

In this study, you will be able to understand the role of the spinal cord and spinal nerves as important communication pathways between the brain and all other parts of the body. The spinal cord is like a lifeline. Any damage to it will result in disturbances in motor activities which will therefore interrupt many of the daily routine activities that are usually undertaken by an individual.

The spinal cord gives off *31 pairs* of nerves along its length and therefore forms an extension network throughout the body. These nerves carry impulses to and from the brain.

When you have grasped the essential functions of the spinal cord and nerves, you should be able to understand some of the problems that may occur in an individual if the cord is diseased or injured by trauma.

SPINAL CORD ANATOMY *Pages 376–80*

Q1.   **List three general functions of the spinal cord.**

_____

_____

Q2.   **The spinal cord is part of which nervous system?**

_____

Q3.   **Complete the exercise below, which describes the anatomy of the spinal cord.**

The spinal cord is about (a) _____ cm in length in the adult and it lies within the

(b) _____ canal of the vertebral column. It is completely surrounded by connective

tissue coverings, called (c) _____ . These have an outermost layer, the

(d) _____ , an inner layer the (e) _____ and a middle layer, the

(f) _____ . The space between the inner and the middle layer is known as the

(g) _____ space. The spinal cord has two enlargements, which are found at the

(h) _____ and (i) _____ regions.

Lumbar puncture *Page 380*

Lumbar puncture is an important procedure that is undertaken for diagnostic purposes or for other medical reasons. As a nurse, you may at some stage be involved in assisting the doctor with this procedure. It is therefore important that you understand what is actually involved. Question 4 should help you to obtain some facts about the procedure of lumbar puncture.

Q4.   **Complete the exercise below, which relates to lumbar puncture.**

A lumbar puncture is usually performed under local anaesthetic and it enables

(a) _____ (name of the specimen) to be obtained for laboratory culture, to detect,

for example, the types of micro-organisms that may be the cause of an infection affecting the

nervous system, such as (b) _____ (inflammation of the meninges).

In the adult, a lumbar puncture is normally performed between the (c) _____ and (d) _____ or (d) _____ and (e) _____ (f) _____ vertebrae. The space into which the needle enters is known as the (g) _____ space. For the purpose of treating an infection, (h) _____ (common group of drugs for treating infection) can be administered via a lumbar puncture. This route by which drugs can be administered, is known as 'intrathecal'.

Q5. **For which reason should a patient lie flat following the procedure of lumbar puncture?**

_____

Q6. **Explain why an epidural is likely to exert its effects on nerves with slower and more prolonged action than a spinal tap.**

_____

_____

Q7. **State one example of a procedure for which an epidural may be used.**

_____

Question 8 should help you to understand the external and internal anatomy of the spinal cord.

Q8. **Match the names of the structures listed in the box below with the description.**

1. Cauda equina 2. Filum terminale 3. Spinal segment 4. Conus medullaris

☐ a. Tapering inferior end of the spinal cord.
☐ b. Any region of the spinal cord from which one pair of spinal nerves arises.
☐ c. Non-nervous extension of pia mater; anchors cord in place.
☐ d. 'Horse's tail'; extension of spinal nerves in lumbar and sacral regions within subarachnoid space.

Q9. **a. Diagram Figure 6.1 below shows a cross section of the spinal cord. Label all the parts (numbered 1–8), using the following terms: sensory nerve root, anterior median fissure, anterior grey horn, posterior grey horn, grey commissure, lateral grey horn, motor nerve root, lateral white column.**

Figure 6.1.
Outline of the spinal
cord, roots, and
nerves.

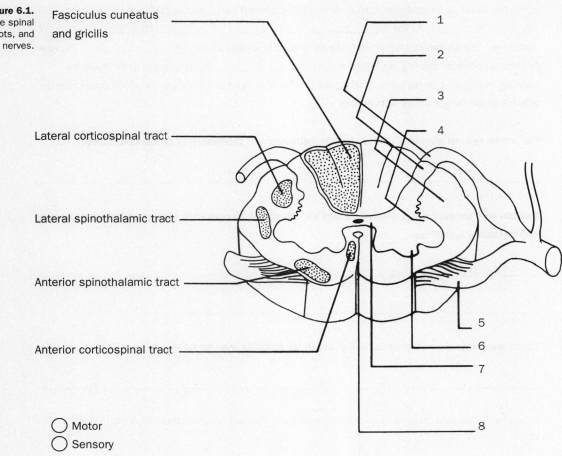

Fasciculus cuneatus
and gricilis

1
2
3
4

Lateral corticospinal tract

Lateral spinothalamic tract

Anterior spinothalamic tract

Anterior corticospinal tract

5
6
7

8

◯ Motor
◯ Sensory

b.   **Complete the exercise below which refers to the internal anatomy of the spinal cord.**

Tracts conduct nerve impulses in the (a) _____ (central? peripheral?) nervous
system. Functionally, they are comparable to (b) _____ in the peripheral nervous
system.

Tracts are located in (c) _____ _____ . They appear white, since
they consist of bundles of (d) _____ nerve fibres. Ascending tracts are all
(e) _____ , conveying impulses between the spinal cord and the (f) _____.
All motor tracts in the cord are (g) _____ (ascending? descending?).

Spinal cord physiology 📖 *Pages 380–9*

Q10.   **Refer to Figure 6.1 and identify the five tracts within the spinal cord. Colour them and beside
each one, write its correct function.**

Q11.   **Complete the exercise below, which gives more detail about the functions of the spinal cord.**

One primary function of the spinal cord is to permit (a) _____ between nerves in the
periphery, such as the arms and legs, and the brain by means of the (b) _____
located in the white column of the cord.

Another function of the cord is to serve as a (c) _____ centre by means of spinal

nerves. These are attached by (d) _____ roots. The (e) _____ root
contains sensory nerve fibres, and the (f) _____ root contains motor fibres.

At this point you could colour the sensory and motor roots on Figure 6.1.

Q12. **Complete the exercise below, which gives more details about the tracts in the spinal cord.**

The name 'lateral corticospinal' indicates that the tract is located in the (a) _____
white column, that it originates in the (b) _____ _____ , and that it
ends in the (c) _____ . The lateral corticospinal tract is descending
(d) _____ , and it is a (e) _____ tract.

The rubrospinal, tectospinal and vestibulospinal tracts are (f) _____ tracts.
These are involved with the control of automatic movements such as the maintenance of
muscle (g) _____ , posture and equilibrium.

Simple reflex arc 📖 *Pages 382–4*

The simplest type of pathway in the spinal cord is known as a **reflex arc**. To understand
how a reflex arc operates, you need to be familiar with all the components that are essential
for such reflex action to take place. When you have read this section in your text, labelled
Figure 6.2 below and answered question 13, you should have grasped the basic principles
of the spinal reflex.

Q13. **Figure 6.2 shows a cross section of the spinal cord and the components that are essential in
a reflex arc. Label A–H using the following terms:**

effector, motor neurone, axon, motor neurone cell body, sensory neurone axon, sensory
neurone cell body, sensory neurone dendrite and synapse.

Note that the letters are arranged in an orderly fashion to indicate the conduction pathway of
a reflex arc. Using arrows, indicate the direction of nerve transmission.

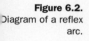

Figure 6.2.
Diagram of a reflex
arc.

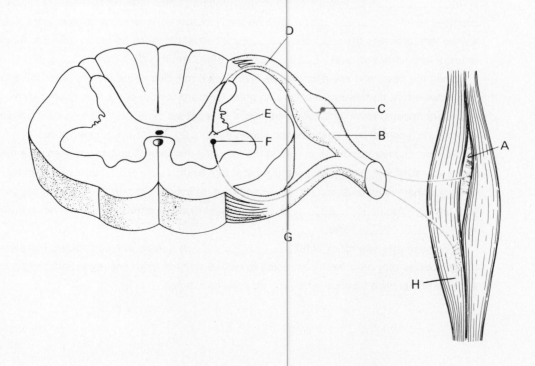

Q14.   Complete this exercise which relates to the reflex arc, as shown in Figure 6.2.

The spinal reflex contains (a) _____ (how many ?) neurones. The neurone that conveys the impulse toward the spinal cord is a (b) _____ neurone; the one that carries the impulse toward the effector is a (c) _____ neurone. This is a (d) _____ (having only one synapse) reflex arc. The synapse, like all somatic synapses, is located in the (e) _____ (CNS? PNS?).

Receptors, in this case located in skeletal muscles, are called (f) _____ _____ . They are sensitive to changes in (g) _____ and therefore, this type of reflex might be called a (h) _____ reflex.

Since sensory impulse enter the cord on the same side as motor impulses leave, the reflex is called (i) _____ . The effector in Figure 16.2 is a (j) _____ . One example of a stretch reflex is the (k) _____ , in which stretching of the patellar tendon initiates the reflex.

Q15.   Complete this exercise describing how tendon reflexes protect tendons. 📖 *Pages 385–6.*

Receptors located in tendons are named (a) _____ _____ . They are sensitive to changes in muscle (b) _____ , as when the hamstring muscles are contracted excessively, pulling on tendons.   When this occurs, association neurones cause (c) _____ of this same muscle, so that the hamstring fibres (d) _____ . Simultaneously, other association neurones fire impulses that stimulate (e) _____ (synergistic? antagonistic?) muscles (such as the quadriceps in this case). These muscles then (f) _____ . The net effect of such a polysynaptic (g) _____ reflex is that the tendons are protected.

Q16.   Contrast stretch, flexor, and crossed extensor reflexes in this learning activity.

A flexor reflex (a) _____ (does? does not?) involve association neurones, and so it is (b) _____ (more? less?) complex than a stretch reflex. A flexor reflex sends impulses to (c) _____ (one? several?) muscle(s), whereas a stretch reflex, such as a knee jerk, activates (d) _____ (one? several?), such as the quadriceps. A flexor reflex is also known as a (e) _____ reflex, and it is (f) _____ .

When the flexor and extensor (biceps and triceps) muscles of the forearm are contracted with equal effort, no movement occurs. In order for movement to occur, it is necessary for extensors (triceps) to be inhibited while flexors (biceps) are stimulated. The nervous system exhibits such control by a phenomenon known as (g) _____ innervation.

Reciprocal innervation also occurs in the following instance. Suppose you step on a nail under your right foot. You quickly withdraw that foot by (h) _____ your right leg, using your hamstring muscles. (Stand up and try it, of course not with a nail.) What happens to your left leg? You (I) _____ it. This is an example of reciprocal innervation involving a (j) _____ reflex.

A crossed extensor reflex is (k) _____ . It may be intersegmental. Therefore, many muscles may have been contracted to extend your left thigh and leg to shift weight to your left side and provide balance, when you stepped on the nail.

Reflexes and neurological impairment 📖 *Pages 388–9*

Although you are not expected to make diagnoses, as nurses you will be involved in assisting patients with different types of neurological problems. In caring for such patients, you should at least understand why they may present you with certain signs and symptoms. Being aware of these would obviously enhance your delivery of care for such a category of patients. You may also sometimes notice such a new problem in your patient when you are carrying out nursing observations, perhaps for different reasons. The table below should enable you to become familiar with normal and abnormal reflexes.

Q17. **Complete the table about reflexes that are indicative of a neurological problem.**

	Patellar reflex	Achilles reflex	Babinski sign
Procedure used to demonstrate reflex	Tap patellar ligament	a.	b.
Nature of positive response	c.	Plantar flexion	d.
Spinal nerve and muscles evaluated by procedure in reflex	e.	f.	Determines if corticospinal tract is myelinated
Cause of negative response	g.	h.	Plantar flexion reflex: all toes curl under; normal after age 1
Cause of exaggerated response	i.	Damage to motor tracts in S1 or S2 segments of cord	j.

Spinal nerves and plexuses 📖 *Pages 389–99*

Having completed the study on the spinal cord, you can now move on to the spinal nerves and plexuses. When you have completed question 18, you should be able to understand the distribution of spinal nerves in the body.

Q18. **Complete this exercise about spinal nerves.**

There are (a) _____ pairs of spinal nerves. They are distributed as follows:

(b) _____ cervical, (c) _____ lumbar, sacral and coccygeal nerves form the (g) _____ _____ .

Spinal nerves are attached by two roots. The posterior root is (h) _____ , the anterior root is (i) _____ , whereas the spinal nerve is (j) _____ .
Individual nerve fibres are wrapped in a connective tissue covering known as (k) _____ .
Groups of nerve fibres are held in bundles (fascicles) by (l) _____ . The entire nerve is wrapped with (m) _____ .

Spinal nerves branch when they leave the intervertebral foramen. These branches are called (n) _____ . Since they are extensions of spinal nerves, rami are (o) _____ (sensory ? motor ? mixed ?). The larger ramus is the (p) _____ and it supplies all the extremity and the ventral and lateral portions of the trunk. The dorsal ramus innervates (q) _____ and (r) _____ of the back.

Q19.   Match the plexus names in the box with the descriptions. 📖 *Figure 13.2a, Page 378.*

1. Brachial 2. Cervical 3. Lumbar 4. Sacral 5. Intercostal

☐ a. Provides the entire nerve supply for the arm.

☐ b. Contains the origin of the phrenic nerve (nerve that supplies the diaphragm).

☐ c. Forms median, radial and axillary nerves.

☐ d. Not a plexus at all, but rather segmentally arranged nerves.

☐ e. Supplies nerves to the scalp, the neck and part of the shoulder and chest.

☐ f. Supplies fibres to the femoral nerve which innervates the quadriceps, so injury to this plexus would interfere with actions such as touching the toes.

☐ g. Forms the largest nerve in the body (sciatic), which supplies the posterior of the thigh and the leg.

Q20.   Match the names of spinal nerves in the box with their descriptions. For each of the statements write the site of origin of the nerve. The first is completed for you.

1. Axillary 2. Inferior gluteal 3. Pudendal 4. Radial 5. Sciatic 6. Musculocutaneous

☐ a. Consists of two nerves, the tibial and common peroneal; supplies the hamstrings, adductors and all muscles distal to the knee. (L4–S3).

☐ b. Supplies the deltoid muscles.

☐ c. Innervates the major flexors of the arm.

☐ d. Supplies most extensor muscles of the forearm, wrist and fingers; may be damaged by extensive use of crutches.

☐ e. Supplies the gluteus maximus muscle.

☐ f. May be anaesthetised in chilbirth, since it innervates external genitalia and the lower part of the vagina.

Q21.   Giving the rationale for each of your answers, suggest how the following structures and functions may be affected if the cord were completely severed just below the C7 spinal nerve.
📖 *Page 378, Figure 13.2a*

a.   Breathing via the diaphragm.

_____

_____

b.   Movement and sensation of the thigh and leg.

_____

_____

c. Movement and sensation of the arm.

_____

_____

d. Use of muscles of facial expression and muscles that move the jaw, tongue and eyeballs.

_____

_____

Q22. Match the terms in the box with the descriptions below.

> **1. Quadriplegia 2. Monoplegia 3. Hemiplegia 4. Paraplegia**

☐   a. Paralysis of one extremity only.
☐   b. Paralysis of both legs.
☐   c. Paralysis of both arms and legs.
☐   d. Paralysis of the arm, leg and trunk on one side of the body.

Q23. Describe the changes associated with transection of the spinal cord.

Hemisection of the cord refers to transection of (a) _____ (half? all?) of the spinal cord.

If the posterior columns (cuneatus and gracilis) and lateral corticospinal tracts on the right side of the cord are severed at level T11–T12, symptoms of loss awareness of muscle sensations (proprioception), loss of touch sensations, and paralysis are likely to occur in the (b) _____ (right arm? right leg? left arm? left leg?).

The period of spinal shock is likely to last for several (c) _____ (days? weeks? years?). During this time, the person is likely to experience (d) _____ , meaning no reflexes. When reflexes gradually return to the injured person, they are likely to return in a specific sequence.

Arrange the reflexes below in order, from first to last, according to their return.

1. Cross extensor reflex.
2. Flexion reflex.
3. Stretch reflex.

_____

Q24. Complete this exercise on shingles.

Shingles is an infection of the (a) _____ nervous sytem. The causative virus is also the agent of (b) _____ (which other disease?). Following recovery from chickenpox, the virus remains in the body in the (c) _____ _____ ganglia. At times, the virus is activated and travels along (d) _____ neurones, causing severe (e) _____ (pain? paralysis?).

Q25.   Match the name of disorders in the box with the definitions below.

> **1. Areflexia 2. Neuritis 3. Poliomyelitis 4. Sciatica 5. Shingles**

☐   a.   Inflammation of a single nerve.

☐   b.   Lack of reflex activity.

☐   c.   Acute inflammation of the nervous system by herpes zoster virus.

☐   d.   Neuritis of a nerve in the posterior of the hip and thigh; often due to a slipped disc in the lower lumbar region.

☐   e.   Also known as infantile paralysis; caused by a virus that may destroy motor cell bodies in the brainstem or in the anterior grey horn of the spinal cord.

You have now completed the second part of your study of the nervous system. If you have found this part of the study difficult, please do not despair. If it is of any consolation, most students do find the nervous system difficult. It is worth discussing the areas you found difficult with your colleagues. Try to use the difficult terms, so that you become familiar with them. Well done!

To check your progress, try the Checkpoints Exercise.

CHECKPOINTS EXERCISE

Arrange the statements in questions 26–29 in the correct sequence.

Q26.   From superficial to deep:

a.   Subarachnoid space.

b.   Epidural space.

c.   Dura mater.

Q27.   From anterior to posterior spinal cord:

a.   Fasciculus gracilis and cuneatus.

b.   Anterior spinothalamic tract.

c.   Central canal of the spinal cord.

Q28.   The plexuses, from superior to inferior:

a.   Lumbar.

b.   Brachial.

c.   Cervical.

d.   Sacral.

Q29.   Structures in a conduction pathway, from origin to termination.

a.   Motor neurone.

b.   Sensory neurone.

c.   Integrative centre.

d.   Receptor.

e.   Effector.

Q30. **Which one of the following tracts is motor?**

a.   Anterior spinothalamic.

b.   Lateral spinothalamic.

c.   Fasciculus cuneatus.

d.   Lateral corticospinal.

e.   Posterior spinocerebellar.

Q31. **Choose the false statement about the spinal cord.**

a.   It has enlargements in the cervical and lumbar areas.

b.   It lies in the vertebral foramen.

c.   It extends from the medulla to the sacrum.

d.   It is surrounded by meninges.

e.   In cross section, an H-shaped area of grey matter can be found.

Q32. **Which one of the following is composed of grey matter?**

a.   Posterior root (spinal) ganglia.

b.   Tracts.

c.   Lumbar plexus.

d.   Sciatic nerve.

e.   Ventral ramus of a spinal nerve.

Q33. **Which is a false statement about the patellar reflex?**

a.   It is called the knee jerk.

b.   It involves a two-neurone, monosynaptic reflex arc.

c.   It results in extension of the leg by contraction of the quadriceps femoris.

d.   It is contralateral.

Q34. **Which one of the following best describes the cauda equina?**

a.   It is another name for the cervical plexus.

b.   It is the inferior extension of the pia mater.

c.   It is a canal running through the centre of the spinal cord.

d.   It is the lumbar and sacral nerves extending below the end of the cord and resembling a horse's tail.

Q35. **Circle 'T' (true) or 'F' (false) for each of the statements below.**

T   F   a. The layer of the meninges that gets its name from its delicate structure, which is much like a spider's web, is the arachnoid.

T   F   b. The two main functions of the spinal cord are that it serves as a reflex centre and it is the site where sensations are felt.

T   F   c. Dorsal roots of spinal nerves are sensory, ventral roots are motor, and spinal nerves are mixed.

T   F   d. A tract is a bundle of nerve fibres inside the central nervous system.

T   F   e. Synapses are present in posterior (dorsal) root ganglia.

T   F   f. After an individual reaches 18 months, the Babinski sign should be negative, as indicated by plantar flexion (curling under of toes and foot).

T   F   g. Visceral reflexes are used diagnostically more often than somatic reflexes, since it is easy to stimulate most visceral receptors.

T   F   h. Transection of the spinal cord at level C6 will result in greater loss of function than transection at level T6.

T   F   i. The ventral root of a spinal nerve contains axons and dendrites of both motor and sensory neurones.

T   F   j. A lumbar puncture is usually performed at about the level of vertebrae L1 to L2, since the cord ends between about L3 and L4.

Answers to questions

Q1.   Processing centre (for reflexes), integration (summing) of afferent or efferent nerve impulses and pathway for those impulses.

Q2.   Central nervous system.

Q3.   a, 42–45; b, vertebral; c, meninges; d, dura mater; e, pia mater; f, arachnoid mater; g, subarachnoid; h, cervical; i, lumbar.

Q4.   a, CSF; b, meningitis; c, 3rd; d, 4th; e, 5th; f, lumbar; g, subarachnoid; h, antibiotics.

Q5.   To minimise leakage of CSF, otherwise this may cause severe headache.

Q6.   The anaesthetic must penetrate epidural tissues and then all three layers of the meninges before reaching the nerve fibres, whereas an anaesthetic in the subarachnoid space needs to penetrate only the pia mater to reach nerve tissue.

Q7.   Childbirth (labour and delivery).

Q8.   4a, 3b, 2c, 1d.

Q9b.   a, central; b, nerves; c, white columns; d, myelinated; e, sensory; f, brain; g, descending.

Q9a and Q10.

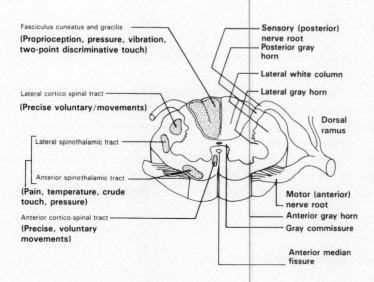

Fasciculus cuneatus and gracilis
(Proprioception, pressure, vibration, two-point discriminative touch)

Lateral cortico spinal tract
(Precise voluntary/movements)

Lateral spinothalamic tract

Anterior spinothalamic tract
(Pain, temperature, crude touch, pressure)

Anterior cortico-spinal tract
(Precise, voluntary movements)

Sensory (posterior) nerve root
Posterior gray horn
Lateral white column
Lateral gray horn
Dorsal ramus
Motor (anterior) nerve root
Anterior gray horn
Gray commissure
Anterior median fissure

Q11. a, Conduction; b, tracts; c, reflex; d, two; e, posterior (dorsal); f, ventral (anterior).

Q12. a, Lateral; b, cerebral cortex; c, spinal cord; d, motor; e, pyramidal; f, extrapyramidal; g, tone.

Q13.

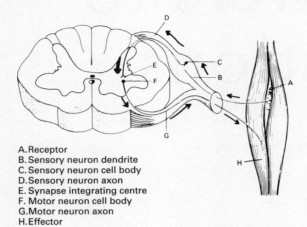

A. Receptor
B. Sensory neuron dendrite
C. Sensory neuron cell body
D. Sensory neuron axon
E. Synapse integrating centre
F. Motor neuron cell body
G. Motor neuron axon
H. Effector

Q14. a, two; b, sensory; c, motor; d, monosynaptic; e, CNS; f, muscle spindles; g, length; h, stretch; i, ipsilateral; j, skeletal muscle; k, knee jerk or patellar reflex.

Q15. a, tendon organ; b, tension; c, inhibition; d, relax; e, antagonistic; f, contract; g, tendon.

Q16. a, does; b, more; c, several; d, one; e, withdrawal; f, ipsilateral (same side of the body); g, reciprocal; h, flexing; i, extend; j, crossed extensor; k, contralateral.

Q17. a, Tap on calcaneal (Achilles) tendon; b, Light stimulation of outer margin of sole of foot; c, Extension of leg; d, Great toe extends, with or without fanning of other toes. Abnormal after age $1\frac{1}{2}$; shows incomplete myelination; e, L2–4 (quadruceps muscles); f, L4–5, S1–3 (gastrocnemius and soleus muscles); g, Chronic diabetes mellitus, neurosyphilis; h, Diabetes neurosyphilis, alcoholism; i, Injury to corticospinal tracts; j, Positive Babinski sign after age $1\frac{1}{2}$ indicates interruption of corticospinal tracts.

Q18. a, 31; b, 8; c, 12; d, 5; e, 5; f, 1; g, cauda equina; h, sensory; i, motor; j, mixed; k, endoneurium; l, perineurium; m, epineurium; n, rami; o, mixed; p, ventral; q, muscles; r, skin.

Q19. 1a, 2b, 1c, 5d, 2e, 3f, 4g.

Q20. 5a (L4–S3), 1b (C5–C6), 6c (C5–C7), 4d (C5–C8), 2e (L5–S2), 3f (S2–S4).

Q21. a. Not affected, since the (phrenic) nerve to the diaphragm originates from the cervical plexus (at C3–C5), higher than the transection. So this nerve continues to receive nerve impulses from the brain.
b. Complete loss of sensation and paralysis since lumbar and sacral plexuses originate below the injury, and therefore no longer communicate with the brain.
c. Most arm functions are not affected. The brachial plexus originates from C5 through T1, so most nerves to the arm (those from C5 through T1) still communicate with the brain.
d. Not affected, since all are supplied by cranial nerves that originate from the brain.

Q22. 2a, 4b, 1c, 3d.

Q23. a, half; b, right leg; c, days to weeks; d, areflexion; 3, 2, 1.

Q24.   a, Peripheral; b, chickenpox; c, dorsal root; d, sensory; e, pain.

Q25.   2a, 1b, 5c, 4d, 3e.

Q26.   b, c, a.

Q27.   b, c, a.

Q28.   c, b, a, d.

Q29.   d, b, c, a, e.

Q30.   d.

Q31.   c.

Q32.   a.

Q33.   d.

Q34.   d.

Q35.   Ta, Fb, Tc, Td, Fe, Tf, Fg, Th, Fi, Fj

Overview and key terms

Brain and cranial nerves

DISORDERS (H)

AGING, DEVELOPMENT (G)

CRANIAL NERVES (P)
- I Olfactory
- II Optic
- III Oculomotor
- IV Trochlear
- V Trigeminal
- VI Abducens
- VII Facial
- VIII Vestivulocochlear
- IX Glossopharyngeal
- X Vagus
- XI Accessory
- XII Hypoglossal

BRAIN

NEUROTRANSMITTERS (E)

PROTECTION (A)
- Meninges
- CSF
- Blood supply
  - BBB

- Brainstem (B)
  - Medulla
  - Pons
  - Midbrain
- Diencephalon (B)
  - Thalamus
  - Hypothalamus
- Cerebrum (C)
  - Structure
  - Functions
- Cerebellum (D)
  - Structure
  - Functions

7. The Brain and Cranial Nerves

Learning outcomes

1. To describe how the brain is protected.

2. To outline the main structures and functions of the brain.

3. To outline the formation and circulation of cerebrospinal fluid (CSF).

4. To describe the blood supply to the brain and the concept of the blood–brain barrier.

5. To identify the various neurotransmitters and their functions in the brain.

6. To list the 12 pairs of cranial nerves.

7. To describe the effects of ageing on the nervous system.

8. To outline patients' problems in relation to the following neurological disorders: cerebrovascular accident, Alzheimer's disease, Parkinson's disease, multiple sclerosis.

9. To define some of the terminologies associated with the central nervous system.

Chapter 14

INTRODUCTION

The brain is the most important organ governing all our bodily movements, our behaviour, our intellect, our memory and our emotions, and above all, it is the organ that puts man ahead of other primates. The brain also contains most of the so-called vital centres, for example centres for regulation of blood pressure, respiration rate, co-ordination of posture and balance.

The brain is related to the *spinal cord* and also to the 12 pairs of *cranial nerves*. In this study, you will discover the various parts of the brain and their functions. You should gain essential knowledge on some important disorders, such as cerebrovascular accident (CVA), Alzheimer's disease, cerebral palsy, multiple sclerosis and Parkinson's disease. This should assist you when you are planning nursing care with this type of disorder.

You may find part of this study very complex, and you are therefore advised to give yourself plenty of time when embarking on this study. You may perhaps need to study only one small section in any period of study.

BRAIN PROTECTION AND COVERINGS 📖 *Pages 405–11*

Q1. **Figure 7.1 shows a sagittal section of the brain and meninges. Study it by identifying all the parts labelled. Write the parts (labelled A–K) against the appropriate letter on the diagram. Then proceed by completing the exercise below.**

a. Structures 1–3 are parts of the _____.

b. Structures 4 and 5 together form the _____.

c. Structure 6 is the largest part of the brain, the _____.

d. The second largest part is structure 7, the _____.

Q2. **List three ways in which the brain is protected.**

_____

Q3. **Name the three layers of the meninges covering the brain and spinal cord. Label the layers on the diagram.**

_____

OVERVIEW OF BRAIN ANATOMY 📖 *Page 405*

Q4. **Complete the following exercise which gives on overview of the brain.**

The brain weighs approximately 1.3 kg and is situated in the (a) _____ cavity. It is divided into right and left halves called (b) _____ and they are both connected by the (c) _____ _____ . The brain is covered by membranes known as (d) _____ . The brain can be divided into four principal parts: diencephalon, (e) _____ cerebellum and (f) _____ .

CEREBROSPINAL FLUID (CSF) 📖 *Pages 405–10*

The brain and spinal cord are nourished and protected by CSF. CSF surrounds the whole brain and is found in the subarachnoid space and central canal of the spinal cord. CSF is closely related to structures called ventricles and sometimes the system is referred to as the ventricular system of the brain. The ventricles form a system consisting of cavities filled with CSF.

When you have worked through question 5, you should understand the ventricular system.

Figure 7.1.
Brain and meninges seen in sagittal section. Parts of the brain are numbered; Letters indicate pathway of cerebrospinal fluid.

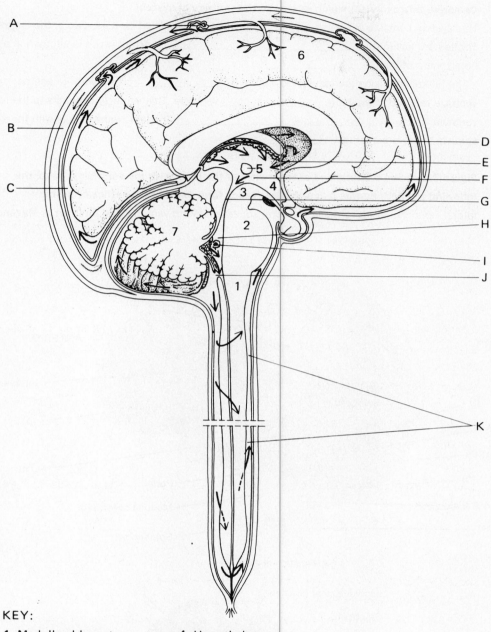

KEY:

1. Medulla oblongata
2. Pons
3. Midbrain
4. Hypothalamus
5. Thalamus
6. Cerebrum
7. Cerebellum

A. Arachnoid villus
B. Cranial venous sinus
C. Subarachnoid space of brain
D. Lateral venticle
E. Interventricular foramen
F. Third ventricle
G. Cerebral aqueduct
H. Fourth ventricle
I. Lateral aperture
J. Median aperture
K. Subarachnoid space of spinal cord

Q5.   **Complete this exercise, which relates to the ventricular system.**

This system consists of (a) _____ (how many?) filled cavities. Two of the largest cavities are called (b) _____ _____ , each of which is situated in a hemisphere of the (c) _____ .

The lateral ventricles are connected via the (d) _____ of Munro, to another ventricle referred to as the (e) _____ ventricle. This ventricle connects to the fourth ventricle via the (f) _____ _____ . The last connection is with the spinal cord via the foramen of (g) _____ .

Q6.   **Figure 7.2 shows a lateral and anterior view of the brain with the ventricles. Label the following (on both figures if appropriate) which form part of the ventricular system:**

lateral ventricles, third ventricle, cerebral aqueduct, fourth ventricle and foramen of Magendie.

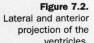

Figure 7.2.
Lateral and anterior projection of the ventricles.

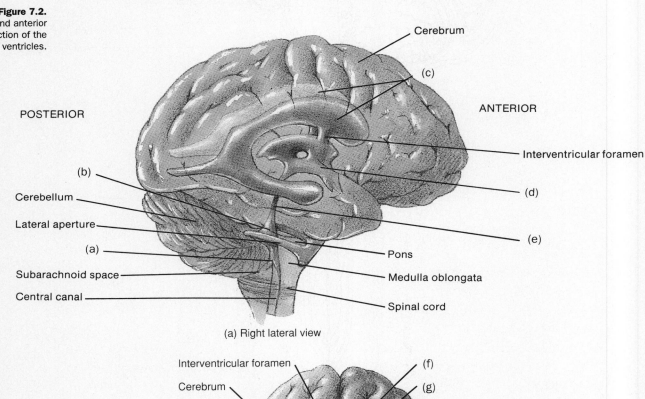

(a) Right lateral view

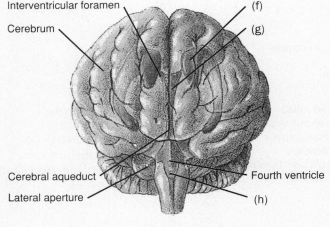

(b) Anterior view

Figure 7.3.
Brain, ventricles, spinal cord and meninges in frontal section.

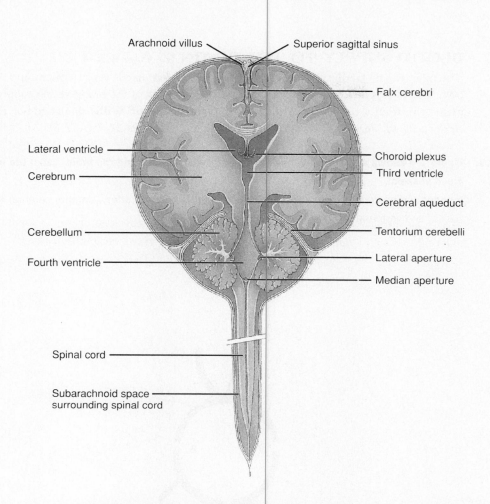

Arachnoid villus
Superior sagittal sinus
Falx cerebri
Lateral ventricle
Choroid plexus
Cerebrum
Third ventricle
Cerebral aqueduct
Cerebellum
Tentorium cerebelli
Fourth ventricle
Lateral aperture
Median aperture
Spinal cord
Subarachnoid space surrounding spinal cord

Now that you understand the basic structures of the ventricles, you can concentrate on CSF.

Q7.   Complete this question, which relates to CSF.

CSF is produced by the (a) _____ _____ which are networks of blood capillaries found in the (b) _____ _____ of each cerebral hemisphere. The amount of CSF secreted is approximately (c) _____ to (d) _____ ml. Reabsorption of CSF takes place through the (e) _____ . If there is an obstruction in the reabsorption of CSF, this may give rise to the condition known as (f) _____ .

Q8.   Check your understanding of the pathway of CSF by listing in order the structures through which it passes. Use key letters on Figure 7.1. Start at the site of formation of CSF.

_____

Q9.   List three main functions of CSF.

_____

_____

BLOOD SUPPLY TO THE BRAIN 📖 *Pages 652–4*

The brain is a metabolically active organ and it therefore needs very large amount of blood flow. This is supplied by a network of blood vessels. Most of the blood vessels supplying the brain arise from a circular network known as the **circle of Willis**. Refer to 📖 *Page 652 (Exhibit 21.6), Page 654 (Figure 21.22) & Page 655 (Exhibits 21.7 & 21.8).*

Q10. **Figure 7.4 shows a posterior view of the blood vessels supplying the brain. Label the following blood vessels:**

anterior and posterior communicating artery, posterior cerebral artery, anterior cerebral artery, basilar and vertebral artery.

Figure 7.4.
The circle of Willis.

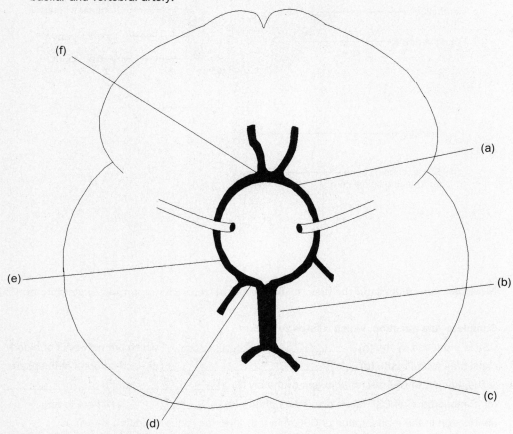

Q11. **Complete the following exercise which relates to blood supply in the brain.**

The right and left internal (a) _____ arteries together with the (b) _____ artery forms the circle of Willis. The (c) _____ artery gives rise to the (d) _____ cerebral arteries. These are connected with internal carotids by (e) _____ _____ arteries. Anterior cerebral arteries are connected by (f) _____ arteries.

Q12. **Giving the rationale for your answer, explain why the brain may be permanently injured if the blood supply is interrupted for four minutes.** 📖 *Page 411.*

_____

_____

Blood–Brain Barrier (BBB) 📖 *Page 411*

When you have answered questions 13–17, you will be able to understand the important function of the BBB.

Q13. **Describe the blood–brain barrier in the exercise below.**

Blood capillaries supplying the brain are (a) _____ (more? less?) leaky than most capillaries of the body. This fact is related to a large number of (b) _____ (gaps? tight?) junctions, as well as an abundance of neuroglia named (c) _____ pressed against the capillaries.

Q14. **What advantages are provided by this membrane?**

_____

_____

Q15. **List two or more substances needed by the brain that do normally cross the BBB.**

_____

Q16. **What problems may result from the fact that some chemicals cannot cross this barrier?**

_____

_____

_____

Q17. **List several substances that may harm the brain and that are able to cross this barrier.**

_____

BRAINSTEM 📖 *Pages 411–8*

Now that you have completed the study of the blood circulation in the brain, it is appropriate to look ot the various structures in the brain. We will start by looking at the **brainstem.**

Q18. **Complete the exercise below on the brainstem.**

The brainstem consists of the _____ , and the _____ .

Q19. **Describe the principal functions of the medulla in this exercise.**

The medulla serves as a (a) _____ pathway for all ascending and descending tracts. Its white matter therefore transmits (b) _____ (sensory? motor? both sensory and motor?) impulses. Included among these tracts, are the triangular (c) _____ tracts, which are the principal (d) _____ (sensory? motor?) pathways. The main fibres that pass through the pyramids are the (e) _____ (spinothalamic? corticospinal?) tracts.

Crossing (or (f) _____) of fibres occurs in the medulla. This explains why movements of your right hand are initiated by motor neurones that originate in the (g) _____ side of your cerebrum. The (h) _____ (axons? dendrites?) of these motor neurones decussate in the medulla to proceed down the right lateral (i) _____ tract.

The medulla contains grey areas as well as white matter. Several important nuclei lie in the medulla. Two of these are synapse points for sensory axons that ascended in the posterior columns of the cord. These nuclei, named (j) _____ and (k) _____ , transmit impulses for sensations of two-point discriminatory touch, (l) _____ , and vibrations.

A hard blow to the base of the skull can be fatal, since the medulla is the site of three vital centres: the (m) _____ centre, regulating the heart; the (n) _____ centre, adjusting the rhythm of breathing; and the (o) _____ centre, regulating the blood pressure by altering the diameter of blood vessels. Some input to the medulla arrives by means of cranial nerves; these nerves may serve motor functions. Which cranial nerves are attached to the medulla? _____ .

Q20   Complete this exercise, which summarises important aspects of the pons.

The name 'pons' means (a) _____ . It serves as a bridge in two ways. It contains longitudinally arranged fibres that connect the (b) _____ and (c) _____ with the upper part of the brain. It has transverse fibres that connect the two sides of the (d) _____ .

Cell bodies associated with fibres in cranial nerves numbered (e) _____ lie in nuclei in the pons. (f) _____ is controlled by the pneumotaxic and apneustic areas of the pons.

Q21.   Complete this exercise, which relates to the reticular activating system.

You maintain a conscious state, or you wake up from sleep, on account of the regions of the brain known as the RAS (write in full) (a) _____ _____ _____. These areas are specially sensitive to sensations such as (b) _____ from the ears and (c) _____ or (d) _____ from the skin. The RAS is part of the reticular formation.

Q22.   Where is the reticular formation located?

_____

_____

Q23.   This exercise relates briefly to the anatomy of the midbrain, the pons and medulla.

Like the pons and medulla, the midbrain is about (a) _____ cm long.

The midbrain is more (b) _____ (anterior and superior? posterior and inferior?) to the pons and medulla.

THALAMUS

Now that you have completed the study of the brainstem, you can proceed to look at the thalamus, which is situated above the brainstem. Question 24 should help you in the study of the thalamus.

Q24. **Complete the exercise below, which relates to the structure of the thalamus.**

The thalamus consists of a pair of (a) _____ structures situated deeply within each (b) _____ hemisphere. The thalamus lies above the (c) _____ and consists mainly of (d) _____ matter.

The thalamus is H shaped. The cross-bar of the H is known as the (e) _____ mass. It passes through the centre of the slit-like (f) _____ ventricle. The two side bars of the H form the lateral walls of the third ventricle.

The thalamus is the principal relay station for (g) _____ (motor? sensory?) impulses. For example, spinothalamic and lemniscal tracts convey general sensations such as pain, (h) _____ , _____ , _____ , and temperature to the thalamus, where they are relayed to the cerebral cortex. Special sense impulses (for vision and hearing) are relayed through the (i) _____ (geniculate? reticular? ventral posterior?) nuclei of the thalamus.

The thalamus (j) _____ (does? does not?) contain nuclei controlling motor functions. However, its principal role is conveying (k) _____ (motor? sensory?) impulses.

HYPOTHALAMUS

The hypothalamus lies below the thalamus and plays an important role in controlling many body activities and is one of the major regulators of homeostasis.

Q25. **List some of the important functions of the hypothalamus.**

_____

_____

_____

_____

Now that you have been introduced to the brainstem, thalamus and hypothalamus, check your progress by completing question 26, below.

Q26. **Check your understanding of the brainstem and the diencephalon by matching them with the descriptions given below.**

> **1. Hypothalamus 2. Medulla 3. Midbrain 4. Pons 5. Thalamus**

☐   a. It is the principal regulator of visceral activities since it acts as a liaison between the cerebral cortex and the autonomic nerves that control the viscera.

☐ b. It is the site of the red nucleus, the origin of rubrospinal tracts concerned with muscle tone and posture.

☐ c. Cranial nerves III–IV attach to this part of the brain.

☐ d. Cranial nerves V–VIII attach to this part of the brain.

☐ e. Cranial nerves VIII–XII attach to this part of the brain.

☐ f. Feelings of hunger, fullness and thirst stimulate centres here, so that you can respond accordingly.

☐ g. All sensations except smell are relayed through here.

☐ h. Regulation of heart, blood pressure, and respiration occurs by centres located here.

☐ i. It constitutes four-fifths of the diencephalon.

☐ j. It lies under the third ventricle, forming its floor.

☐ k. It forms most of the side walls of the third ventricle.

☐ l. Tumour in this region could compress the cerebral aqueduct and cause internal hydrocephalus.

☐ m. The olivary and vestibular nuclei associated with equilibrium and posture control are located here.

☐ n. Mammillary bodies and supraoptic and preoptic regions are located here.

CEREBRUM 📖 *Pages 418–26*

The **cerebrum** forms the main bulk of the brain and consists of several structures that you will encounter in this study.

Q27. Complete this exercise about the cerebrum.

The outer layer of the cerebrum is called the (a) _____ _____ . It is composed of (b) _____ matter. This means that it contains mainly (c) _____ . Its thickness is between 2 and (d) _____ mm.

The surface of the cerebrum forms folds that are called (e) _____ . The deep grooves between the folds are known as (f) _____ , whilst the shallow grooves are called (g) _____ .

The cerebrum is divided into two halves, called (h) _____ . Connecting them is a band of (i) _____ matter called the (j) _____ _____ .
You can note this structure in 📖 *Page 417, Figure 14.9.*

The falx cerebri is composed of (k) _____ _____ (nerve fibres? dura mater?). It is located in between the cerebral hemispheres. At its superior and inferior margins, the falx is dilated to form channels for venous blood flowing from the brain; these enclosures are called (l) _____ _____ (at least two anatomical locations).

Understanding the functions of the cerebrum

To understand the functions of the cerebrum, you really need to be able to locate some of the lobes and specific anatomical locations in those lobes. Figure 7.5 should assist you in this study.

Q28. Figure 7.5 shows a right lateral view of the lobes and fissures of the cerebrum. Label A–H by using the following terms:

frontal lobe, occipital lobe, parietal lobe, temporal lobe, central sulcus, lateral cerebral sulcus, precentral gyrus and post central gyrus.

Figure 7.5.
Right lateral view of
lobes and fissures
of the cerebrum.

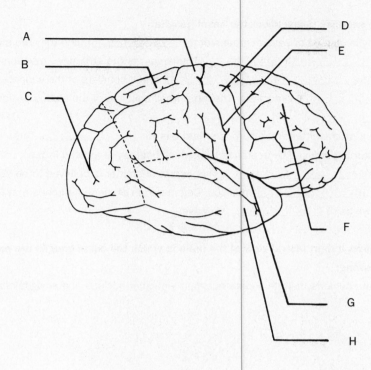

A

B

C

D

E

F

G

H

Q29.   Match the three types of white matter fibres in the box with the correct descriptions.

| 1. Association 2. Commissural 3. Projection |

- a. The corpus callosum contains these fibres and connects the two cerebral hemispheres.
- b. Sensory and motor fibres passing between cerebrum and other parts of the CNS are this type of fibre; the internal capsule is an example.
- c. These fibres transmit impulses among different areas of the same hemispheres.

Basal ganglia 📖 *Pages 421–2 & 429*

The basal ganglia are important structures in terms of their functions, for it is recognised that if they are affected as a result of degeneration or other diseases, many bodily motor activities will be disturbed. Apart from physical symptoms, behavioural symptoms may also become apparent. A classical mental disturbance, believed to be associated with a disorder of the basal ganglia, is that of **schizophrenia**. In this study you should note that the neurotransmitter **dopamine** is essential for the proper functioning of the basal ganglia.

Q30.   Complete the exercise below about the basal ganglia.

The basal ganglia consist of several groups of (a) _____ and they are situated in the (b) _____ _____ . The largest of the structures mentioned in (a) above is the (c) _____ _____ and it consists of the caudate nucleus and the (d) _____ nucleus. The latter itself consists of the globus pallidus and the (e) _____ .

The main neurotransmitter in the corpus striatum is (f) _____ . This neurotransmitter is produced by neurones whose cell bodies are located in the (g) _____ _____ . This neurotransmitter is believed to be involved in movement of (h) _____ muscles. Degeneration of these neurones may lead to the condition known as (i) _____ disease.

Q31.   Figure 7.6 shows a right lateral view of the brain in which the basal ganglia are exposed. Label the following:

head of caudate nucleus, tail of caudate nucleus, lenticular nucleus and amygdaloid body.

Figure 7.6.
Diagram of right
lateral view of brain.

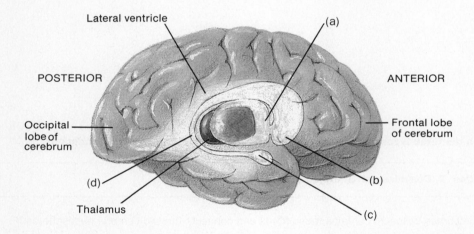

Limbic system 📖 *Pages 422–3*

The limbic system is a very complex system that consists of several areas of grey matter. It also consists of portions of the cerebrum, thalamus and hypothalamus. Note the specific structures of this system in 📖 *Page 422, Figure 14.13.*

Q32.   What are the main functions of the limbic system in relation to behaviour?

_____

_____

Q33. For what reason is it believed that the limbic system may play a role in memory?

_____

_____

Q34. Explain why the limbic system is sometimes called the 'visceral' or 'emotional' brain.

_____

_____

Functional areas of the cerebral cortex 📖 *Pages 423–4*

Read the section on functional areas of the cerebral cortex and then answer questions 35–37.

Q35. On Figure 7.5, indicate the functional areas of the cerebral cortex. Choose those areas from the list mentioned beneath the diagram.

Q36. The exercise below should help you to draw two important generalisations about brain functions.

In general, the anterior of the cerebrum is more involved with (a) _____ (motor? sensory?) control, whereas the posterior of the cerebrum is more involved with (b) _____ (motor? sensory?) functions.

As a general rule, (c) _____ (primary? association?) sensory areas receive sensations and (d) _____ sensory areas are involved with interpretation and memory of sensations.

Q37. Check your understanding of the functional areas of the cerebral cortex by completing this matching exercise. Answers may be used more than once.

> **1. Frontal eye field 2. Gnostic area 3. Motor speech area (Broca's) 4. Primary auditory area**
> **5. Primary motor area 6. Primary olfactory area 7. Primary somesthetic area 8. Primary visual area**

☐   a. In the occipital lobe.

☐   b. In the postcentral gyrus.

☐   c. Receives sensations of pain, touch, pressure and temperature.

☐   d. In the parietal lobe.

☐   e. In the temporal lobe; permits hearing.

☐   f. Integrates general and special sensations to form a common thought about them.

☐   g. In precentral gyrus of the frontal lobe; controls specific muscles or groups of muscles.

☐   h. In the frontal lobe; translates thoughts into speech.

☐   i. Controls smell.

☐   j. Controls scanning movements of eyes, such as searching for a name in a telephone directory.

Speech 📖 *Page 425*

Speech is very important for communication. As a nurse, you should be aware that speech defects may occur, if certain parts of the brain are damaged. For example, in many patients with cerebrovascular accident (CVA), also known as stroke, speech may be affected. Question 38 will assist you to understand the control of speech.

Q38. Complete this exercise about the control of speech.

Language areas are located in the (a) _____ (which side?) cerebral hemisphere. This is true for most (b) _____ (persons who are right-handed? persons, regardless of handedness?)

The term aphasia refers to inability to (c) _____ . Fluent aphasia means inability to (d) _____ (articulate or form? understand?). Word blindness refers to inability to understand (e) _____ (spoken? written?) words, whereas word deafness is inability to understand (f) _____ .

Brain wave and electroencephalogram (EEG) 📖 *Pages 425–6*

Nerve cells generate action potentials and added together from the millions of nerves in the brain produce the so called **brain waves**. Question 39 gives an overview of the types of brain waves.

Q39. Identify the type of brain waves associated with each of the following situations.

1. Alpha 2. Beta 3. Delta 4. Theta

☐ a. Occur in persons experiencing stress and in certain brain disorders.

☐ b. Lowest frequency brain waves, normally occurring when adult is in deep sleep; presence in awake adult indicates brain damage.

☐ c. Highest frequency waves, noted during periods of mental activity.

☐ d. Present when awake but resting, these waves are intermediate in frequency between alpha and delta waves.

CEREBELLUM 📖 *Pages 427–8*

The cerebellum is the second largest portion of the brain, and its main function is to ensure the smooth co-ordination of motor activities of skeletal muscles. This therefore allows for precision of movement. When you have worked through questions 40–43, you should understand some aspects of cerebellar functions.

Q40. Outline the anatomical location of the cerebellum.

_____

_____

Q41. Briefly describe the structure of the cerebellum.

_____

_____

_____

Q42. Describe the functions of the cerebellum, using the following key terms: co-ordinated movements, posture, equilibrium, emotions.

_____

_____

Q43. Name the three cerebellar peduncles and in each case indicate the structure that connects it to the cerebellum.

_____

_____

_____

NEUROTRANSMITTERS

You have already met neurotransmitters when you studied the chapter on nervous tissue. In the study to follow you will meet several types of neurotransmitters. **Remember** that some neurotransmitters are also recognised as hormones.

Q44. Complete the exercise below which relates to neurotransmitters.

Neurotransmitters bind to their (a) _____ to cause either the quick opening or the (b) _____ of (c) _____ (specific? or non specific?) channels in the membrane, resulting in fast or (d) _____ synaptic transmission.

Chemically most neurotransmitters are (e) _____ (large lipid? small? water-soluble?) molecules.

Q45. Match the neurotransmitter or neuromodulator from the box with the description that best fits.

| 1. Acetylcholine 2. Dopamine 3. Gamma aminobutyric acid 4. Serotonin 5. Endorphins, enkephalins and dynorphins 6. Substance P |

☐ a. Released at neuromuscular junctions and by many neurones, including those of pyramidal tracts.

☐ b. Produced by neurones that degenerate in Parkinson's disease.

☐ c. The most common inhibitory neurotransmitter in the brain.

☐ d. Made by neurones involved with emotional responses and automatic movements of skeletal muscles.

☐ e. Morphine-like chemicals that are the body's 'natural painkillers'.

☐ f. Concentrated in brainstem neurones, this chemical helps control sleep, temperature, and mood.

☐ g. Produced by neurones that are destroyed in Alzheimer's disease.

☐ h. Transmit pain-related impulses.

Q46. From the list of neurotransmitters or neuromodulators in question 45, identify those that are either amino acids (AA), biogenic amines (B), or neuropeptides (N).

_____

_____

Q47. Complete the following exercise which relates to enzymes that break down neurotransmitters.

Acetylcholine is destroyed by the enzyme (a) _____. A group of neurotransmitters known as catecholamines that include (b)_____ , _____ , _____ (three of them) are destroyed by two enzymes, namely COMT, which stands for (c) _____ and (d) _____ .

CRANIAL NERVES 📖 *Pages 431–5 and Figure 14.18 (Page 432)*

In recognising functions of the **cranial** nerves, you should be able to understand some of the symptoms experienced by individuals, when those nerves are affected by diseases or injury. Read the section on cranial nerves and then answer question 48.

Q48. Complete this exercise about cranial nerves.

Cranial nerves, of which there are (a) _____ pairs, form part of the (b) _____ nervous system. (c) _____ (how many?) pairs of cranial nerves are attached to the brainstem. They leave the brain via the (d) _____ of the (e) _____ .

The cranial nerves are numbered by roman numerals in the order that they leave the cranium, thus the most anterior is the (f) _____ nerve and the most posterior is the (g) _____ nerve.

Q49. To check your understanding of the functions of the cranial nerves, fill in the gaps in the following table, by identifying the number, name or function of the appropriate nerves.

Number	Name	Functions
(a)	Olfactory	(b)
(c)	(d)	Vision (not pain or temperature of the eye).
III	(e)	(f)
(g)	Trochlear	(h)
V	(i)	(j)
(k)	(l)	Stimulates lateral rectus muscle to abduct eye; proprioception.
(m)	Facial	(n)
(o)	(p)	Hearing: equilibrium
IX	(q)	(r)
(s)	Vagus	(t)
XI	(u)	(v)
(w)	(x)	Supplies muscles of the tongue with motor and sensory fibres.

Q50. Check your understanding of cranial nerves by completing this exercise. Write the name of the correct cranial nerve following the related description.

a. Differs from all other cranial nerves in that it originates from the brainstem and from the spinal cord: _____ .

b. Eighth cranial nerve (VIII): _____ .

c. Is widely distributed into the neck, thorax and abdomen: _____.

d. Senses toothache, pain under a contact lens, wind on the face: _____.

e. The largest cranial nerve; has three parts (opthalmic, maxillary and mandibular): _____ .

f. Controls contraction of the muscle of the iris, causing constriction of pupil: _____ .

g. Innervates muscles of facial expression: _____ .

h. Two nerves that contain taste fibres and autonomic fibres to salivary glands: _____ , _____ .

i. Three purely sensory cranial nerves: _____ , _____ , _____ .

Q51. Write the number (from the table above) of the cranial nerve related to each of the following disorders.

☐ a. Bell's palsy.

☐ b. Anosmia.

☐ c. Blindness.

☐ d. Strabismus and diplopia.

☐ e. Vertigo.

☐ f. Inability to shrug shoulders or turn head.

☐ g. Trigeminal neuralgia.

☐ h. Paralysis of vocal cords; loss of sensation of many organs.

Q52. Complete the following exercise which relates to the VIII cranial nerve.

The VIII cranial nerve consists of two branches: the (a) _____ , which is responsible for balance and equilibrium, and the (b) _____ , which is resposible for hearing.

Injury to the (c) _____ can lead to (d) _____ (described as feeling dizzy or head turning), whilst injury to the (e) _____ may cause (f) _____ (ringing in the ears) or (g) _____ .

AGEING AND THE NERVOUS SYSTEM 📖 *Page 431*

The normal process of ageing may in many cases lead to the degeneration of neurones, thereby affecting many neurological functions. This process is inevitable and unfortunately many elderly people will be affected, and consequently may lose all their independence and will have to be looked after by their families or the state. Carers need to be aware of the possible physical and mental problems faced by the elderly as a result of neuronal dysfunction. Many of those affected will also have various degrees of dementia.

The elderly population is growing, and many elderly will reach the ripe old age of 90 and above. Therefore the demands for health care provisions will increase dramatically.

Q53. Briefly explain the effects of ageing on the nervous system and suggest how these may affect an elderly individual.

_____

_____

_____

_____

Some interesting neurological disorders 📖 *Pages 438–40*

In this study, you are not expected to know an exhaustive list of neurological disorders. What is more important is for you to grasp the basic principles of **pathophysiology** and how these may affect the individual.

You will be introduced to four of the commonest nervous disorders. They are cerebrovascular accident (CVA), multiple sclerosis, Alzheimer's disease and Parkinson's disease. Apart from multiple sclerosis, the other three diseases mentioned above are very common in the elderly.

As nurses you will encounter some of these patients in your care. It is therefore imperative that you have some knowledge of the possible causation of these disorders, how they may affect the individuals (e.g. signs and symptoms) and also their management. When you have read the section Disorders: homeostatic imbalances in 📖 *Pages 438–40,* answer questions 54–57.

Q54. Complete this exercise on CVA.

CVA stands for (a) _____ , also known as (b) _____ and is the most common brain disorder. It may be caused as a result of reduced blood supply to the brain, thus resulting in (c) _____ or as a result of bleeding, commonly referred to as (d) _____ from a blood vessel in the pia mater or brain.

Another cause of CVA is the blockage of a blood vessel in the brain with blood clots, which could have been transferred to the brain from other parts of the body, and this is referred to as (e) _____ . Possible reasons for the development of blood clots, also known as (f) _____ may be damage to the lining of a blood vessel.

Q55. **List some of the risk factors that may give rise to the development of CVA.**

_____

_____

Q56. **Complete this exercise about Parkinson's disease.**
This condition involves a decrease in the neurotransmitter (a) _____ . It is normally produced by cell bodies located in the substantia nigra, which is part of the (b) _____ . Axons from the substantia nigra travel to the (c) _____ _____ (you have already studied this structure), where dopamine is released. Dopamine is an (d) _____ (excitatory? inhibitory?) neurotransmitter.

The most common sign of parkinsonism is (e) _____ . Briefly explain how tremor and muscle rigidity are related to a low level of dopamine.

_____

_____

Voluntary movements may be slower than normal; this is the condition known as (f) _____ . It would seem reasonable to administer dopamine in order to treat parkinsonism, but this is not done because dopamine cannot cross the (g) _____ _____. However, to relieve symptoms of parkinsonism, the drug (h) _____ is administered, as it is a (i) _____ of dopamine. Anticholinergic medications may provide some relief, especially that of (j) _____ and rigidity.

Q57. **Complete this exercise, which briefly describes the condition of multiple sclerosis.**
Multiple sclerosis affects (a) _____ (which part of the neurones?) within the (b) _____ nervous system. At sites along the nerves where myelin is destroyed, many scars or (c) _____ form; this is the basis for the name 'multiple sclerosis'.

Initial symptoms are most likely to occur around age (d) _____. Multiple sclerosis affects (e) _____ (motor? sensory? both motor and sensory?) neurones. The first symptoms of MS are usually muscle (f) _____ and the individual may be unable to control his/her bladder and this may give rise to urinary (g) _____ .

There is some evidence that MS may be caused by a (h) _____ infection that precipitates an (i) _____ response. It is for this reason that drugs belonging to the group known as (j) _____ are sometimes administered to MS sufferers.

Q58. Match the name of the disorders in the box with the related descriptions.

1. Cerebral palsy 2. Cerebrovascular accident 3. Dyslexia 4. Multiple sclerosis 5. Neuralgia 6. Parkinsonism 7. Poliomyelitis 8. Reye's syndrome 9. Tay-Sachs disease 10. Transient ischaemic attack

☐ a. Degeneration of myelin sheath to form hard plaques in many regions, causing loss of motor and sensory function.

☐ b. Degeneration of dopamine-releasing neurones in the basal ganglia; characterised by tremor or rigidity of muscles.

☐ c. Temporary cerebral dysfunction caused by interference of blood supply to the brain.

☐ d. Most common brain disorder; also called stroke.

☐ e. Characterized by difficulty in handling words and symbols, for example, reversal of letters (b for d); cause unknown.

☐ f. Attack of pain along an entire nerve, for example tic douloureux.

☐ g. A disease of children causing swelling of brain cells and fatty infiltration of liver; usually follows viral infection, especially if aspirin is taken.

☐ h. Inherited disease, especially among Jewish populations, due to excessive lipids in the brain cells; affects infants.

☐ i. Of viral origin; often affects only the respiratory system; when nervous system involved, affects movement, but not sensation.

☐ j. Motor disorder caused by damage during fetal life, birth, or infancy; not progressive; apparent mental retardation but often actually only speaking or hearing disability.

You have now completed the study on the brain and cranial nerves. We hope you have enjoyed this study, despite the complexities of this system. If you did find it difficult, do not worry, because with patience and perseverance, things will eventually fall into place. You will reap the benefits when you can actually see the relevance and the application of such study in your nursing practice.

To check your progress, you can attempt the Checkpoints Exercise.

CHECKPOINTS EXERCISE

Q59. Which one of the following is not located in the medulla?

a. Nucleus cuneatus and nucleus gracilis.

b. Cardiac centre, which regulates the heart.

c. Site of decussation of pyramidal tract.

d. The olive.

e. Origin of cranial nerves V and VIII.

Q60. Which one of the following is a function of the postcentral gyrus?

a. Controls specific groups of muscles, causing their contraction.

b. Receives general sensations from skin, muscles and viscera.

c. Receives olfactory impulses.

d. Primary visual reception area.

e. Somesthetic association area.

Q61. Which one of the following structures does not contain CSF?

a.   Subdural space.

b.   Ventricles of the brain.

c.   Central canal of the spinal cord.

d.   Subarachnoid space.

Q62. Which one of the following is likely to occur if the accessory nerve is damaged?

a.   Inability to turn the head or shrug the shoulders.

b.   Loss of normal speech function.

c.   Hearing loss.

d.   Anosmia.

Q63. Which one of the following is not a function of the hypothalamus?

a.   Control of body temperature.

b.   Release of chemicals (regulating factors) that affect release or inhibition of hormones.

c.   Principal relay station for sensory impulses.

d.   Involved in maintaining sleeping or waking state.

Q64. Which one of the following is likely to occur as a result of damage to the occipital lobe?

a.   Loss of hearing.

b.   Loss of vision.

c.   Loss of ability to smell.

d.   Paralysis.

e.   Loss of feeling in muscles (proprioception).

Q65. Which one of the following is a false statement?

a.   Multiple sclerosis is a progressive disorder that gets worse with time.

b.   Cerebral palsy is a progressive disorder that gets worse with time.

c.   About 70% of cerebral palsy individuals appear to be mentally retarded, but, in fact, this may be a reflection of inability to speak or walk well.

d.   Poliomyelitis may affect motor nerves, but does not affect sensations.

Q66. Which one of the following is not a catecholamine?

a.   Acetylcholine.

b.   Adrenaline.

c.   Noradrenaline.

d.   Dopamine.

Q67. **Circle 'T' (true) or 'F' (false) for each of the following statements.**

T   F   a. The thalamus, hypothalamus, and cerebellum are all developed from the forebrain.

T   F   b. Endorphins, enkephalins and dopamine are all chemicals that are considered the body's own pain killers.

T   F   c. The language areas are located in the cerebellar cortex.

T   F   d. Cranial nerves I, III, and VIII are purely sensory nerves.

T   F   e. The limbic system functions in the control of emotional aspects of behaviour.

T   F   f. GABA, serotonin and acetylcholine may all function as excitatory transmitter substances.

T   F   g. Delta brain waves have the lowest frequency of the four kinds of waves produced by normal individuals.

PATIENT SCENARIO

Derek Johnson, aged 65, is admitted to a medical rehabilitation ward, following a stroke (cerebrovascular accident). Nursing assessment reveals that he suffers from a right hemiplegia. He is conscious, although he appears to be disorientated. He is also dysphasic and is incontinent of urine and faeces. Nursing observations of pulse and respiratory rate and his skin colour indicate that they are within normal limits, but his blood pressure is elevated at 220/120 mmHg. He also appears to be overweight. The yellowish discoloration of his fingertips suggests that he is a heavy smoker.

Q68. **Suggest which part of Mr Johnson's brain has been affected.**

_____

_____

_____

_____

Q69. **What is the likely explanation for his hemiplegia on the right side of his body?**

_____

_____

_____

_____

Q70. Briefly explain why Mr Johnson is dysphasic.

_____

_____

_____

_____

Q71. Discuss the care of Mr Johnson during the acute phase.

_____

_____

_____

Q72. Suggest the likely factor that could have lead to Mr Johnson's cerebrovascular accident.

_____

_____

_____

Q73. Mr Johnson has made significant progress and he will be able to resume most of his daily activities. He prefers to be very independent. With regard to health education, what advice should you give to Mr Johnson?

_____

_____

_____

_____

QUESTIONS FOR FURTHER DISCUSSION

Q1. Giving the rationale for your answer, discuss as many as possible of the complications that could affect Mr Johnson's progress.

Q2. In your answer to question 1, suggest how these complications may be prevented (whenever appropriate) through nursing management.

Q3. Discuss all the facilities (you should include the primary health care team and other agencies) that are available in the community and can therefore provide care that will assist Mr Johnson in maintaining optimum health.

CEREBROVASCULAR ACCIDENT

Cerebrovascular accident (CVA) is the most common disease of the nervous system and is ranked as the third leading cause of death in the developed countries. CVA is more common in persons between 75 and 85 years of age, although a person of any age group can be affected.

There are three main causes of CVA: **thrombosis, embolism,** and **haemorrhage.** Thrombosis is the most common cause of CVA and the most common cause of thrombosis is **atherosclerosis**. Many factors may give rise to atherosclerosis. They include diabetes mellitus, obesity, high serum cholesterol and lipids, cigarette smoking and stress.

Embolism is the second most common cause of CVA.

Haemorrhage usually occurs as a result of ruptured aneurysm (area of weakness in a blood vessel). There are other factors that may contribute to the development of CVA, and these are hypertension, or the use in women of oral contraceptive pills. Whatever the cause of CVA, the most important altered physiology in the brain is that of oxgygen lack, leading to anoxia. The area most likely to be damaged is the **internal capsule**. This affects both the upper motor neurones fibres and the sensory fibres.

Symptoms depend on how much of the brain has been damaged. Therefore, patients may be unconscious, semi-conscious or conscious (alertness may be diminished). They may suffer with hemiplegia (paralysis initially flaccid, but as a result of increased muscle tone becoming spastic–rigid) or hemiparesis (weakness) on the side of the body opposite to the damage. There may be problems with vision, which may include diplopia (double vision) or blurred vision. Dysphasia or aphasia (disorder of language) may occur, especially if the left hemisphere is affected. There may be urine or faecal incontinence.

An approach to minimise limb and muscle problems is to use the so called Bobath technique. This is performed by assessing muscle tone, posture and movement and then providing sensations that will evoke a response in keeping with the normal movements.

Answers to questions

Q1.   a, brainstem; b, diencephalon; c, cerebrum; d, cerebellum.

Q2.   Skull bones, meninges and cerebrospinal fluid.

Q3.   Dura mater, pia mater and arachnoid.

Q4.   a, cranial; b, hemispheres; c, corpus callosum; d, meninges; e, brainstem; f, cerebrum.

Q5.   a, four; b, lateral ventricles; c, cerebrum; d, foramen; e, third; f, cerebral aqueduct; g, foramen of Magendie.

Q6.   a, foramen of Magendie; b, fourth ventricle; c, lateral ventricle; d, third ventricle; e, cerebral aqueduct; f, lateral ventricle; g, third ventricle; h, foramen of Magendie.

Q7.   a, choroid plexuses; b, lateral ventricle; c, 80; d, 150; e, arachnoid villi; f, hydrocephalus.

Q8.   D, E, F, G, H, I, J, K, C, A, B.

Q9.   Serves as shock absorber for the brain and the cord. Provides nutrients. Provides an optimal chemical environment for accurate neuronal signalling.

Q10.   a, anterior cerebral; b, basilar; c, vertebral; d, posterior cerebral; e, posterior communicating; f, anterior communicating.

Q11.   a, Carotid; b, basilar; c, basilar; d, posterior; e, posterior communicating; f, anterior communicating.

Q12.   The brain will be deprived of oxygen and glucose. In the absence of oxygen, the lysosomes in the brain rupture and release their enzymes, which bring about the destruction of brain cells.

Q13.   a, less; b, tight; c, astrocytes.

Q14.   Most substances that otherwise could be harmful to the brain cells are prevented from entering the brain.

Q15.   Glucose, oxygen, water, sodium and potassium ions.

Q16.   Antibiotics or other chemotherapeutic agents will not be able to reach the brain cells if they are needed, for example in a severe infection of the meninges or the brain. This may be true in the treatment of meningitis, for example. This situation is remedied by giving the medication intrathecally (injection given via a lumbar puncture). This was explained in Chapter 6.

Q17. Alcohol, caffeine, nicotine and heroin.

Q18. Midbrain, pons and medulla.

Q19. a, Conduction; b, both sensory and motor; c, pyramidal; d, motor; e, corticospinal; f, decussation; g, left; h, axons; i, corticospinal; j, cuneatus; k, gracilis (order for j and k not important); l, proprioception; m, cardiac; n, respiratory; o, vasomotor.

Cranial nerves are VIII, IX, X, XI, XII.

Q20. a, Bridge; b, spinal cord; c, medulla; d, cerebellum; e, V–VII and part of VIII; f, respiration.

Q21. a, Reticular activating system; b, sound; c, temperature; d, pain.

Q22. Medulla, pons and midbrain, as well as portions of the diencephalon (thalamus and hypothalamus) and spinal cord.

Q23. a, 2.5; b, anterior and superior.

Q24. a, Oval; b, cerebral; c, midbrain; d, grey; e, intermediate; f, third; g, sensory; h, touch, pressure, proprioception (order of answer is not important); i, geniculate; j, does; k, sensory.

Q25. Controls and integrates autonomic nervous system such as in contraction of smooth muscles and secretions of various glands. Regulates body temperature. Controls the feeling of rage and aggression. Regulates food intake (satiety and hunger centres). Controls thirst. Releases releasing factors, which stimulate anterior pituitary secretion. Controls arousal and consciousness.

Q26. 1a, 3b, 3c, 4d, 2e, 1f, 5g, 2h, 5i, 1j, 5k, 3l, 3m, 1n.

Q27. a, Cerebral cortex; b, grey; c, cell bodies; d, 4; e, gyri; f, fissures; g, sulci; h, hemispheres; i, white; j, corpus callosum; k, dura mater; l, superior and inferior sagittal sinuses.

Q28. A, post central gyrus; B, parietal lobes; C, occipital lobes; D, precentral gyrus; E, central sulcus; F, frontal lobe; G, lateral cerebral sulcus; H, temporal lobe.

Q29. 2a, 3b, 1c.

Q30. a, Nuclei; b, cerebral hemisphere; c, corpus callosum; d, lenticular; e, putamen; f, dopamine; g, substantia nigra; h, skeletal; i, Parkinson's disease.

Q31. a, lenticular nucleus; b, head of caudate nucleus; c, amygdaloid body; d, tail of caudate nucleus.

Q32. Has primary functions in emotions such as pain, pleasure, anger, rage, fear, sorrow, sexual feeling and affection.

Q33. Because lesions in parts of the limbic system cause memory impairment. People with such damage cannot commit anything to memory.

Q34. This is explained in the answer to question 32.

Q35.

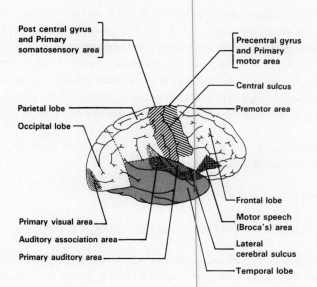

Post central gyrus and Primary somatosensory area

Precentral gyrus and Primary motor area

Central sulcus

Parietal lobe

Premotor area

Occipital lobe

Frontal lobe

Primary visual area

Motor speech (Broca's) area

Auditory association area

Lateral cerebral sulcus

Primary auditory area

Temporal lobe

Q36. a, Motor; b, sensory; c, primary; d, association.

Q37. 8a, 7b, 7c, 7d, 4e, 2f, 5g, 3h, 6i, 1j.

Q38. a, Left; b, persons, regardless of handedness; c, speak; d, understand; e, written; f, spoken.

Q39. 4a, 3b, 2c, 1d.

Q40. Situated in the posterior part of the cranial cavity. It is posterior to the medulla and pons and inferior to the occipital lobes of the cerebrum.

Q41. 📖 *Page 427.*

Q42. Controls skeletal muscle contractions required for skilled movements, co-ordination, posture and balance.

Q43. Inferior cerebellar peduncle – connects the cerebellum to the medulla at the base of the brainstem and spinal cord. Middle cerebellar peduncle – connects the cerebellum to the cord. Superior cerebellar peduncle – connects the cerebellum to the midbrain.

Q44. a, Receptors; b, closing; c, specific; d, slow; e, water soluble.

Q45. 1a, 2b, 3c, 2d, 5e, 4f, 1g, 6h.

Q46. b, B; c, AA; d, B; e, N; f, B; h, N.

Q47. a, Acetylcholine; b, adrenaline, noradrenaline, dopamine (order of answer is not important); c, catechol-O-methyl-transferase; d, monoamine oxidase.

Q48. a, 12; b, peripheral; c, 10; d, foramina; e, skull; f, olfactory; g, hypoglossal.

Q49. a, I; b, Smell; c, II; d, Optic; e, Oculomotor; f, Movement of eyelid and eyeball, accommodation of lens for near vision and constriction of pupil; proprioception; g, IV; h. Movement of eyeball; proprioception; i, Trigeminal; j, Chewing; conveys sensation for touch, pain and temperature; proprioception; k, VI; l, Abducens; m, VII; n, Facial expression and secretion of saliva and tears; proprioception and taste; o, VIII; p, Vestibulocochlear; q, Glossopharyngeal; r, Secretion of saliva; taste and regulation of blood pressure; proprioception; s, X; t, Smooth muscle contraction and relaxation; Secretion of digestive fluids; sensation from organs supplied; proprioception; u, Accessory; v, Swallowing movements; movement of head; proprioception; w, XII; x, Hypoglossal.

Q50. a, Accessory; b, vestibulocochlear; c, vagus; d, trigeminal; e, trigeminal; f, oculomotor; g, facial; h, facial, glossopharyngeal; i, olfactory, optic, vestibulocochlear.

Q51. a, VII; b, I; c, II; d, III; e, VIII; f, XI; g, V; h, X.

Q52. a, Vestibular; b, cochlear; c, vestibular; d, vertigo; e, cochlear; f, tinnitus; g, deafness.

Q53. The total number of nerve cells decreases; conduction velocity slows down; the time required for a typical reflex increases; voluntary motor movements slow down. Impaired hearing, known as presbycusis, may occur. Although the cause is not established, a disease such as Parkinson's may occur as a result of old age (most common motor disorder in the elderly).

Q54. a, Cerebrovascular accident; b, stroke; c, ischaemia; d, haemorrhage; e, thrombosis; f, thrombi.

Q55. High blood pressure; high blood cholesterol; atherosclerosis, which may in fact lead to high blood pressure; diabetes mellitus; smoking; obesity; excessive alcohol intake.

Q56. a, Dopamine; b, midbrain; c, basal ganglia; d, inhibitory; e, tremor.
Explanation – Lack of inhibitory DA causes a double-negative effect; extra unnecessary movement occurs (tremor), which may then interfere with normal movement (rigidity).
f, Bradykinesia; g, blood–brain barrier; h, L-dopa; i, precursor; j, tremor.

Q57. a, myelin sheath; b, central; c, scleroses; d, 33; e, both motor and sensory; f, weakening; g, incontinence; h, viral; i, immune; j, immunosuppressants.

Q58. 4a, 6b, 10c, 2d, 3e, 5f, 8g, 9h, 7i, 1j.

Q59. e. **Q60.** b. **Q61.** a. **Q62.** a. **Q63.** c. **Q64.** b. **Q65.** b. **Q66.** a.

Q67. Ta, Fb, Fc, Fd, Te, Ff, Tg.

Q68. It is likely to be the left side of his brain, since you know that nerves of the pyramidal tract cross over (decussate) in the medulla. This means that the left cerebral hemisphere controls movements on the right side of the body and vice versa. The clues to this question are that Derek is suffering from right hemiplegia and he is also dysphasic.

Q69. This has been explained above.

Q70. Dysphasic means having difficulty with speech. The speech centre (Broca's area) of most individuals, regardless of handedness, is believed to be situated in the left hemisphere. Evidence for this is that upper motor neurone diseases or trauma affecting the left cerebral hemisphere is usually accompanied by speech problems. This is very common in stroke patients who have suffered damage to the left cerebral hemisphere. Obviously, the other sign is a right hemiplegia.

Q71. Care in the acute phase:

Maintaining airway

It is essential that Mr Johnson's breathing is monitored. Although he is conscious initially, his condition could deteriorate, and he could be at risk of inhaling his secretions, food or fluid. In the early stage, the swallowing or cough reflex may be affected. He should be placed in the most comfortable position that will allow for maximum pulmonary ventilation. Check for possible obstruction with dentures. If Mr Johnson is very disorientated, it is preferable to remove the dentures and keep them in a safe place, until he is more alert.

Assessment for possible neurological complications

Assess for neurological complications, such as intracranial pressure (blood pressure increases – vasomotor involvement), whilst pulse rate decreases (cardiac centre involvement). Check the rate and depth of respiration. Monitor pupil size and reaction to light. If intracranial pressure occurs, the pupils become unequal (dilate on the affected side) and unresponsive to light. Fixed dilated pupil is an extremely serious prognostic sign.

Positioning in bed

In order to prevent problems such as joint stiffness, foot drop and bent knee, Mr Johnson should be properly positioned in bed and all care given to the limbs. Various aids may be used, such as bed-cradle, to take the weight of the bed clothes and thus allow Mr Johnson free movements. The physiotherapist will encourage passive limb movements at first, but these may be followed by active exercises. The nurse can assist by providing some of the exercises whenever appropriate.

Activities

Since Mr Johnson is conscious, he may not want to be on bedrest, but it is important to encourage him to comply. He should be given careful explanations as to why he requires bedrest.

Communication

Communication may be a problem, as Mr Johnson is dysphasic. He may be very distressed as he is not able to let you know what he wants or does not want. It is often worse for the first few days. The nurse should be very patient and understanding and not rush Mr Johnson when he is trying to communicate verbally. Do let him know that you can comprehend his conversation. Mr Johnson should be reassured that as he makes progress, his speech will improve. There may be excessive salivation, especially if there is severe paralysis on the side of the face. This may also interfere with communication. Ensure that paper tissues are available for Mr Johnson to wipe his mouth.

Prevention of decubitus ulcers

As Mr Johnson is incontinent of both faeces and urine, it is important that he is kept clean and dry, to prevent the problems of pressure sores, which could give rise to decubitus ulcers. Mr Johnson should be encouraged to change position frequently, and the nurse should assist him in doing so.

Q72. From the case history, it is suggested that Mr Johnson might be a heavy smoker and that he is also hypertensive. The assumptions to be made are as follows: smoking could have been a contributing factor and this could have led to atherosclerosis. In turn, the atherosclerosis probably gave rise to hypertension. Hypertension precipitated the development of either a thrombus or a haemorrhage.

Q73. With regard to the health education, any advice given should take into consideration Mr Johnson's circumstances and also his life-style. If he is smoking, he should be strongly advised to cut down or give it up. It is important that he has the appropriate support from the multidisciplinary team. The health visitor can play a vital role in supporting Mr Johnson in the community. As he is overweight, he would have been seen by the dietician with regard to losing weight. The nurse can reinforce the recommended regimen for his diet. He should also be encouraged to take daily exercises as his health allows.

He should receive instructions with regard to taking any medications regularly and as has been prescribed, especially if he is prescribed antihypertensive medication. He should also be given information on the importance of reporting any illness which may be due to side effects of the medication he is taking. For example, he could develop postural hypotension. To refresh your memory on postural hypotension, please refer to question 14 in Chapter 1.

Overview and key terms

Sensory, motor and integrative system

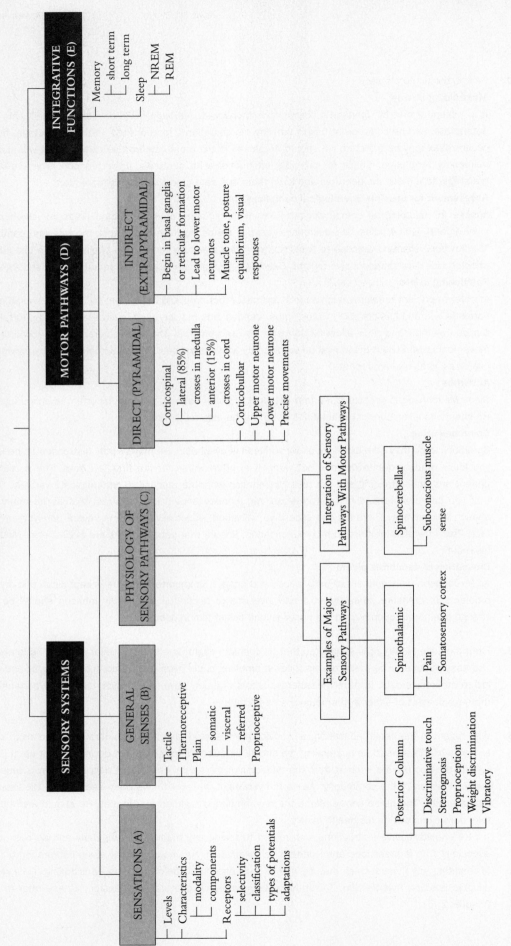

8. Sensory, Motor and Integrative Systems

Learning outcomes

1. To define a sensation and list the characteristics of sensations.

2. To describe the classification of receptors.

3. To list the location and function of the receptors for tactile sensations (touch, pressure, vibration), thermoreceptive sensations (heat and cold) and pain.

4. To distinguish somatic, visceral, referred and phantom pain.

5. To outline the functions of proprioceptive receptors.

6. To outline the neuronal components and functions of the posterior column–medial lemniscus and the spinothalamic and spinocerebellar pathways.

7. To describe the integration of sensory input and motor output.

8. To compare the location and functions of the direct and indirect motor pathways.

9. To explain how the basal ganglia and cerebellum are related to motor responses.

10. To compare integrative functions, such as memory, wakefulness and sleep.

Chapter 15

INTRODUCTION

The last three chapters have introduced you to the components of the nervous system, and mainly how neurones are organised in the brain, spinal cord and spinal and cranial nerves.

In this chapter you will be exposed to the specific nerve pathways that include the general senses (touch, pain and temperature), the motor pathway for voluntary and involuntary movements and other integrative systems such as memory and sleep.

Your study will begin with a quick review of the basic functions of the nervous system.

SENSATIONS 📖 *Pages 444–6*

Q1. **Recall the three basic functions of the nervous system by listing the three statements in sequence.**

a. Receiving _____ input.

b. _____ information.

c. Transmitting _____ impulses to _____ or _____ .

Understanding sensations 📖 *Pages 444–6*

In our day-to-day life experiences, if we are fortunate to be healthy, we take many things, such as all our sensations of things around us, for granted. Life would be very dull if we were deprived of some of these sensations.

In answering question 2, you will be able to understand how important sensations are for homeostasis.

Q2. **For a moment, visualise what your life would be like if you were unable to experience any sensations. List the three types of sensations that you believe you would miss most.**

_____ , _____ , _____ .

Now write a sentence describing how your health and safety might be endangered by lack of ability to perceive sensations.

_____

_____

Q3. **Complete this activity about levels of sensation.**

(a) _____ (perception? sensation?) is the awareness (either conscious or unconscious) of stimuli, such as the act of seeing a dog, whereas (b) _____ is the conscious awareness and interpretation of sensation, such as the recognition of that dog as a labrador and not a rottweiler.

Q4. **Identify levels of sensation by matching the parts of the nervous system listed in the box with the descriptions below.**

> **1. Brainstem 2. Cerebral cortex 3. Spinal cord 4. Thalamus**

☐ a. Immediate reflex action is possible without involvement of the brain.

☐ b. Involves subconscious motor reactions, such as those that facilitate balance and equilibrium.

☐ c. Offers a general (or 'crude') awareness of local sensations and type of sensations, such as awareness of pressure within the leg or that something is being heard; offers no specifics.

☐ d. Gives precise information about sensations, such as distinguishing Beethoven from Berlioz from Bach, as well as memories of hearing a particular musical work.

Q5. **Is it possible for sensation to be experienced despite an interruption in the sensory input, such as the cutting of a nerve?**

Using an appropriate example, explain your answer.

_____

_____

_____

_____

_____

Characteristics of sensations 📖 *Pages 444–5*

Q6. **Complete this exercise on the characteristics of sensations.**

The quality that makes the sensation of pain different from the sense of touch or that makes hearing different from vision is called the (a) _____ of sensation. Any single sensory neurone carries sensations of (b) _____ _____ (one modality? many modalities?). Different modalities of sensations are distinguished precisely at the level of the (c) _____ (which part of the brain?). We are not constantly aware that our clothes are rubbing against our skin. This is known as the characteristic of (d) _____ . This type of receptor adapts most slowly: (e) _____ (pain? pressure? smell? touch?). Explain how such slow adaptation is advantageous to you.

_____

Describe what is meant by the **selectivity** of receptors.

_____

Is selectivity absolute? Explain.

_____

Components of sensation 📖 *Pages 444–5*

For a sensation to arise, four events must occur. Question 7 should help you to appreciate the components of sensation.

Q7.   Arrange in correct order the components in the pathway of sensation.

> **A. Conduction B. Stimulation C. Transduction D. Translation**

1. _____ 2. _____ 3. _____ 4. _____

Now match each of these components of sensation with the correct description below.

☐ a. Activation of a neurone.

☐ b. Stimulus generator potential.

☐ c. Generator potential nerve impulse; impulse is conveyed along a first order neurone into the spinal cord or brainstem up to a higher level of the brain.

☐ d. Nerve impulse sensation; usually occurs in the cerebral cortex.

Sensory receptors 📖 *Pages 445–6*

There are many types of receptors in the body; some are simple whilst many are complex. In answering questions 8–12, you should grasp the basics of sensory receptors.

Q8.   Briefly differentiate between simple and complex receptors.

_____

_____

Q9.   Identify the class of receptor that fits each description.

> **E. Exteroceptor I. Interoceptor P. Proprioceptor**

☐ a. These receptors inform you that you are hungry or thirsty; they also inform your brain of the need for adjustment of blood pressure.

☐ b. Your ears, eyes and receptors in your skin for pain, touch, hot and cold are of this type.

☐ c. With your eyes closed, you can tell your exact body position, thanks to these receptors.

Q10.   Fill in the types of receptors based on the nature of the stimulus detected.

a. You can maintain balance by means of inner ear _____ receptors sensitive to change in position.

b. Different tastes and smells are distinguished with the help of _____ receptors in the nose and mouth.

c. _____ receptors inform you of the temperature around you.

Q11. **Choose the descriptions associated with general (G) or special (S) receptors.**

☐   a. These are numerous and widespread in the body.

☐   b. Relatively complex receptors are of this type.

☐   c. Sight, hearing, smell and taste involve receptors of this type.

☐   d. Sensations of the skin (cutaneous) are of this type.

Q12. **Contrast generator potential (GP) with receptor potential (RP) by completing this table.**

	GP	RP
Triggers action potential (yes or no)	a.	b.
Most receptors for (general? special?) senses of this type	c.	d.
(Always excitatory? always inhibitory? excitatory or inhibitory?)	e.	f.

General senses 📖 *Pages 446–51*

Q13. **List six examples of cutaneous sensations.**

_____

_____

Q14. **Complete the following exercise about tactile sensations.**

The tactile sensations are: (a) _____ , _____, _____,

_____, _____ (answer in any order that you wish).

These sensations are all sensed by (b) _____ receptors. Receptors for these

sensations are (c) _____ (evenly? unevenly?) distributed throughout the skin of the

body.

(d) _____ (Discriminative? Light?) touch refers to ability to determine that

something has touched the skin, but its precise location, shape, size or texture cannot be

distinguished.

In general, pressure receptors are more (e) _____ (superficial? deep?) in

location than touch receptors. Sensations of (f) _____ result from rapid repetition of

sensory impulses from tactile receptors.

Q15. **Match the names of the receptors in the box with the correct descriptions. Please note that**
you may have to use some of the numbers more than once.

---

1. Corpuscles of touch 2. Hair cells of the inner ear 3. Joint kinesthetic receptors 4. Lamellated (Pacinian) corpuscles 5. Muscle spindles 6. Nociceptors 7. Tendon organs 8. Type I cutaneous mechanoreceptors 9. Type II cutaneous mechanoreceptors

---

☐   a. Egg-shaped masses located in dermal papillae, especially in fingertips, palms of hands and soles of feet.

☐   b. Onion-shaped structures sensitive to pressure and high-frequency vibration.

☐   c. Slowly adapting touch receptors (two answers).

☐   d. Proprioceptors (four answers).

☐   e. May respond to any type of stimulus if the stimulus is strong enough to cause tissue damage.

☐   f. Respond to chemicals released from injured tissue, such as prostaglandins and kinins.

☐   g. Type Ia and type II fibres that are sensitive to stretch.

☐   h. Sensitive to tension; monitor the force of muscle contraction.

Q16.   Figure 8.1 shows a section of the skin. Identify the four receptors (labelled A–D).

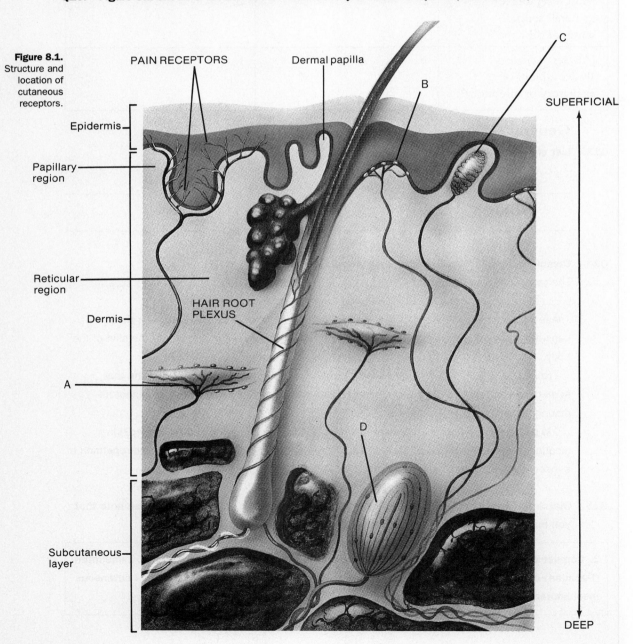

Figure 8.1. Structure and location of cutaneous receptors.

Pain sensation 📖 *Page 448*

Q17. **a. Differentiate between visceral and somatic pain.**

_____

_____

b. Differentiate between general and spinal anaesthesia.

_____

_____

Nursing application

Q18. **Explain why an individual who is to undergo surgery under general anaesthetic must fast for a couple of hours.**

_____

_____

_____

Many individuals often experience pain which is said to be 'referred pain'. This is because the pain is felt in a location perhaps quite distant from the organ that is affected. When you have completed question 19, you should understand the term 'referred pain'.

Q19. **Complete the exercise below, which refers to 'referred pain'.**

Pain impulses that originate in the heart, for example in a myocardial infarction, commonly referred to as a 'heart attack', enter the spinal cord at the same level as do sensory fibres from the skin covering the (a) _____ . This level of the cord is about
(b) _____ to (c) _____ .

Refer to 📖 *Page 449, Figure 15.2*. Note that some liver and gallbladder pain is felt in a region quite distant from these organs, that is in the (d) _____ region. These organs lie just inferior to the dome-shaped (e) _____ , which is supplied by the phrenic nerve from the (f) _____ plexus. A painful gallbladder can send impulses to the cord via the phrenic nerve, which enters the cord at the same level (about C (g) _____ or C (h) _____) as nerves from the neck and shoulder. So gallbladder pain is said to be (i) _____ to the neck and shoulder area.

Proprioceptive sensations 📖 *Pages 448–51*

Q20.   Name the three main proprioceptors and their locations.

_____

Q21.   What is the name of the efferent neurone to intrafusal muscle fibre?

_____

Physiology of sensory pathways 📖 *Pages 451–4*

The most important information to be gained from the study that follows is that most **sensory** nerves ascend to the brain and cross over to the **opposite side** in the spinal cord or the brainstem before ascending to the **thalamus.** Thus, the left brain controls the right side of the body and vice versa.

Q22.   Check that you understand the pathway of sensation by arranging the statements below in the correct order.

a.   These cross to the opposite side of the spinal cord or brain stem and ascend to the thalamus.

b.   These reach the spinal cord or brainstem.

c.   These pass to the somatosensory region of the cerebral cortex and also travel (via collaterals) to the cerebellum and reticular formation.

_____   _____   _____

To assist you in understanding pathways and the route that they take to reach the brain, you are invited to study Figure 8.2 and then to complete questions 23 and 24.

Q23.   Complete this question, which should help you to understand sensory reception in the cerebral cortex.

Picture the brain as roughly similar in shape to a small, rounded loaf of bread. The crust would be comparable to the cerebral (a) _____ . Suppose you cut a slice of bread in midloaf that represents the **postcentral** gyrus. It looks somewhat like the 'slice' or section of brain shown at the top of Figure 8.2. Locate the Z on that Figure. This portion (next to the (b) _____ fissure) receives sensations from the (c) _____ (face? hand? hip? foot?). Refer to 📖 *Page 453, Figure 15.6* for extra help.

Suppose a person suffered a loss of blood supply (CVA or 'stroke') to the area of the brain marked X in Figure 8.2. Loss of sensation in the (d) _____ (face? hand? leg?) area would result. Damage to the area marked W is located on the temporal lobe. The letters W, X, Y, and Z are marked on the (e) _____ side of the brain.

If a friend stands and faces you, the right side of your friend's brain will be in your left field of view. What effects would brain damage to the area Y of the postcentral gyrus have? Loss of (f) _____ (sensation? movement?) to the (g) _____ (face? hand? foot?) on the (h) _____ side of the body.

Figure 8.2.
gram of the central
nervous system.

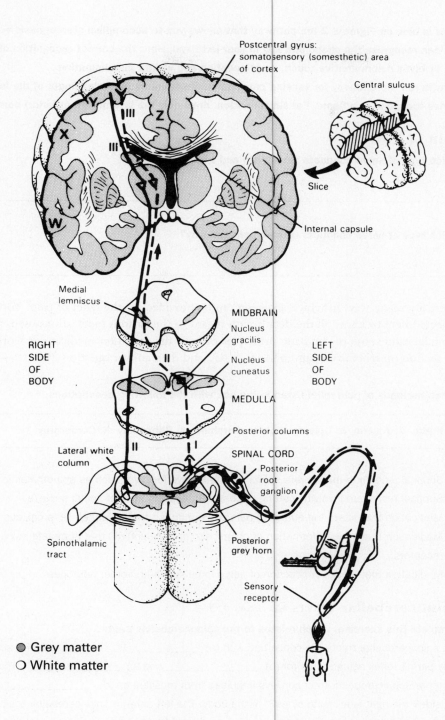

Postcentral gyrus:
somatosensory (somesthetic) area
of cortex

Central sulcus

Slice

Internal capsule

Medial
lemniscus

MIDBRAIN

Nucleus
gracilis

Nucleus
cuneatus

RIGHT
SIDE
OF
BODY

LEFT
SIDE
OF
BODY

MEDULLA

Posterior columns

Lateral white
column

SPINAL CORD

Posterior
root
ganglion

Spinothalamic
tract

Posterior
grey horn

Sensory
receptor

● Grey matter
○ White matter

Q24. On Figure 8.2, draw a sensory pathway indicating the first, second, and third order neurones
as I, II, III. Try to impress yourself and do it from memory. Of course, if you have problems,
check your text.

Q25. Define the term stereognosis.

Q26. Draw in blue on Figure 8.2 the pathway that allows you to accomplish stereognosis so that you can recognise the shape of a key in your left hand. Hint: the correct recognition of the key involves discriminative touch, proprioception and weight discrimination.

Draw in red the pathway for sensing pain and temperature as the index finger of the left hand comes too close to a flame. For simplification, draw only the lateral (not anterior) component.

Pain 📖 *Page 452*

Q27. Which type of nerve conducts acute pain and why?

_____

Q28. Which type of nerve conducts chronic pain and why?

_____

There are many ways in which analgesia can be provided for the relief of pain. You are not expected here to know all the details with regard to the various medications used, but only to understand some of the basic principles of how the common medications work. Read the section on relief from pain in 📖 *Page 452* and then answer question 29.

Q29. Match methods of pain relief listed in the box with the following descriptions.

1. Anaesthetic 2. Aspirin 3. Opioids such as morphine 4. Rhizotomy 5. Cordotomy

☐　a. Surgical technique that severs spinal cord pathways for pain, such as spinothalamic tracts.
☐　b. Surgical technique involving cutting of posterior (sensory) root of spinal nerve/s.
☐　c. Medication that alters the quality of pain perception, so that pain feels less noxious.
☐　d. Medication that inhibits formation of chemicals (prostaglandins) that stimulate pain receptors.
☐　e. Medication that blocks conduction of nerve impulses in first-order neurones.

Spinocerebellar tracts 📖 *Pages 453–4*

Q30. Complete this exercise, which relates to the spinocerebellar tracts.

The spinocerebellar tracts are concerned with (a) _____ muscle and joint sense. They permit reflex adjustments for (b) _____ and (c) _____ . The left posterior spinocerebellar tract conveys impulses from muscles on (d) _____ (the left side? the right side? both sides?) of the body. The left anterior spinocerebellar tract conveys impulses from the muscles on (e) _____ of the body.

Integration of sensory input and motor output 📖 *Page 454*

If there is to be a **motor** response from the CNS, you already know that there should be a **sensory** input. But do all sensory inputs trigger a motor response?

Read the section on integration and sensory input and motor output and then answer question 31.

Q31. **The linking of sensory to motor response occurs at different levels in the central nervous system. Indicate which is the highest level required for each of these responses.**

---
1. Basal ganglia 2. Cerebellum 3. Cerebral cortex 4. Spinal cord

---

☐   a. Quick withdrawal of a hand when it touches a hot object.

☐   b. Unconscious responses to proprioceptive impulses to permit smooth, co-ordinated movements (two answers).

☐   c. Playing the piano or writing a letter.

Physiology of motor pathways 📖 *Pages 454–61*

Motor pathways arise from the motor cortex. They are responsible for conducting all motor impulses via **efferent** neurones to the appropriate muscles for voluntary movements.

To understand motor pathways, you will need to refer to Figure 8.3 and then complete the relevant exercise.

Q32. **Refer to Figure 8.3 and complete this exercise about motor control.**

This 'slice' or section of the brain containing the primary motor cortex is located in the

(a) _____ lobe. Area P in this Figure controls (b) _____ (sensation? movement?) to the (c) _____ (left? right?) (arm? leg? side of the face?). Motor neurones in area P would send impulses to the pons to activate cranial nerve

(d) _____ to facial muscles. If there is damage to the area R, this may result in

(e) _____ (type of paralysis) paralysis of the (f) _____ (left? right?) foot.

Q33. **Show the route of impulses along the principal pyramidal pathway by listing in correct sequence the structures that comprise the pathway. If you have difficulty with this exercise, refer to 📖 *Page 455, Figure 15.8*.**

a. Anterior grey horn (lower motor neurone).

b. Midbrain and pons.

c. Effector (skeletal muscle).

d. Internal capsule.

e. Lateral corticospinal tract.

f. Medulla, decussation site.

g. Precentral gyrus (upper motor neurone).

h. Ventral root of spinal nerve.

_____ _____ _____ _____

_____ _____ _____

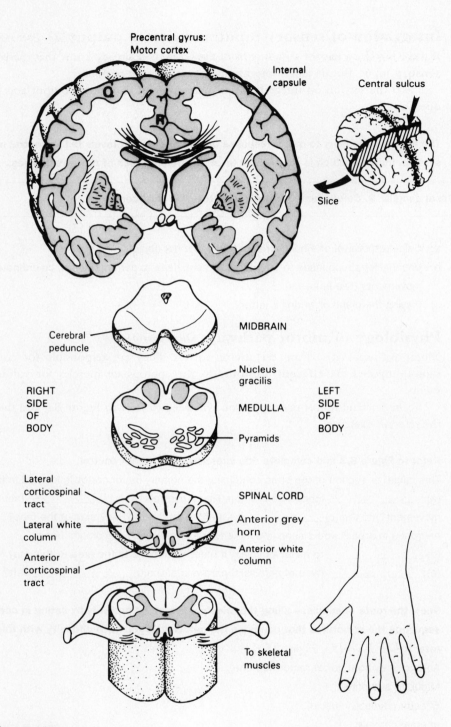

Figure 8.3. Diagram of the central nervous system.

● Grey matter
○ White matter

Q34. Now draw this pathway on Figure 8.3. Show the control of muscles in the left hand by means of neurones in the lateral corticospinal pathway (pyramidal tract). Label the upper and lower neurones.

Q35. Complete this exercise contrasting anterior with lateral corticospinal tracts.

Only about (a) _____ % of the upper motor neurones pass through anterior corticospinal tracts; (b) _____ % pass through the large (c) _____ corticospinal (pyramidal) tracts.

Left anterior corticospinal tracts consist of axons that originated in upper motor neurones on the (d) _____ side of the motor cortex.

Q36. Give an anatomical explanation for the fact that a six-month-old baby cannot be expected to walk.

_____

_____

Q37. State the functions of corticobulbar tracts.

_____

_____

Q38. Complete this exercise on upper motor neurones and lower motor neurones.

Upper motor neurones are located in the (a) _____ , whereas lower motor neurones are in (b) _____ or (c) _____ .

Destruction of (d) _____ motor neurones results in spastic paralysis since the brain is not controlling movements. Flaccid paralysis results from damage of (e) _____ motor neurones. Why are lower motor neurones called the 'final common pathway'?

Damage to the basal ganglia 📖 *Page 457*

You have already met the basal ganglia in a previous study and you were also introduced to the disease known as Parkinson's disease, which occurs as a result of dysfunction of the **basal ganglia**. Another condition that can occur as a result of basal ganglia dysfunction is Huntington's chorea.

Q39. Complete this exercise, which relates to the dysfunction of the basal ganglia.

(a) _____ disease involves changes to basal ganglia associated with a decrease in the neurotransmitter (b) _____ . Signs of this condition are (c) _____ (jerky movements and facial twitches? muscle rigidity and tremors?). A predominant sign of Huntington's disease is jerky movements or 'dance', known as (d) _____ related to loss of neurones that make the inhibitory transmitter named (e) _____ . Signs of this progressive condition are most likely to be first noted at about the age of (f) _____ .

A child of a parent with Huntington's disease has (g) _____ chance of having this condition.

Integrative functions 📖 *Pages 461–5*

The last section in this study is the integrative functions of the cerebellum. Though poorly understood, these functions are nevertheless important for humans.

Q40. **List three types of activities that require complex integration processes by the brain.**

_____

Q41. **Define the terms: learning, memory and engram.**

_____

_____

_____

Q42. **Which parts of the brain are thought to be associated with memory?**

_____

_____

Q43. **Complete this exercise on memory.**

Looking up a phone number, dialing it, and then quickly forgetting it is an example of (a) _____ memory. One theory of such memory is that the phone number is remembered only as long as a (b) _____ neuronal circuit is active.

Repeated use of a telephone number can commit it to long-term memory. Such reinforcement is known as memory (c) _____ . (d) _____ (Most? Very little?) of the information that comes to conscious attention goes into long-term memory, since the brain is selective about what it retains.

Some evidence indicates that (e) _____ memory involves electrical and chemical events rather than anatomical changes. Supporting this idea is the fact that chemicals used for anaesthesia and shock treatments interfere with (f) _____ memory.

Q44. **Explain the possible relationship of RNA and long-term memory.**

_____

_____

Sleep and wakefulness 📖 *Pages 462–4*

Q45. Complete this exercise about sleep and wakefulness.

(a) _____ rhythm is a term given to the usual daily pattern of sleep and wakefulness in humans. Whether you are awake or asleep depends upon whether the reticular formation, also known as the (b) _____ system (RAS) is active. The RAS has two principal parts: the (c) _____ portion is responsible for your waking from a deep sleep, and the (d) _____ portion helps you to maintain a conscious state.

List three types of sensory input that can stimulate the RAS: _____ ,

_____ , _____ .

Stimulation of the reticular formation leads to (e) _____ activity of the cerebral cortex, as indicated by (f) _____ recordings of brain waves. Continued feedback between the RAS, the (g) _____ , and the (h) _____ maintains the state called consciousness. Inactivation of the RAS produces a state known as (i) _____ .

Q46. Complete this activity, which should help you to understand sleep.

There are two kinds of sleep, referred to as REM, which stands for (a) _____

_____ _____ and NREM, which stands for (b) _____

_____ _____ _____ . (c) _____ sleep is required first in order for (d) _____ sleep to occur. In (e) _____ sleep, a person gradually progresses from stage (f) _____ into deep sleep. Alpha waves are present in stage(s) (g) _____ (1? 3 and 4?), whereas slow delta waves characterise stage(s) (h) _____ (1? 3 and 4?) sleep.

REM sleep is also called (i) _____ sleep, since it follows, but is much more active than, the deep stage of sleep. Respirations and pulse are much (j) _____ over their levels in stage 4; alpha waves are present as in stage (k) _____ sleep. Dreaming occurs during (l) _____ (stages 1–4 of NREM? REM?) sleep. Periods of REM and NREM sleep alternate throughout the night in about (m) _____ minute cycles. During the early part of an 8-hour sleep period REM periods last about (n) _____ minutes; they gradually increase in length until the final REM period which lasts (o) _____ minutes.

You have now completed this part of the study on the nervous system. Give yourself a pat on the back. We hope that you found this study interesting, though somewhat complex, but such is the nature of the nervous system.

You may wish to check you progress, by attempting the Checkpoints Exercise.

CHECKPOINTS EXERCISE

Q47. Which one of the following sensations is not conveyed by the posterior column–medial lemniscus pathway?

a. Pain and temperature.

b. Proprioception.

c. Fine touch, two-point discrimination.

d.   Vibration.

e.   Stereognosis.

Q48.   Which one of the following is the false statement about REM sleep?

a.   Infant sleep consists of a higher percentage of REM sleep than does adult sleep.

b.   Dreaming occurs during this type of sleep.

c.   The eyes move rapidly behind closed lids during REM sleep.

d.   EEG readings are similar to those of stage 4 of NREM sleep.

e.   REM sleep occurs periodically throughout a typical 8-hour sleep period.

Q49.   Which one of the following is the false statement about pain receptors?

a.   They may be stimulated by any type of stimulus, such as heat, cold or pressure.

b.   They have a simple structure with no capsule.

c.   They are characterized by a high level of adaptation.

d.   They are found in almost every tissue of the body.

e.   They are important in helping to maintain homeostasis.

Q50.   Arrange the answers in the correct sequence, for the levels of sensation, from those causing the simplest, least precise reflexes to those causing the most complex and precise responses.

a.   Thalamus.

b.   Brainstem.

c.   Cerebral cortex.

d.   Spinal cord.

_____ _____ _____ _____

Q51.   Arrange the answers in the correct sequence, for the pathway for conduction of most of the impulses for voluntary movement of muscles.

a.   Anterior grey horn of the spinal cord.

b.   Precentral gyrus.

c.   Internal capsule.

d.   Location where decussation occurs.

e.   Lateral corticospinal tract.

_____ _____ _____ _____ _____

Q52. **Circle 'T' (true) or 'F' (false) for each of the following statements.**

T   F   a. In general, the left side of the brain controls the right side of the body.

T   F   b. Stimulation of pressure receptors can result in the sensation of pain.

T   F   c. The final common pathway consists of upper motor neurones.

T   F   d. Circadian rhythm pertains to the complex feedback circuits involved in producing co-ordinated movements.

T   F   e. Sight, hearing, smell and pressure are all special senses.

T   F   f. Pain in the diaphragm, liver or gallbladder may seem to be felt in the shoulder and neck region, since the phrenic nerve enters the cord at the same levels (C3–C5) as cutaneous nerves of the shoulder and neck.

T   F   g. The neurone that crosses to the opposite side in sensory pathways is usually the second order neurone.

T   F   h. Muscle spindles, tendon organs, joint kinesthetic receptors are all examples of proprioceptive receptors.

T   F   i. Damage to the left lateral spinothalamic tract would be most likely to result in loss of awareness of pain and vibration sensations in the left side of the body.

T   F   j. Conscious sensations, such as those of sight and touch, can only occur in the cerebral cortex.

T   F   k. Pain experienced by an amputee as if the amputated limb were still there is an example of phantom pain.

T   F   l. Damage to the final common pathway will result in flaccid paralysis.

Answers to questions

Q1.   a, sensory; b, integrating, associating and storing; c, motor effect, muscles, glands.

Q2.   Pain, change in body temperature, seeing or hearing.

Q3.   a, sensation; perception.

Q4.   3a, 1b, 4c, 2d.

Q5.   Yes. An example is pain that is often felt by patients who have had an amputation. This is often referred to as 'the phantom limb pain'.

Q6.   a. Modality; b, one modality; c, cerebral cortex; d, adaptation; e, pain.

Protects you by continuing to provide warning signals of painful stimuli.

Vigorous response of each type of receptor to a specific type of stimulus, such as touch receptor response to mechanical energy.

No. Receptors may respond somewhat to other types of stimuli.

Q7.   1, B; 2, C; 3, A; 4 D.

Ba, Cb, Ac, Dd.

Q8.   Simple receptors are associated with general senses, whilst complex receptors are associated with special senses.

Q9.   Ia, Eb, Pc.

Q10.   a, mechano; b, chemo; c, thermo.

Q11.   Ga, Sb, Sc, Gd.

Q12.   a, Yes; b, No; c, General (such as pain. Hint: remember G as in 'generator for general senses'); d, Special (such as vision); e, Always excitatory; f, Excitatory or inhibitory.

Q13.   Touch, pressure, vibration, cold, heat and pain.

Q14. a, Touch, pressure, vibration, itch, tickle; b, mechano; c, unevenly; d, light; e, deep; f, vibration.

Q15. 1a, 4b, 8 and 9 for c, 2,3,5 and 7 for d, 6e, 6f, 5g, 7h.

Q16. A, Type II cutaneous mechanoreceptor (end organ of Ruffini); B. Type I cutaneous mechanoreceptor (tactile or Merkel disc); C, Corpuscle of touch (Meissner's corpuscle); D, Lamellated (Pacinian corpuscle).

Q17. a. Visceral pain results from stimulation of receptors in the viscera, whereas somatic pain arises as a result of stimulation of receptors in the skin, skeletal muscle, joints and tendons.

b. General anaesthesia removes sensations including pain and also produces unconsciousness and sometimes muscular relaxation. Spinal anaesthesia is a form of local anaesthesia, usually involving injection of a drug via a lumbar puncture into the subarachnoid space.

Q18. This is to reduce the risk of vomiting, therefore preventing aspiration of stomach content and saliva into the airway, which could lead to asphyxiation.

Q19. a, Medial aspects of left arm; b, T1; c, T4; d, shoulder and neck region; e, diaphragm; f, cervical; g, C3; h, C4; i, referral.

Q20. Muscle spindles, tendon organs, joint kinesthetic receptors.

Q21. Gamma motor neurone.

Q22. b, a, c.

Q23. a, Cortex; b, longitudinal; c, foot; d, face; e, right; f, sensation; g, hand; h, left.

Q24.

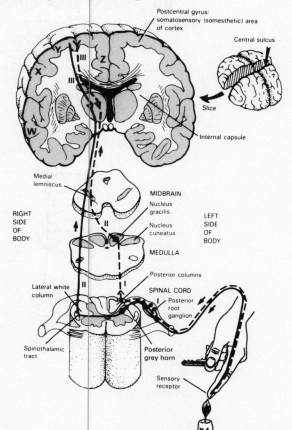

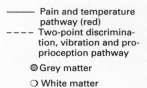

Q25. The ability to recognise an object such as a key in the hand by its size, weight, shape and texture.

Q26. See 📖 *Page 451, Figure 15.4.*

Q27. Acute pain is conducted by type A fibre because it is myelinated. You know that myelin speeds up conduction.

Q28. Chronic pain is conducted by type C fibre and this is because it is unmyelinated.

Q29. 5a, 4b, 3c, 2d, 1e.

Q30. a, Subconscious; b, posture; c, muscle tone; d, left side; e, both sides.

Q31. 4a, 1 and 2 for b, 3c.

Q32. a, Frontal; b, movement; c, left side of the face; d, VII; e, spastic; f, left.

Q33. g, d, b, f, e, a, h, c.

Q34.

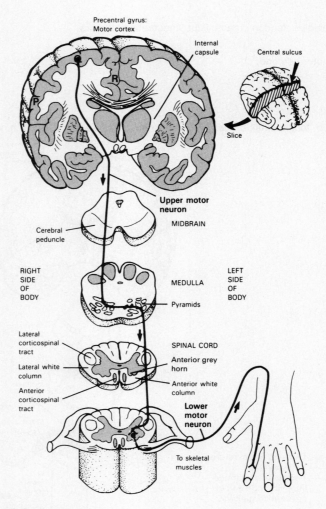

Precentral gyrus:
Motor cortex

Internal
capsule

Central sulcus

Slice

**Upper motor
neuron**

MIDBRAIN

Cerebral
peduncle

RIGHT
SIDE
OF
BODY

LEFT
SIDE
OF
BODY

MEDULLA

Pyramids

Lateral
corticospinal
tract

SPINAL CORD

Lateral white
column

Anterior grey
horn

Anterior
corticospinal
tract

Anterior white
column

**Lower
motor
neuron**

To skeletal
muscles

● Grey matter
○ White matter

Q35. a, 15; b, 85; c, lateral; d, left.

Q36. Myelination of axons in the corticospinal tracts is not complete until after the first 12 months of life.

Q37. These tracts synapse with neurones of all cranial nerves with motor functions (III–VII and IX–XII). They control voluntary movements of the head and neck.

Q38. a, motor cortex; b, brainstem; c, anterior grey matter of spinal cord; d, upper; e, lower.

This is because these neurones which are activated by input from a variety of sources, must function for any movement to occur.

Q39. a, Parkinson's; b, dopamine; c, muscle rigidity and tremors; d, chorea; e, GABA; f, 40; g, 50/50.

Q40. Memory, sleep and wakefulness and emotional responses.

Q41. *Learning* – the ability to acquire knowledge or a skill through instruction or experience.

Memory – the ability to recall thoughts.

Engram – the change in the brain that represents an experience which is committed to memory.

Q42. The association cortex of the frontal, parietal, occipital and temporal lobes; parts of the limbic system, especially the hippocampus and amygdaloid nucleus; and the diencephalon.

Q43. a, short-term; b, reverberating; c, consolidation; d, very little; e, short-term; f, long-term.

Q44. It is believed that RNA is important for long-term memory. There is evidence that if RNA is inhibited, long-term memory does not occur.

Q45. a, Circadian; b, reticular activity system; c, thalamus; d, pons and midbrain.
Three types of sensory input that can stimulate the RAS: light, sound, touch, impulse from the cerebral cortex.
e, Increased; f, electroencephalograph; g, cerebral cortex; h, spinal cord; i, sleep.

Q46. a, Rapid eye movement; b, non-rapid eye movement; c, NREM; d, REM; e, NREM; f, 1 to 4; g, 1; h, 3 and 4; i, paradoxical; j, increased; k, 1; l, REM; m, 90; n, 5–10; o, 50.

Q47. a.

Q48. d.

Q49. a.

Q50. d, b, a, c.

Q51. b, c, d, e, a.

Q52. Ta, Tb, Fc, Fd, Fe, Tf, Tg, Th, Fi, Tj, Tk, Tl.

Overview and key terms

The special senses

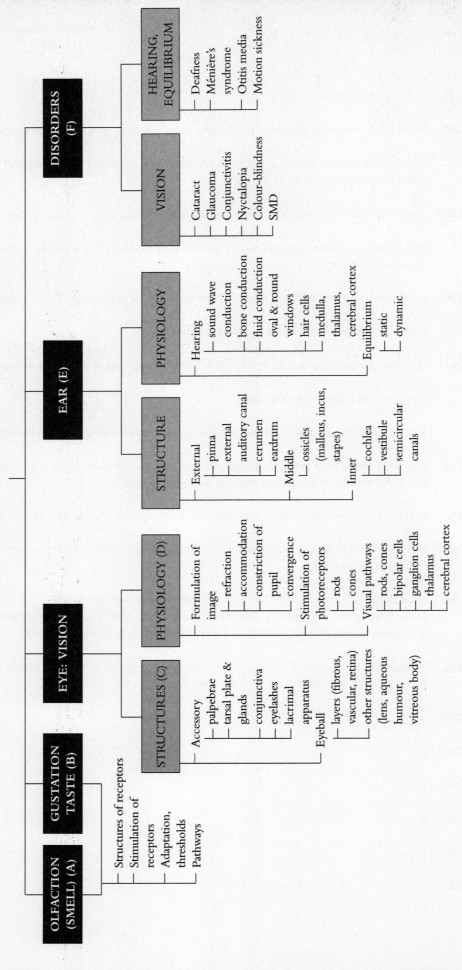

OLFACTION (SMELL) (A)

GUSTATION TASTE (B)

- Structures of receptors
- Stimulation of receptors
- Adaptation, thresholds
- Pathways

EYE: VISION

STRUCTURES (C)
- Accessory
  - palpebrae
  - tarsal plate & glands
  - conjunctiva
  - eyelashes
  - lacrimal apparatus
- Eyeball
  - layers (fibrous, vascular, retina)
  - other structures (lens, aqueous humour, vitreous body)

PHYSIOLOGY (D)
- Formulation of image
  - refraction
  - accommodation
  - constriction of pupil
  - convergence
- Stimulation of photoreceptors
  - rods
  - cones
- Visual pathways
  - rods, cones
  - bipolar cells
  - ganglion cells
  - thalamus
  - cerebral cortex

EAR (E)

STRUCTURE
- External
  - pinna
  - external auditory canal
  - cerumen
  - eardrum
- Middle
  - ossicles (malleus, incus, stapes)
- Inner
  - cochlea
  - vestibule
  - semicircular canals

PHYSIOLOGY
- Hearing
  - sound wave conduction
  - bone conduction
  - fluid conduction
  - oval & round windows
  - hair cells
  - medulla, thalamus, cerebral cortex
- Equilibrium
  - static
  - dynamic

DISORDERS (F)

VISION
- Cataract
- Glaucoma
- Conjunctivitis
- Nyctalopia
- Colour-blindness
- SMD

HEARING, EQUILIBRIUM
- Deafness
- Ménière's syndrome
- Otitis media
- Motion sickness

9. The Special Senses

Chapter 16

INTRODUCTION

This chapter will introduce you to the special senses of smell, taste, vision, hearing and equilibrium. These structures all contain receptors, but they are somewhat more complex.

As nurses, understanding the functions of such structures as the eyes and the ears should make you aware of the problems faced by patients or individuals whose hearing and vision is severely affected. Just imagine all those little things in life that we usually take for granted, such as seeing a smiling face or hearing a sympathetic reassuring voice. What would the world be like if suddenly an individual was to lose these senses?

It is hoped that in this study, you will grasp some of the basic principles of the various sense organs and how individuals may be affected if they become dysfunctional. We start this study by looking at the sense of smell.

OLFACTORY SENSATIONS 📖 *Pages 468–9*

Q1. **Describe olfactory receptors in this exercise.**

Receptors for smell are located in the (a) _____ portion of the nasal cavity.

Receptors consist of (b) _____ (what types of neurones?) neurones, which are located between (c) _____ cells. The distal end of each olfactory receptor cell consists of dendrites that have cilia known as olfactory (d) _____ . The olfactory (Bowman's) glands in the nose produce (e) _____ , which acts as a solvent for odorant (f) _____ .

Since smell is a (g) _____ sense, receptors in olfactory hair membranes respond to different chemical molecules, leading to a (h) _____ _____ and (i) _____ _____ . Adaption to smell occurs (j) _____ (slowly? rapidly?) at first and then happens at a much slower rate.

Q2. **Complete this exercise about the nerves associated with the nose.**

Upon stimulation of olfactory hairs, impulses pass to cell bodies and axons; the axons of these olfactory cells form cranial nerves (a) _____ , the olfactory nerves. These pass from the nasal cavity to the cranium to terminate in the olfactory (b) _____ located just inferior to the (c) _____ lobes of the cerebrum.

Neurones in the olfactory bulb then convey impulses along the olfactory (d) _____ directly to the (e) _____ . Note that olfaction is one sense that (f) _____ (does? does not?) involve the thalamus.

What is the effect of the projection of sensations of smell and taste to the limbic system?

The olfactory pathway just described transmits sensations for the (g) _____ (general? special?) sense of smell. General senses, such as irritation of the nose by pepper leading to sniffles or tears, are carried primarily by cranial nerve (h) _____ , the facial nerve.

Q3. **Briefly explain why an individual who has a cold cannot taste his food?**

_____

_____

GUSTATORY SENSATIONS: TASTE 📖 *Pages 469–71*

Q4.   **Complete the following exercises which describes the receptors for taste.**

Receptors for taste, or (a) _____ sensation, are located in taste buds. These receptors are protected by a (b) _____ formed of supporting cells, as well as the (c) _____ cells that produce the supporting cells. Within each taste bud are about (d) _____ (number?) gustatory receptor cells with gustatory (e) _____ that project from a taste bud pore. The life span of each gustatory receptor cell is about (f) _____ .

Taste buds are located on elevated projections of the tongue called (g) _____ . The largest of these are located in a V-formation at the back of the tongue. These are (h) _____ papillae. (i) _____ papillae are mushroom-shaped and located on the sides and tip of the tongue. Pointed (j) _____ papillae cover the (k) _____ of the tongue, and these (l) _____ (do? do not?) contain many taste buds.

Q5.   **Complete the following exercise about taste.**

There are only four primary taste sensations: (a) _____ , _____ , _____ , _____ , (do not worry about the order). The taste buds at the tip of the tongue are most sensitive to (b) _____ and (c) _____ tastes, whereas the posterior portion is most sensitive to (d) _____ taste.

The four primary tastes are modified by (e) _____ sensations to produce the wide variety of 'tastes' experienced. If you have a cold, you may not be able to discriminate the usual variety of tastes, largely because of loss of the sense of (f) _____ .

The threshold for smell is quite (g) _____ (high? low?), meaning that (h) _____ (a large? only a small?) amount of odour must be present in order for smell to occur. The threshold varies for the four primary tastes; the threshold for (i) _____ is lowest, while the thresholds for (j) _____ (two tastes) are highest.

Taste impulses are conveyed to the brainstem by cranial nerves (k) _____ , (l) _____ and (m) _____ (give your answer in the order from lowest to highest nerve); from there nerve messages travel to the lower parts of the brain, including the thalamus, (n) _____ , and the (o) _____ system, and finally stimulate the cerebral cortex.

Now that you have completed olfactory and gustatory sensations, you can move on to study the eye and vision.

VISUAL SENSATIONS: ANATOMY 📖 *Pages 471–82*

It is as well to start this part of the study by becoming familiar with the structures that form the eye. Figure 9.1 shows a transverse cross section of the eyeball. Label all the parts (A–S).

Figure 9.1.
Transverse cross section of the eyeball.

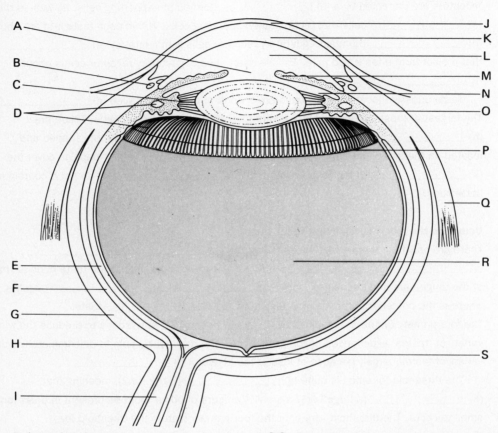

Colour the three layers of the eye. Look at 📖 *Page 474, Figure 16.5* and check your answers. Examine your own eye in a mirror, and with the help of Figure 9.1, identify the following accessory structures in the box below.

---

1. Conjunctiva 2. Eyebrow 3. Eyelashes 4. Lacrimal glands 5. Palpebrae 6.Tarsal glands

7. Tarsal plate

Please note that for the lacrimal glands, you need to refer only to the diagram of the eye.

Q6. **To check your understanding of those structures mentioned above, complete the following exercise, which relates to descriptions of those structures.**

a. Eyelid: _____.

b. Thick fold of connective tissue that forms much of the eyelid: _____.

c. Covers the orbicularis oculis muscle; provides protection: _____.

d. Short hairs; infection of glands at the base of these hairs is a stye: _____ .

e. Located in superolateral region of orbit; secrete tears: _____.

f. Secrete oil; infection is a chalazion: _____.

g. Mucous membrane lining the eyelids and covering the anterior surface of the eye:

_____.

Q7. **Complete this exercise on accessory eye structures.**

Lacrimal glands produce (a) _____ as a result of (b) _____
(sympathetic? parasympathetic?) stimulation. Glands normally produce (c) _____ml
per day of tears. Tears also contain a bactericidal enzyme called (d) _____ .
Lacrimal fluid (e) _____ and moistens the eyeball. Tears are drained away by
passing into the (f) _____ canal and then into the (g) _____
_____ (two words).

Each eye is moved by (h) _____ (how many?) extrinsic muscles; these are
innervated by cranial nerves (i) _____ , (j) _____, and
(k) _____ (give your answer in the right sequence from lowest to highest nerve).

The eye sits in the bony socket known as the (l) _____ with only the anterior
(m) _____ of the eyeball exposed.

Q8. **Explain why corneal transplant is one of the most successful types of transplant?** 📖 *Page 473.*

_____

_____

Q9. **What is the name of the instrument that is used to view the retinal blood vessels?**

_____

Q10. **What is the name given to the location where the central retinal artery enters the eye?**

_____

Lens and cavities of the eye 📖 *Pages 477–8*

Q11. **Complete the following exercise, which describes the lens and the cavities of the eye.**

The lens is composed of (a) _____ arranged in layers, much like an onion. It is
normally (b) _____ (its appearance?). A loss of transparency of the lens occurs in
the condition called (c) _____ .

The lens is held in position by the (d) _____ _____ (two words).
The lens divides the eye into anterior (e) _____ and vitreous (f) _____ .
The posterior cavity is filled with (g) _____ body, which has a jelly-like consistency.
This body helps to hold the (h) _____ in place. Vitreous body is formed during
embryonic life and (i) _____ (is? is not?) replaced in later life.

The anterior cavity is subdivided by the (j) _____ into two chambers. The larger
chamber is the (k) _____ chamber. A watery fluid called the (l) _____
humour is present in the anterior cavity. This fluid is formed by the (m) _____
processes, and it is normally replaced every 90 minutes.

Aqueous fluid is produced by the (n) _____ _____ (two words). It
provides nutrients and (o) _____ (vital for all living cells) and removes wastes from
the lens and (p) _____ . If it is increased, it may give rise to (q) _____

which, if not treated, can cause damage to the (r) _____ resulting in

(s) _____ .

Now that you have studied the accessory structures and the macroscopic structures of the eye, it is appropriate to look at the inner detail of the eye, such as the retina and the photoreceptor cells.

Q12. **Contrast the two types of photoreceptor cells by writing 'R' for rods or 'C' for cones before the related descriptions.**

☐ a. About 6 million in each eye; most concentrated in the central fovea of the macula lutea.

☐ b. Over 120 million in each eye; located mainly in peripheral regions of the eye.

☐ c. Sense colour and acute (sharp) vision.

☐ d. Used for night vision.

Q13. **Complete this exercise that describes the retina.**

After light strikes the back of the retina, nerve impulses pass anteriorly through three zones of neurones. First is the region of rods and cones, or (a) _____ zone; next is the

(b) _____ layer; most anterior is the (c) _____ layer. Axons of the ganglion layer converge to form the optic nerve. This nerve exits from the eye at the point known

as the (d) _____ disc, or (e) _____ _____(two words). The name indicates that no image formation can occur here, since no rods or cones are present.

Q14. **What functions do amacrine and horizontal cells serve?**

_____

Q15. **Check your progress on the study of the eye, by completing the exercise below. Match the structures of the eye mentioned in the box with the descriptions below.**

> **1. Central fovea 2. Choroid 3. Ciliary muscle 4. Cornea 5. Iris 6. Lens 7. Optic disc 8. Pupil 9. Retina 10. Sclera 11. Canal of Schlemm**

☐ a. 'White of the eye'.

☐ b. Normally clear; if cloudy, it is a cataract.

☐ c. Blind spot; area in which there are no cones or rods.

☐ d. Area of sharpest vision; area of densest concentration of cones.

☐ e. Anteriorly located, avascular coat responsible for about 75% of all focusing done by the eye.

☐ f. Consists of a pigmented epithelium and a neural portion; if these two portions separate (detach), blindness may occur.

☐ g. Brown–black layers prevent reflection of light rays; also nourish the eyeball, since it is vascular.

☐ h. A hole; appears black, like a circular doorway leading into a dark room.

☐ i. Regulates the amount of light entering the eye; coloured part of the eye.

☐ j. Attaches to the lens by means of radially arranged fibres called suspensory ligaments.

☐ k. Located at the junction of iris and cornea; drains aqueous humour.

Image formation on the retina 📖 *Pages 479–82*

Q16. Briefly outline how an image is formed on the retina to include the following processes: refraction of light, accommodation of the lens, constriction of the pupil, convergence of the eyes.

_____

_____

_____

_____

_____

Q17. Complete the following exercise about formation of an image on the retina.

Bending of light rays so that images focus exactly upon the retina is a process known as

(a) _____ . The (b) _____ (cornea? lens?) accomplishes most of the refraction within the eye. Explain why you think this is so?

_____

_____

Q18. Explain why the objects that we see are right side up even though refraction produces inverted images on your retina.

_____

_____

_____

Q19. Complete this question, which is a further explanation of accommodation.

A (a) _____ (concave? convex?) lens will bend light rays so that they converge and finally intersect. The lens in each of your eyes is (b) _____ (shape?).

When you bring your finger toward your eye, light rays from your finger must converge

(c) _____ (more? less?) so that they will focus on your retina. Thus, for near vision, the anterior surface of your lens must become (d) _____ (more? less?) convex. This occurs by a thickening and bulging of the lens caused by (e) _____ of the

(f) _____ muscles. In fact, after long periods of close work, such as reading, you may experience eye strain.

The near point of vision for a young adult is (g) _____ cm, whilst in a 70-year old it is (h) _____ cm. This difference is due to the loss of (i) _____ in the (j) _____ (which structure?) with ageing.

Refraction and accommodation

Some people need to wear glasses in order for accommodation of vision to be corrected, enabling them to see objects and images clearly. The exercise below should help you to understand some of the errors in refraction and accommodation.

Q20. **Describe errors in refraction and accommodation in this exercise.**

The normal or (a) _____ eye can refract rays from a distance of (b) _____ metres and form a clear image on the retina.

In the nearsighted or (c) _____ eye, images focus (d) _____ (in front of? behind?) the retina. This may be due to an eyeball that is too (e) _____ (long? short?). Corrective lenses should be slightly (f) _____ (shape?) so that they refract rays less and allow them to focus farther back on the retina.

The farsighted person can see (g) _____ (near? far?) well, but has difficulty seeing (h) _____ (near? far?) without the aid of corrective lenses. The farsighted or (i) _____ person requires (j) _____ lenses. After about the age 40, most persons lose the ability to see near objects clearly.

Q21. **Underline the correct response for each of the statements.**

a. Both accommodation of the lens and constriction of the pupil involve (extrinsic? intrinsic?) muscles, whereas convergence of the eyes involves (extrinsic? intrinsic?) muscles.

b. The pupil (dilates? constricts?) in the presence of bright light; the pupil (dilates? constricts?) in stressful situations when sympathetic nerves stimulate the iris.

Q22. **List the three principal processes that are necessary for vision to occur.**

a. _____ .

b. _____ .

c. _____ .

Q23. **Complete this exercise, which relates to photoreceptors and photopigments.**

The basis for the names **rods** and **cones** rests in the shape of the outer segments of these cells, that is, the segment closest to the (a) _____ (which structure in the eye?). Photopigments such as rhodopsin are located in the (b) _____ segment. On the other hand, the nucleus, Golgi complex and mitochondria are found in the (c) _____ segment.

There are (d) _____ (how many?) types of photopigment found in the human retina. Rhodopsin is the photopigment found in (e) _____ . There are (f) _____ (how many?) types of photopigment in cones.

Any photopigment consists of two parts: retinal and opsin. Retinal is a vitamin (g) _____ derivative and is formed from carotenoids. What is the function of retinal?

Q24. List some of the foods that contain carotene.

_____

Q25. Explain how carotenoids in foods may help to prevent nyctalopia?

_____

_____

Q26. Imagine that you enter a dark room. You will be staying in the room for a while. In answering the question below, you should be able to understand the physiological changes that take place in the rods of your eye.

In order to see in dim light (as in a dark room), you use (a) _____ (rods? cones?). Rods produce a pigment called (b) _____ (or visual purple). In bright light, this chemical is broken down very (c) _____ (rapidly? slowly?), so as you enter the dark room, your rods lack sufficient rhodopsin to see in the dark.

During the short time that you are stumbling around in darkness, rhodopsin can form in the following manner. An enzyme converts retinal from its *trans* form to its (d) _____ form, which fits well with a glycoprotein named (e) _____ to produce rhodopsin.

As soon as you have sufficient rhodopsin present in the rods, stimulation of the rods by a dim light present in the room will begin breaking down rhodopsin. This is a rapid but stepwise process, ultimately resulting in the cleavage of rhodopsin into two parts: again the glycoprotein (f) _____ and the (g) _____ (*cis*? *trans*?) form of retinal. As a result of this process, a (h) _____ impulse develops, and a nerve impulse then passes to your brain informing you of what you have seen in the dim light, such as silhouettes of people also present in the room. What you are experiencing in the dark room is (i) _____ (dark? light?) adaptation in which visual sensitivity increases very slowly.

Your vision becomes increasingly better after a few more minutes in the dim light, since you continue to form rhodopsin. But should you step outside, the bright light will (j) _____ rhodopsin so rapidly and completely that you will have to start the dark-induced synthesis of rhodopsin all over again once you go back into the dark room.

Q27. Complete this exercise, which deals with the function of cones.

Cones contain pigments that do require bright light for breakdown. Three different pigments are present, sensitive to three colours: (a) _____ , _____ and _____. A person who is red–green colour-blind lacks some of the cones receptive to two colours, (b) _____ and (c) _____ , and so cannot distinguish between these colours. This condition occurs more often in (d) _____ (which sex?).

Q28. **Describe the conduction pathway for vision by arranging these structures in sequence. Write the letters in the correct order on the lines provided. Also indicate the four points where synapsing occurs by placing an asterisk (*) between the letters.**

1. Bipolar cells.

2. Cerebral cortex.

3. Ganglion cells.

4. Optic nerve.

5. Optic chiasma.

6. Optic tract.

7. Photoreceptor cells.

8. Thalamus.

_____ _____ _____ _____ _____ _____ _____ _____

Q29. **Answer these questions about the visual pathway of the brain. You may find** 📖 *Page 486, Figure 16.25* **useful.**

Hold your left hand up high and to the left, so that you can still see it. Your hand is in the (a) _____ visual field of your left eye, and in the (b) _____ visual field of your right eye.

Due to refraction, the image of your hand will be projected onto the (c) _____ (left? right?) lower portion of the retinas of your eyes. All nerve fibres from these areas of your retinas reach the (d) _____ (left? right?) side of your thalamus and cerebral cortex.

Damage to the right optic tract, right side of the thalamus or right visual cortex would result in loss of sight of the (e) _____ (left? right?) visual fields of each eye.

This concludes the study on the eye. We hope that you have enjoyed it! To check your progress, you may wish to do the Checkpoints Exercise.

CHECKPOINTS EXERCISE

For questions 30–34, arrange the answers in the correct sequence.

Q30. **Layers of the eye, from superficial to deep:**

a. Sclera.

b. Retina.

c. Choroid.

_____ _____ _____

Q31. **From anterior to posterior:**

a. Vitreous body.

b. Optic nerve.

c. Cornea.

d. Lens.

_____ _____ _____ _____

Q32. **Pathway of aqueous humour, from site of formation to destination:**

  a.   Anterior chamber.

  b.   Scleral venous sinus.

  c.   Ciliary body.

  d.   Posterior chamber.

  _____ _____ _____ _____

Q33. **Pathway of tears, from site of formation to entrance to the nose:**

  a.   Lacrimal gland.

  b.   Lacrimal duct.

  c.   Nasolacrimal duct.

  d.   Surface of conjunctiva.

  e.   Lacrimal punctae and lacrimal glands.

  _____ _____ _____ _____

Q34. **From anterior to posterior:**

  a.   Anterior chamber.

  b.   Iris.

  c.   Lens.

  d.   Posterior cavity.

  e.   Posterior chamber.

  _____ _____ _____ _____

Q35. **Which one of the following is not a correct statement about rods?**

  a.   There are more rods than cones in the eye.

  b.   Rods are concentrated in the fovea and are less dense around the periphery.

  c.   Rods enable you to see in dim (not bright) light.

  d.   Rods contain rhodopsin.

  e.   No rods are present at the optic disc.

Q36. **Choose the false statement about the lens of the eye.**

  a.   It is biconvex.

  b.   It is avascular.

  c.   It becomes more rounded (convex) as you look at distant objects.

  d.   Its shape is changed by contraction of the ciliary muscle.

  e.   Change in curvature of the lens is called accommodation.

Q37. **Circle 'T' (true) or 'F' (false) for each of the statements.**

T   F   a. Parasympathetic nerves stimulate the circular iris muscle to constrict the pupil, whereas sympathetic nerves cause dilatation of the pupil.

T   F   b. Convergence and accommodation are both results of contraction of the smooth muscle of the eye.

T   F   c. Both the aqueous body and vitreous humour are replaced constantly throughout your life.

PATIENT SCENARIO

Mrs Freda Goodwin, aged 70, is admitted to the surgical ward for planned abdominal surgery. She is blind in the right eye. She has cataract of the left eye and her vision is very blurred. She has a patch covering the left eye because of severe irritation as a result of conjunctivitis.

She is prescribed chloramphenicol ointment three times daily for the left eye.

She is extremely anxious, as the hospital environment is a new experience for her. She wishes to remain independent, as she is ambulant. However, due to her present condition, this may be difficult.

Q38. **Discuss how you would help Mrs Goodwin to settle on the ward, so as to allay her fear and anxiety and to reassure her of her safety.**

_____

_____

_____

_____

_____

Q39. **Whilst on the ward, a junior nurse wishes to gain clinical experience in instilling eye ointment in Mrs Goodwin's left eye. Giving reasons for your answer, how should you prepare the junior nurse for this procedure?**

_____

_____

_____

_____

QUESTION FOR DISCUSSION

1. Up until the time prior to surgery, Mrs Goodwin wishes to care for herself (e.g. going to the toilet, washing and bathing). How should you assist Mrs Goodwin in order that she remains independent and free from frustration?

THE EAR (HEARING AND EQUILIBRIUM) 📖 *Pages 487–98*

Another important organ of sensation is the ear. It is responsible for hearing and equilibrium. In this study you will meet some of the important structures of the ear and also their functions.

We will start this study by referring to a diagram of the ear and identifying the main anatomical structures.

Q40. **Figure 9.2 shows a cross section of the ear. Label all the parts indicated (A–N). O and P are already labelled. Please note that M, N, O and P are in a cross section of the cochlea.**

Figure 9.2.
Diagram of the ear in frontal section.

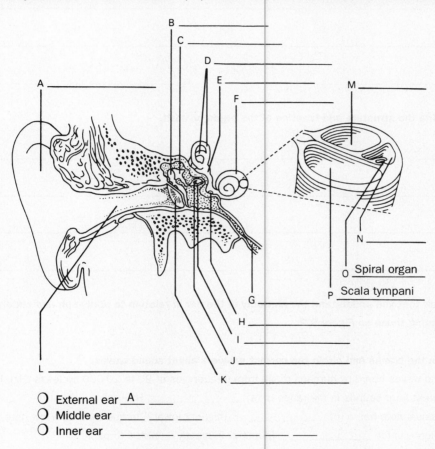

B _____
C _____
D _____
E _____
F _____
A _____
M _____
N
O Spiral organ
P Scala tympani
G _____
H _____
I _____
J _____
K _____
L _____

○ External ear _A_ ___
○ Middle ear ___ ___ ___
○ Inner ear ___ ___ ___ ___ ___ ___

The ear can be divided into three parts: external, middle and inner ear. Write the letters (as identified in the diagram) that correspond to each part illustrated in Figure 9.2.

Q41. **Select the structures in the box that best fit the descriptions below. Please note you will not use all the answers.**

1. Auricle (pinna) 2. Oval window 3. Auditory tube 4. Round window 5. Incus 6. Stapes 7. Malleus 8. Tympanic membrane

☐ a. Tube used to equalise pressure on either side of tympanic membrane.

☐ b. Eardrum.

☐ c. Structure on which stapes exerts piston-like action.

☐   d. Ossicle adjacent to eardrum.

☐   e. Anvil-shaped ear bone.

☐   f. Portion of the external ear shaped like the flared end of a trumpet.

Q42. **Outline the structure of the bony labyrinth.** 📖 *Page 490*

_____

_____

_____

_____

Q43. **Outline the structure and function of the organ of Corti.**

_____

_____

_____

_____

Q44. **Check that you understand the anatomy of the ear in relation to perilymph and endolymph by colouring these on Figure 9.2.**

Q45. **Fill in the blanks and circle the correct answers about sound waves.**

Sound waves heard by humans range from frequencies of 20 to 20 000 cycles/s (Hz). Humans can best hear sounds in the range of (a) _____ Hz.

A musical note has a (b) _____ (higher? lower?) frequency than a low note, so frequency is (c) _____ (directly? indirectly?) related to pitch.

Sound intensity (loudness) is measured in units called (d) _____ . Normal conversation is at a level of about (e) _____ dB, whereas sounds at

(f) _____ dB can cause pain.

Q46. **Complete the exercise below, which outlines some of the processes of hearing. You may find** 📖 *Page 493, Figure 16.20* **helpful.**

Sound waves travel through the (a) _____, _____, _____ and strike the (b) _____ _____. Sound waves are magnified by the action of the (c) _____ in the middle ear.

The ear bone named (d) _____ strikes the oval window, setting up waves in (e) _____ (endolymph? perilymph?). This pushes on the floor of the upper scala

(f) _____. As a result, the cochlear duct is moved, and so is the perilymph in the lower canal, the scala (g) _____ . The pressure of the perilymph is finally expanded by bulging out the (h) _____ window.

As the cochlear duct moves, tiny hair cells embedded in the floor of the duct are stimulated. These hair cells are part of the (i) _____ organ; its name is based on its spiral arrangement on the (j) _____ membrane all the way around the two coils of the cochlear duct.

As spiral organ hair cells are moved by waves in endolymph, hairs move against the gelatinous (k) _____ membrane. This movement generates receptor potentials in hair cells that excite nearby sensory neurones of the (l) _____ branch of the cranial nerve (m) _____ . The pathway continues to the brainstem, (n) _____ (relay centre), and finally to the (o) _____ lobe of the cerebral cortex.

Q47. **Check your understanding of the pathway of fluid conduction by placing the following structures in the correct sequence. Write the letters on the line provided.**

> **1. Basilar membrane 2. Cochlear duct 3. Oval window 4. Round window 5. Scala tympani**
> **6. Scala vestibuli 7. Vestibular membrane**

_____ _____ _____ _____ _____ _____ _____

Q48. **Contrast receptors for hearing and for equilibrium in this summary of the inner ear** 📖 *Pages 493–4.*

Receptors for hearing and equilibrium are all located in the (a) _____ ear. All consist of supporting cells and (b) _____ cells that are covered by a (c) _____ membrane.

In the spiral organ, which senses (d) _____ , the gelatinous membrane is called the (e) _____ membrane. Hair cells move against this membrane as a result of (f) _____ (sound waves? change in body position?).

In the macula, located in the (g) _____ (semicircular canals? vestibule?), the gelatinous membrane is embedded with calcium carbonate crystals called (h) _____. These respond to gravity in such a way that the macula is the main receptor for (i) _____ (static? dynamic?) equilibrium. An example of such equilibrium occurs as you are aware of your (j) _____ (position while lying down? change in position? on a careering roller coaster?).

In the semicircular canals the gelatinous membrane is called the (k) _____. Its shape is (l) _____ (flat? like an inverted cup?). The cupula is part of the (m) _____ (crista? saccule?) located in the ampulla. Change in direction (as in a roller coaster) causes (n) _____ to bend hairs in the cupula. Cristae in semicircular canals are therefore receptors primarily for (o) _____ (static? dynamic?) equilibrium.

Q49.   Outline the role of the cerebellum in the maintenance of equilibrium.

_____

_____

_____

_____

Now that you have grasped the essential physiology of vision and hearing, you can review some of the disorders of the eye and the ear 📖 *Pages 498–9*. When you have done this, you can answer question 50.

Q50.   Match the name of the disorder with the description.

> **1. Blepharitis 2. Cataract 3. Conjunctivitis 4. Glaucoma 5. Hyperacusia 6. Keratitis**
> **7. Ménière's syndrome 8. Myopia 9. Myringitis 10. Presbyopia 11. Strabismus 12. Tinnitus**
> **13. Vertigo**

☐   a. Condition requiring corrective lenses to focus distant objects.

☐   b. Excessive intraocular pressure resulting in blindness; second most frequent cause of blindness.

☐   c. Ringing in the ears.

☐   d. Pink eye.

☐   e. Abnormally sensitive hearing.

☐   f. Inflammation of the eardrum.

☐   g. Inflammation of the eyelid.

☐   h. Disturbance of the inner ear with excessive endolymph.

☐   i. Loss of the transparency of the lens.

☐   j. Farsightedness due to loss of elasticity of lens, especially after the age of 40.

☐   k. Inflammation of the cornea.

☐   l. Sense of spinning or whirling.

☐   m. Condition where the eyes focus on different points.

This completes the study on the ear. We hope that you have enjoyed it! You may wish to check your progress by attempting the Checkpoints Exercise.

CHECKPOINTS EXERCISE

Q51.   Arrange the answers below in sequence of the pathway of sound waves and resulting mechanical action.

a.   External auditory canal.

b.   Stapes.

c.   Malleus and incus.

d.   Oval window.

e.   Tympanic membrane.

_____ _____ _____ _____ _____

Q52.   Infections in the throat (pharynx) are most likely to lead to ear infections in the following manner.

a.   External auditory meatus to the external ear.

b.   Auditory (eustachian) tube to the middle ear.

c.   Oval window to the inner ear.

d.   Round window to the inner ear.

Q53.   Choose the false statement about the middle ear.

a.   It contains three ear bones called ossicles.

b.   Infection here is called otitis media.

c.   It functions in conduction of sound from the external ear to the inner ear.

d.   The cochlea is located here.

Q54.   Choose the false statement about the semicircular canals.

a.   They are located in the inner ear.

b.   They sense acceleration or changes in position.

c.   Nerve impulses arising here are conveyed to the brain by the vestibular branch of cranial nerve VIII.

d.   There are four semicircular canals in each ear.

e.   Each canal has an enlarged portion called an ampulla.

Answers to questions

Q1.   a, superior; b, bipolar; c, supporting; d, hairs; e, mucus; f, gases; g, mechanical; h, generator potential; i, nerve impulse; j, rapidly.

Q2.   a, I; b, bulb; c, frontal; d, tracts; e, cerebral cortex; f, does not.
Awareness of certain smells, such as nasty odours or the fragrance of flowers or perfume, may lead to emotional stress; g, special; h, VII.

Q3.   This is because taste is a chemical sensation and therefore food requires to dissolve first before it can be tasted.

Q4.   a, gustatory; b, capsule; c, basal; d, 50; e, hairs; f, 10 days; g, papillae; h, circumvallate; i, fungiform; j, filliform; k, anterior; l, do not.

Q5.   a, sweet, sour, bitter and salty; b, sweet; c, salty; d, bitter; e, olfactory; f, smell; g, low; h, only a small; i, bitter; j, sweet and salt; k, VII; l, IX; m, X; n, hypothalamus; o, limbic.

Q6.   a, 5; b, 7; c, 2; d, 3; e, 4; f, 6; g, 1.

Q7.   a, tears; b, parasympathetic; c, 1; d, lysozyme; e, lubricates; f, lacrimal; g, nasal cavity; h, 6; i, III; j, IV; k, VI, l, orbit; m, one-sixth.

Q8.   The cornea is avascular and does not contain antibodies.

Q9.   Ophthalmoscope.

Q10.   Optic disc.

Q11.   a, protein; b, clear; c, cataract; d, suspensory ligament; e, cavity; f, chamber; g, vitreous; h, retina; i, is not; j, iris; k, posterior; l, aqueous; m, ciliary; n, choroid plexuses; o, oxygen; p, cornea; q, glaucoma; r, retina; s, blindness.

Q12.   Ca, Rb, Cc, Rd.

Q13.   a, photoreceptor; b, bipolar; c, ganglion; d, optic; e, blind spot.

Q14.   They modify signals transmitted along optic pathways.

Q15.   10a, 6b, 7c, 1d, 4e, 9f, 2g, 8h, 5i, 3j, 11k.

Q16.   Light rays enter the eye; they are refracted at the anterior and posterior surfaces of the cornea. They are further refracted by the lens, so that they focus on the retina. The image focused on the retina is inverted. In order for the image to be sharp, it must fall on the central fovea. This is achieved by the alteration in the shape of the lens. For example, for near vision, the ciliary muscles contract, pulling the ciliary processes and the choroid toward the lens. This causes the lens to shorten and thicken, and hence it bulges, which increases the focusing power. For far vision, the lens is flattened as the suspensory ligament is taut and the ciliary muscles are relaxed. The clear retinal image is also assisted by constriction of the pupil.

Finally, there is convergence of the eyes, brought about by the extrinsic eye muscles; this directs the two eye-balls toward the object to be viewed.

Q17. a, Refraction; b, cornea.
The density of the cornea differs considerably from the air anterior to it.

Q18. The brain learned early in our lives how to 'turn' images so that what we see corresponds with the locations of objects we touch.

Q19. a, Convex; b, biconcave; c, more; d, more; e, contraction; f, ciliary; g, 10; h, 4; i, elasticity; j, lens.

Q20. a, Emmetropic; b, 6; c, myopic; d, in front of; e, long; f, concave; g, far; h, near; i, hypermetropic; j, convex.

Q21. a. intrinsic, extrinsic.
b. constricts, dilates.

Q22. a. Formation of an image on the retina.
b. Stimulation of photoreceptor so that a light stimulus is converted into an electrical stimulus (receptor potential and nerve impulses).
c. Transmission of the impulse along neural pathways to the thalamus.

Q23. a, choroid; b, outer; c, inner; d, 4; e, rods; f, 4; g, vitamin A.
The function of retinal is to absorb light.

Q24. Carrots, broccoli, spinach.

Q25. They lead to the production of retinal, which is a compound in rods and cones.

Q26. a, rods; b, rhodopsin; c, rapidly; d, *cis*; e, opsin; f, opsin; g, *trans*; h, generator; i, dark; j, destroy.

Q27. a, yellow to red, green and blue; b, red; c, green; d, males.

Q28. 7*, 1*, 3, 5, 4, 6*, 8*, 2.

Q29. a, Temporal; b, nasal; c, right; d, right; e, left.

Q30. a, c, b.

Q31. c, d, a, b.

Q32. c, d, a, b.

Q33. a, b, d, e, c.

Q34. a, b, e, c, d.

Q35. b.

Q36. c.

Q37. Ta, Fb, Fc.

Q38. It is important to realise that Mrs Goodwin will have problems with communication, as she is not able to see the nurse and everything else in her new environment. The nurse should introduce herself and give her name. She should talk in a normal manner, i.e. her usual tone of voice. She should let her presence be known every time that she approaches Mrs Goodwin. The nurse should also let the patient know when she is leaving the room.

Every opportunity should be taken to introduce Mrs Goodwin to the other patients. She should decribe the layout of the ward and all the facilities that Mrs Goodwin will be using.

The nurse should keep the immediate area clear and in the way that it has been described to Mrs Goodwin. The nurse should also provide a description of important objects on Mrs Goodwin's locker or table, by describing the location in terms of a clock, for example 'the jug of water is at 3 o'clock on the locker'. This strategy can also be applied to her food when it is presented to her.

Clear instructions should be given as to the use of the 'call nurse button' system. Additional information should also be provided, for example on the different tones for the fire alarm.

Q39. You may take this opportunity to check the junior nurse's knowledge on the anatomy of the eye. It should be emphasised that this is a 'clean' procedure and that every precaution should be taken so as to reduce the risk of the infection spreading to the patient's other eye and also to other patients and staff. The junior nurse should also be introduced to the relevant procedure, e.g the one established within her health authority.

The junior nurse may be allowed to undertake this procedure, if she feels confident with the technique. If not, it may be more appropriate for the junior nurse to observe the demonstration of the procedure by the senior nurse. The following steps should be taken:

1. Prepare the patient psychologically by giving the appropriate information with regard to the procedure that will be undertaken.
2. Wash and dry hands thoroughly.
3. Prepare the necessary equipment and take it to the bedside.
4. Sit the patient comfortably, or if preferred, she may lie supine with the head supported with pillows.
5. Clean the eyes with clean cotton balls, before instilling the ointment if this is necessary.
6. Ask the patient to tilt her head back and look up; bring the lower lid down gently and apply the ointment. The patient should be asked not to blink, or at least resist blinking for a few seconds. The patient should also be informed that she may have a nasty taste in the mouth, as some of the medication finds its way towards the nasolacrimal duct.
7. On completion of the procedure, dispose of the unwanted materials and wash and dry hands thoroughly. Ensure that the patient is comfortable.

Q40. A, Auricle; B, Malleus; C, Incus; D, Semicircular canals; E, Vestibule; F, Cochlea; G, Auditory (eustachian) tube; H, Round window; I, Oval window; J, Stapes; K, Tympanic membrane; L, External auditory canal; M, Scala vestibuli; N, Cochlear duct.

External ear: A, L.
Middle ear: B, C, J.
Inner ear: D, E, F, M, N, O, P.

Q41. 3a, 8b, 2c, 7d, 5e, 1f.

Q42. The bony labyrinth consists of a series of cavities within the petrous portion of the temporal bone. It is divided into three parts: (1) the semicircular canals, (2) the vestibule, and (3) the cochlea. The bony labyrinth is lined with periosteum, and contains a fluid called perilymph. There are three semicircular canals. One end of each canal has a swelling called an ampulla. The cochlea is a spiral canal that surrounds a bony core called the modiolus.

Q43. The organ of Corti is the organ of hearing. It contains about 16 000 hair cells, which are the receptors for auditory sensations. There are two groups of hair cells: inner and outer hair cells. Hair cells have long hair-like processes at their apical ends. They extend into the endolymph of the cochlear duct. The basal ends of the hair cells synapse with fibres of the cochlear branch of the vestibulocochlear nerve (VIII). In contact with the hair cells is the tectorial membrane.

Q45. a, 1000 to 4000; b, higher; c, directly; d, decibels; e, 45; f, 115–120.

Q46. a, External auditory canal; b, tympanic membrane; c, ossicles; d, stapes; e, perilymph; f, vestibuli; g, tympani; h, round; i, spiral; j, basal; k, tectorial; l, cochlear; m, VIII; n, thalamus; o, temporal.

Q47. 3, 6, 7, 2, 1, 5, 4.

Q48. a, inner; b, hair; c, gelatinous; d, hearing; e, tectorial; f, sound waves; g, vestibule; h, otoliths; i, static; j, position while lying down; k, cupola; l, like an inverted cup; m, crista; n, endolymph; o, dynamic.

Q49. The cerebellum receives sensory information from the utricle and saccule, and sends nerve impulses to the motor area of the cerebellum and this can cause a decrease or increase of impulses to specific skeletal muscles to maintain equilibrium.

Q50. 8a, 4b, 12c, 3d, 5e, 9f, 1g, 7h, 2i, 10j, 6k, 13l, 11m.

Q51. a, e, c, b, d.

Q52. b.

Q53. d.

Q54. d.

Overview and key terms

The autonomic nervous system (ANS)

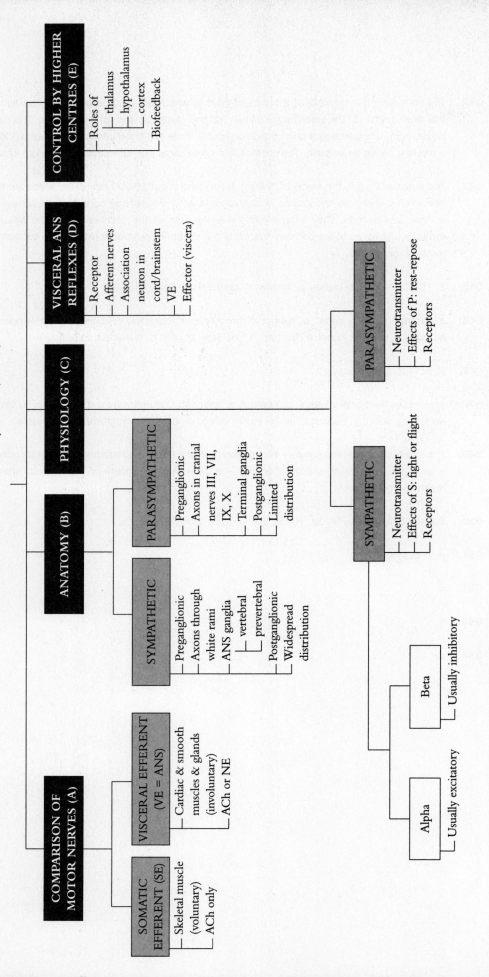

10. The Autonomic Nervous System

Learning outcomes

1. To compare the structural and functional differences between the somatic and autonomic nervous systems.

2. To list the components forming the autonomic nervous system.

3. To compare the structure and function of the parasympathetic and sympathetic nervous systems.

4. To explain the relationship of the hypothalamus to the autonomic nervous system.

Chapter 17

INTRODUCTION

The last system to be discussed in this study of the nervous system is the autonomic nervous system. This is the system that is not under our control. For example, it regulates the heart rate, blood pressure, glandular secretion and digestion.

The autonomic nervous system consists of two parts, the sympathetic and the parasympathetic systems. The autonomic nervous system also controls many of the physiological changes associated with stress.

As a nurse, you will encounter many problems in patients, in which the functions of the autonomic nervous system are altered. And indeed there are many stress-related illnesses. Understanding the structure and function of the autonomic nervous system will enable you to cope with such problems as anxiety and stress in yourself and your patients. You will also be able to appreciate the actions of some of the medications used for this system.

For questions 1–4, see 📖 *Page 503*

Q1.   Name the two divisions of the autonomic nervous system.

_____

Q2.   Why is the autonomic nervous system (ANS) so named, and is it entirely independent of higher control centres? Explain.

_____

_____

Q3.   Contrast the somatic and autonomic nervous systems in the table below.

	Somatic	Autonomic
Sensations and movements are mostly (conscious? unconscious?)	a.	b.
Types of tissue innervated by efferent nerves	Skeletal muscle	c.
Efferent neurones, excitatory (E), inhibitory (I), or both (E+I)	d.	e.
Examples of sensations (input)	f.	Mostly visceral sensory (such as changes in CO_2 level of blood, stretching of visceral wall)
Number of neurones in efferent pathway	g.	h.
Neurotransmitter(s) released by motor neurones	Acetylcholine (ACh)	i.

Q4. **Many visceral organs have dual innervation by the autonomic system.**

a. What does dual innervation mean?

b. How do the sympathetic and parasympathetic divisions work in harmony to control the viscera?

ANATOMY OF THE ANS 📖 *Pages 503–9*

Q5. **Complete this exercise describing the structural differences between visceral efferent and somatic efferent pathways.**

Between the spinal cord and effector, somatic pathways include (a) _____ neurone(s), whereas visceral pathways require (b) _____ neurone(s), known as the preganglionic and (c) _____ neurones.

Somatic pathways begin at (d) _____ (all? only certain?) levels of the cord, whereas visceral routes begin at (e) _____ (all? only certain?) levels of the cord.

Q6. **Contrast preganglionic with postganglionic fibres in this exercise.**

Consider the sympathetic division first. Its preganglionic cell bodies lie in the lateral grey segments (a) _____ to (b) _____ of the cord. For this reason, the sympathetic division is also known as the (c) _____ outflow. Preganglionic axons are (d) _____ (think of the covering of some axons) and therefore they appear white. These axons may branch to reach a number of different (e) _____ where they synapse. These ganglia contain (f) _____ (which type?) neurones' cell bodies whose axons proceed to the appropriate organ. Postganglionic axons are (g) _____ (which colour?) since they do not have a (h) _____ covering.

Parasympathetic preganglionic cell bodies are located in two areas. One is the (i) _____ , from which axons pass out in cranial nerves (j) _____ , _____ , _____ and _____ (give the correct sequence of the nerves). A second location is the (k) _____ (anterior? lateral?) grey horns of segments (l) _____ through (m) _____ of the cord.

Based on the location of (n) _____ (pre? post?)-ganglionic neurone cell bodies, the parasympathetic division is also known as the (o) _____ outflow. The axons of these neurones extend to the (p) _____ (same? different?) autonomic ganglia from those in sympathetic pathways. These postganglionic cell bodies send out short (q) _____ (grey? white?) axons to innervate the viscera.

Most viscera (r) _____ (do? do not?) receive fibres from the sympathetic and the parasympathetic divisions. However, the origin of these divisions in the CNS and the pathways taken to reach viscera (s) _____ (are the same? differ?).

Q7.   Contrast these two types of ganglia. Choose from the words that are in parentheses.

	Posterior root ganglia	Autonomic ganglia
Contains neurones that are (afferent? efferent?)	a.	b.
Contains (somatic? visceral? both?) neurones	c.	d.
Synapsing (does? does not?) occur here	e.	f.

Q8.   Complete the table contrasting types of autonomic ganglia.

	Sympathetic trunk	Prevertebral	Terminal
Sympathetic or parasympathetic	a.	Sympathetic	b.
Alternate name	Paravertebral ganglia or vertebral chain	c.	d.
General location	e.	f.	Close to or in the walls of effectors

More facts about the sympathetic division 📖 *Page 507, Figure 17.2*

Q9.   Trace with your finger the route of a preganglionic neurone. Now describe the pathway common to all sympathetic preganglionic neurones by listing the structures below in the correct sequence.

a.   Ventral root of spinal nerve.
b.   Sympathetic trunk ganglion.
c.   Lateral grey of spinal cord (between T1 and L2).
d.   White ramus communicans.

———— ———— ———— ————

The questions below should test your understanding of pre- and postganglionic fibres relating to the sympathetic nervous system.

Q10.   Suppose you could walk along the route of nerve impulses in sympathetic pathways. Start at the sympathetic trunk ganglion. It may be helpful to refer to 📖 *Page 507, Figure 17.2* and use it as a 'map'.

What is the shortest possible path you could take to reach a synapse to a postganglionic neurone cell body? (a) _____ . You could then ascend and/or descend the sympathetic chain to reach trunk ganglia at other levels. This is important, since sympathetic preganglionic cell bodies are limited in location to (b) _____ and

(c) _____ levels of the cord, yet the sympathetic trunk extends from

(d) _____ to (e) _____ levels of the vertebral column. Sympathetic fibres must be able to reach these distant areas to provide the entire body with sympathetic innervation.

Now 'walk' the sympathetic nerve pathway to sweat glands, blood vessels, or hair muscles in the skin or extremities. Again trace this route on 📖 *Page 507, Figure 17.2.* Preganglionic neurones synapse with postganglionic cell bodies in sympathetic trunk ganglia (at the level of entry or after ascending or descending). Postganglionic fibres then pass through (f) _____ , which connect to (g) _____ , and then convey impulses to skin or extremities.

Some preganglionic fibres do not synapse as described above, but pass on through trunk ganglia without synapsing there. The course runs through (h) _____ nerves to (i) _____ ganglia. Follow their route as they synapse with postganglionic neurones whose axons form (j) _____ en route to the viscera.

Prevertebral ganglia are located only in the (k) _____ . In the neck, thorax and pelvis the only sympathetic ganglia are those of the trunk (refer to 📖 *Page 506, Figure 17.1*). As a result, cardiac nerves, for example, contain only (l) _____ (preganglionic? postganglionic?) fibres, as indicated by broken lines in the figure.

A given sympathetic preganglionic neurone is likely to have many branches; these may take any of the paths you have just 'walked'. Once a branch synapses, it (m) _____ (can? cannot?) synapse again, since any autonomic pathway consists of just (n) _____ (preganglionic? postganglionic?) neurones.

Q11. **Figure 10.1 (next page) shows a preganglionic neurone at level T5 of the spinal cord. One axon is identified as far as the white ramus. Complete the pathway by showing how the axon may branch and synapse, eventually to innervate the three organs: the heart, a sweat gland in the skin of the thoracic region and the stomach. Draw the preganglionic fibre in solid lines and the postganglionic fibres in broken lines.**

PARASYMPATHETIC NERVOUS SYSTEM 📖 *Page 508*

Now that you are familiar with the sympathetic nervous system, you can proceed to study the parasympathetic nervous system. The parasympathetic nervous system is somewhat simpler than the sympathetic nervous system. This system also contains pre- and postganglionic fibres, but you will see that there are differences in their secretions of neurotransmitters.

Q12. **Name the two parasympathetic outflows.**

_____

Cranial outflow

The cranial outflow has five components: four pairs of ganglia and the plexuses associated with the vagus (X) nerve. The four pairs of cranial parasympathetic ganglia innervate structures in the head and are located close to the organs they innervate. Test your understanding of the cranial outflow by completing question 13.

Figure 10.1.
Typical sympathetic
pathway beginning
at level T5 of the
cord.

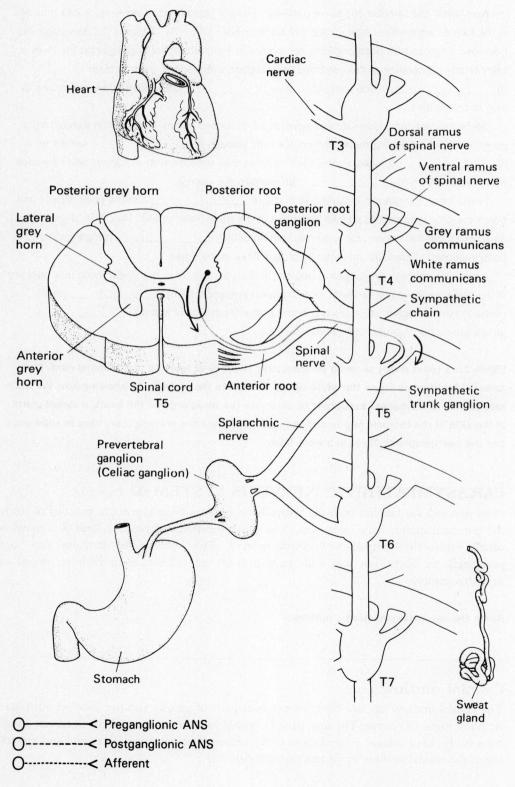

Heart

Cardiac
nerve

T3

Dorsal ramus
of spinal nerve

Ventral ramus
of spinal nerve

Posterior grey horn

Posterior root

Posterior root
ganglion

Lateral
grey
horn

Grey ramus
communicans

White ramus
communicans

Sympathetic
chain

T4

Spinal
nerve

Anterior
grey
horn

Spinal cord
T5

Anterior root

Sympathetic
trunk ganglion

T5

Splanchnic
nerve

Prevertebral
ganglion
(Celiac ganglion)

T6

Stomach

T7

Sweat
gland

O———————< Preganglionic ANS

O- - - - - - - -< Postganglionic ANS

O- - - - - - - - - -< Afferent

Q13.   Complete the table about the cranial portion of the parasympathetic system.

Cranial nerve		Name of terminal ganglion	Structures innervated
Number	Name		
a.	b.	c.	Iris and ciliary muscle of eye
d.	e.	1. Pterygopalatine	1. f.
		2. Submandibular	2. g.
h.	Glossopharyngeal	i.	j.
k.	l.	Ganglia in cardiac and pulmonary plexuses and in abdominal plexuses	m.

If you have grasped the basic structures of the sympathetic and parasympathetic division of the autonomic nervous system, you should be able to complete question 14 below.

Q14.   Write 'S' if the description applies to the sympathetic division of the ANS and 'P' if it applies to the parasympathetic division, and 'P' and 'S' if it applies to both.

☐   a.   Also called the thoracolumbar outflow.

☐   b.   Has long preganglionic fibres leading to terminal ganglia and very short postganglionic fibres.

☐   c.   Coeliac and superior mesenteric ganglia are sites of postganglionic neurone cell bodies.

☐   d.   Sends some preganglionic fibres through the cranial nerves.

☐   e.   Has some preganglionic fibres synapsing in the vertebral chain (trunk).

☐   f.   Has a more widespread effect in the body, affecting more organs.

☐   g.   Has some fibres running in grey rami to supply sweat glands, hair muscles and blood vessels.

☐   h.   Has fibres in white rami (connecting the spinal nerve with the vertebral chain).

☐   i.   Contains fibres that supply viscera with motor impulses.

☐   j.   The only division to supply the kidneys and adrenal glands.

Q15.   Which two glands in the body do not contain postganglionic fibres? Explain.

_____

_____

PHYSIOLOGICAL EFFECTS OF THE ANS 📖 *Pages 509–12*

Q16. **Complete this question about sympathetic and parasympathetic innervation.**

Most viscera receive both sympathetic and parasympathetic innervation, known as

(a) _____ innervation of the ANS. List exceptions here: sympathetic only:

(b) _____ ;

parasympathetic only: (c) _____

Figure 10.2.
Diagram of autonomic and somatic neurones, neurotransmitters and receptors. Note that neurotransmitters and receptors are relatively enlarged.

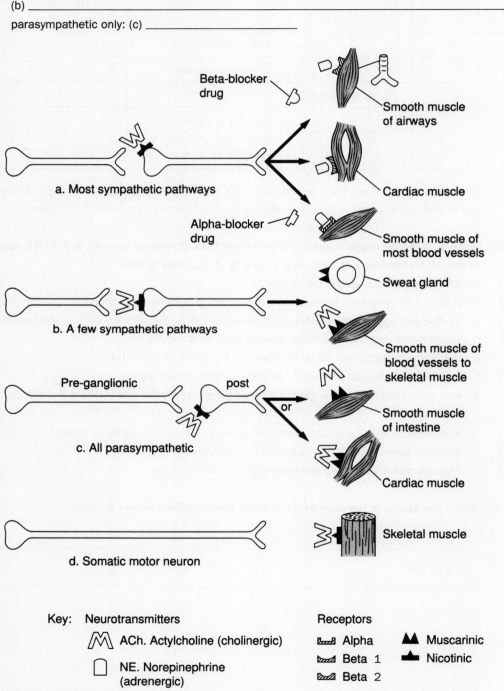

Q17. **Fill in the blanks to indicate which neurotransmitters are released by sympathetic (S) or parasympathetic (P) neurones or by somatic neurones. You may find Figure 10.2 helpful. Choose the neurotransmitter in the box.**

> **1. Acetylcholine (cholinergic) 2. Norepinephrine/noradrenaline or possibly epinephrine/adrenaline**

☐   a. All preganglionic neurones (both S and P) release this neurotransmitter.
☐   b. Most S postganglionic neurones.
☐   c. A few S postganglionic neurones, namely those to sweat glands and some blood vessels.
☐   d. All P postganglionic neurones.
☐   e. All somatic neurones.

Q18.   Complete this activity summarising the effects of autonomic neurotransmitters.

Axons that release the transmitter acetylcholine are known as (a) _____ . Those that release noradrenaline are called (b) _____ . Most sympathetic nerves are said to be (c) _____ , whereas all parasympathetic nerves are (d) _____ .

During stress, the (e) _____ division of the ANS prevails, so stress responses are primarily (f) _____ (adrenergic? or cholinergic?) responses.

Another source of noradrenaline as well as adrenaline is the gland known as the (g) _____ . Therefore, chemicals released by this gland (as in stress) will mimic the action of the (h) _____ division of the ANS.

Q19.   Complete this exercise relating to the fate of ANS neurotransmitters and the overall effects of the two divisions of the ANS.

Acetylcholine is destroyed by the enzyme (a) _____ . Noradrenaline is broken down by **two** enzymes known as (b) _____ and (c) _____ .

The ANS neurotransmitter that has a more lasting effect is (d) _____ (acetylcholine? noradrenaline?). This fact provides one explanation for the longer-lasting effects of (e) _____ (sympathetic/adrenergic? parasympathetic/cholinergic?) neurones.

State two other rationales for the more lasting and widespread effects of the sympathetic system:

f. _____

_____

g. _____

_____

Cholinergic and adrenergic receptors 📖 *Pages 510–11*

To understand why some drugs can interfere with the functions of the parasympathetic and sympathetic nervous systems, you need to be aware of the role of the receptors. A drug interacts with a receptor when the latter has the 'right shape'. This is similar to the 'lock and key' model. The interaction between the drug and receptor can bring about opening and closing of specific channels for various ions, or it can activate specific enzymes. If the interaction of the drug and receptor does promote a specific physiological response, the drug is referred to as an **agonist**; on the other hand, if no response occurs, it is then said to be an **antagonist**. These terms are discussed in Chapter 22.

When you have worked through questions 20–22, you should have gained the desired knowledge on receptors.

Q20. **Complete this exercise on cholinergic and adrenergic receptors.**
There are two types of **cholinergic** receptors, and they are called (a) _____ and (b) _____ receptors (the order of your answer does not matter).(c) _____ receptors are found on both (d) _____ and (e) _____ postganglionic neurones. (f) _____ receptors are found on all muscles and glands innervated by parasympathetic (g) _____ axons.

Cholinergic sympathetic (h) _____ fibres innervate most sweat glands and (i) _____ (type of muscle) muscles in blood vessels, and they also have (j) _____ receptors. Both muscarinic and nicotinic receptors are activated by the neurotransmitter called (k) _____ .

Q21. **Does nicotine activate muscarinic receptors?**

_____

Q22. **Acetylcholine can activate both nicotinic and muscarinic receptors – true or false?**

_____

Q23. **Complete this exercise, which relates to adrenergic receptors.**
There are two types of adrenergic receptors for noradrenaline and adrenaline and they are called (a) _____ and beta receptors. They are only found on (b) _____ structures innervated by (c) _____ postganglionic axons. These effectors are stimulated by (d) _____ . In general, alpha receptors are (e) _____ (type of function).

Q24. **Refer to Figure 10.2 and complete this exercise on neurotransmitters and related receptors. The symbol S denotes *sympathetic* and P indicates *parasympathetic*. Where the words are in parentheses, underline the right response for the statement.**
First identify all nicotinic receptors in the figure. Notice that these receptors are found on cell bodies of (P postganglionic neurones? S postganglionic neurones? autonomic effector cells? somatic effector cells (skeletal muscles)?).

In other words, nicotinic receptors are all sites for action of the neurotransmitter (a) _____ (acetylcholine? noradrenaline? either acetylcholine or noradrenaline?). Activation of nicotinic receptors is (b) _____ (always? sometimes? never?) excitatory.

On what other types of receptors can ACh act? (c) _____ . Identify these receptors on the figure. As you do, notice that these receptors are found on all effectors stimulated by (d) _____ (P? S?) postganglionic neurones. In addition, muscarinic receptors are found on a few S effectors, such as (e) _____ . Activation of muscarinic receptors is (f) _____ (always? sometimes? never?) excitatory. For example, as P nerves (vagus) release ACh to a muscarinic receptor in cardiac muscle, heart activity (g) _____ (increases? decreases?), but when P nerves (vagus) release ACh to a muscarinic receptor in the wall of the stomach or intestine, gastrointestinal activity (h) _____ (increases? decreases?).

Explain what accounts for the names nicotinic and muscarinic for ACh receptors. The names are based on the fact that the action of (i) _____ on these receptors is mimicked by the action of (j) _____ on nicotinic receptors and by a poison named (k) _____ from mushrooms on muscarinic receptors.

Alpha and beta receptors are found only on effectors innervated by (l) _____ (P? S?) nerves; these effectors are stimulated by (m) _____ (ACh? noradrenaline and adrenaline?). Noradrenaline and adrenaline are categorised as (n) _____ neurotransmitters.

Clinical application: Tom receives word that his brother has been seriously injured in a car accident. Among other immediate physiological responses, his skin appears to go pale. This physiological response is explained below. Refer to 📖 *Page 512, Exhibit 17.3.*

Which type of receptor is found in the smooth muscle of blood vessels of the skin? (o) _____ (alpha? beta₁? beta₂?). Alpha receptors are usually (p) _____ (excitatory? inhibitory?). As sympathetic (the stress system) nerves release noradrenaline, the smooth muscle of blood vessels is excited, causing them to (q) _____ (constrict/narrow? dilate/widen?). As a result, blood flows (r) _____ (into? out of?) skin, and the skin looks pale.

Q25. Complete this exercise, which relates to the effects of certain medications that mimic the body's own neurotransmitters.

A beta₁ stimulator mimics (a) _____ (ACh? noradrenaline?), causing the heart rate and strength of contraction to (b) _____ (increase? decrease?). Give the name of one such drug: (c) _____ .

Such a drug has a structure that is close enough to the shape of noradrenaline that it can 'sit on' the beta₁ receptor as noradrenaline would and activate it. A beta blocker also has a shape similar to that of noradrenaline and so can sit on (d) _____ receptors. Name one such drug: (e) _____ . However, this drug cannot activate the receptor, but simply prevents noradrenaline from doing so. So a beta blocker (f) _____ (decreases? increases?) the heart rate and force of contraction.

Other drugs, known as anticholinergics, can take up residence on ACh receptors so that ACh being released from vagal nerve stimulation cannot exert its normal effects. A person taking such a medication may exhibit a (g) _____ (increased? decreased?) heart rate.

Q26. Complete this additional exercise on further effects of medications on ANS nerves.

What types of receptors are located on the smooth muscle of bronchi and bronchioles? (a) _____ (alpha? beta₁? beta₂?). The effect of the sympathetic stimulation of lungs is to cause (b) _____ (dilatation? constriction?) of airways, making breathing (c) _____ (easier? more difficult?) during stressful times.

The effect of noradrenaline on the smooth muscle of the stomach, intestines, bladder and uterus is also (d) _____ (contraction? relaxation?), so that during stress, the body (e) _____ (decreases? increases?) the activity of these organs and can focus on more vital activities, such as heart contractions. From a question above, you may recognise that the sympathetic response during stress causes many blood vessels, such as those in the skin, to (f) _____ . Prolonged stress may therefore lead to (g) _____ (high? low?) blood pressure. One type of medication used to lower blood pressure is an alpha (h) _____ (blocker? stimulator?), since it tends to dilate these vessels and 'pool' blood in non-essential areas like skin, thereby avoiding the heart with blood flow.

Understanding some of the physiological responses of sympathetic reactions 📖 *Pages 511–12*

The so-called 'fight and flight' response occurs in time of stress, and also during physical exercise, and is governed by sympathetic stimulation. This causes various physiological changes to take place. Question 27 should help you to understand how these responses take place.

Q27. Use arrows to show whether parasympathetic (P) or sympathetic (S) fibres stimulate (↑) or inhibit (↓) each of the following activities. Use a dash (–) to indicate that there is no parasympathetic innervation. The first one is done for you.

a.   P__↓__   S__↑__   Dilatation of the pupil.

b.   P_____   S_____   Heart rate and blood flow to coronary (heart muscle) blood vessels.

c.   P_____   S_____   Salivation and digestive organ contractions.

d.   P_____   S_____   Erection of the genitalia.

e.   P_____   S_____   Dilatation of the bronchioles for easier breathing.

f.   P_____   S_____   Contraction of the bladder and relaxation of the internal urethral sphincter, causing urination.

g.   P_____   S_____   Contraction of the pili of hair follicles, causing hair to stand on end.

h.   P_____   S_____   Contraction of the spleen, which transfers some of its blood to the general circulation, causing an increase in blood pressure.

i.   P_____   S_____   Release of adrenaline and noradrenaline from the adrenal medulla.

j.   P_____   S_____   Coping with stress, fight-or-flight response.

Q28. Differentiate between sympathetic and parasympathetic actions on the liver.

_____

_____

_____

Visceral autonomic reflexes 📖 *Pages 512–13*

Q29.   **Which types of neurones stimulate autonomic neurones? (somatic afferents? visceral afferents? either somatic or visceral afferents?)**

_____

Q30.   **List five of the integrating centres that relate to the visceral reflex arc.**

_____

Q31.   **Arrange in correct sequence the structures in the pathway for a painful stimulus at your fingertip to cause a visceral (autonomic) reflex, such as sweating.**
  a.   Association neurone in the spinal cord.
  b.   Nerve fibre in the grey ramus.
  c.   Pain receptor in the skin.
  d.   Cell body of postganglionic neurone in the trunk ganglion.
  e.   Cell body of preganglionic neurone in the lateral grey of the cord.
  f.   Nerve fibre in the anterior root of the spinal nerve.
  g.   Nerve fibre in the white ramus.
  h.   Fibre in the spinal nerve in the brachial plexus.
  i.   Sweat gland.
  j.   Sensory neurone.

____ ____ ____ ____ ____ ____ ____ ____ ____

Q32.   **Complete the statements below.**
Most visceral sensations (a) _____ (do? do not?) reach the cerebral cortex, so most visceral sensations are at (b) _____ (conscious? subconscious?) levels. Hunger and nausea are exceptions.

Control by higher centres 📖 *Pages 513–14*

Q33.   **Which structure is the major control and integration centre for the ANS?**

_____

Q34.   **Which parts of the hypothalamus control the sympathetic nervous system, and which control the parasympathetic nervous system?**

You have now completed the study on the autonomic nervous system. We hope that you have found it interesting. To check your progress, you can attempt the Checkpoints Exercise.

CHECKPOINTS EXERCISE

Please note that questions 35–39 have multiple answers.

Q35.   Choose all true statements about the vagus.

a.   Its autonomic fibres are sympathetic.

b.   It supplies ANS fibres to viscera in the thorax and abdomen, but not in the pelvis.

c.   It causes the salivary glands and other digestive glands to increase their secretions.

d.   Its ANS fibres are mainly preganglionic.

e.   It is a cranial nerve originating from the medulla.

Q36.   Which activities are characteristic of the stress response, or fight-or-flight reaction?

a.   The liver breaks down glycogen to glucose.

b.   The heart rate decreases.

c.   Kidneys increase urine production, since blood is shunted to the kidneys.

d.   There is increased blood flow to the genitalia, causing an erect state.

e.   Hairs stand on end, due to contraction of arrector pili muscles.

f.   In general, the sympathetic system is active.

Q37.   Which fibres are classified as autonomic?

a.   Any visceral efferent nerve fibre.

b.   Any visceral afferent nerve fibre.

c.   Nerves to salivary glands and sweat glands.

d.   Pain fibres from an ulcer in the stomach wall.

e.   Sympathetic fibres carrying impulses to blood vessels.

f.   All nerve fibres within cranial nerves.

g.   All parasympathetic nerve fibres within cranial nerves.

Q38.   Which of the following structures contain some sympathetic preganglionic nerve fibres?

a.   Splanchnic nerves.

b.   White rami.

c.   Sciatic nerve.

d.   Cardiac nerves

e.   Ventral roots of spinal nerves.

f.   The sympathetic chains.

Q39.   Which are structural features of the parasympathetic system?

a.   Ganglia close to the CNS and distant from the effector.

b.   The craniosacral outflow.

c.   Distributed throughout the body, including the extremities.

d.   Supplies nerves to blood vessels, sweat glands and adrenal gland.

e.   Has some of its nerve fibres passing through lateral (paravertebral) ganglia.

Q40.   Which one of the following axons is not cholinergic?

a.   Parasympathetic preganglionic.

b.   Parasympathetic postganglionic

    c.   Sympathetic preganglionic

    d.   Sympathetic postganglionic to sweat glands.

    e.   Sympathetic postganglionic to heart muscle.

Q41.   Which region of the cord contains no preganglionic cell bodies at all?

    a.   Sacral.

    b.   Lumbar.

    c.   Cervical.

    d.   Thoracic.

Q42.   Which one of the statements about postganglionic neurones is false?

    a.   They all lie entirely outside the CNS.

    b.   Their axons are unmyelinated.

    c.   They terminate in visceral effectors.

    d.   Their cell bodies lie in the lateral grey matter of the cord.

    e.   They are very short in the parasympathetic system.

Answers to questions

Q1. Sympathetic and parasympathetic.

Q2. It was thought to be autonomous (self-governing). However, it is regulated by brain centres such as the hypothalamus, medulla and with input from the limbic system and other parts of the cerebellum.

Q3. a, Conscious; b, Unconscious/automatic; c, Cardiac muscle, smooth muscle and most glands; d, E; e, E or I; f, Special senses, general somatic senses of proprioceptors, and possibly visceral sensory, as when pain of appendicitis or menstrual cramping causes a person to curl up (flexion of thighs, legs); g, One (from spinal cord to effector); h, Two (pre- and postganglionic); i, ACh or noradrnaline and adrenaline.

	Somatic	Autonomic
a. Sensations and movements are mostly (conscious/ unconscious/automatic?)	Conscious	Unconscious/automatic
b. Types of issue innervated by efferent nerves	Skeletal muscle	Cardiac muscle, smooth muscle, and most glands
c. Efferent neurones are excitatory (E), inhibitory (I), or both (E or I)	E	E or I
d. Examples of sensations (input)	Special senses, general somatic senses or proprioceptors, and possibly visceral sensory, as when pain of appendicitis or menstrual cramping causes a person to curl up (flexion of thighs, legs)	Mostly visceral sensory (such as changes in CO_2 level of blood or stretching of visceral wall)
a. Number of neurones in efferent pathway	One (from spinal cord to effector)	Two (pre- and postganglionic)
f. Neurotransmitter(s) released by motor neurones	Acetylcholine (ACh)	ACh or norepinephrine (NE) and epinephrine

Q4. a. Most viscera are innervated by both the parasympathetic and sympathetic system.
b. One division excites and the other division inhibits the organ's activity.

Q5. a, 1; b, 2; c, postganglionic; d, all; e, only certain.

Q6. a, T1; b, L2; c, thoracolumbar; d, myelinated; e, ganglia; f, postganglionic; g, grey; h, myelin. i. brainstem. j, III, VII, IX, X; k, anterior; l, S2; m, S4; n, pre; o, craniosacral; p, different; q, grey; r, do; s, differ.

Q7. a, afferent; b, efferent; c, both; d, visceral; e, does not; f, does.

Q8.   a, Sympathetic; b, Parasympathetic; c, Collateral or prevertebral (coeliac, superior and inferior mesenteric); d, Intramural (in walls of viscera); e, In vertical chain along both sides of vertebral bodies from base of skull to coccyx; f, In three sites anterior to spinal cord and close to major abdominal arteries.

	Sympathetic Trunk	Prevertebral	Terminal
a. Sympathetic or parasympathetic	Sympathetic	Sympathetic	Parasympathetic
b. Alternate name	Paravertebral ganglia or vertebral chain	Collateral or prevertebral (ceilac, superior and inferior mesenteric)	Intramural (in walls of viscera)
c. General location	In vertical chain along both sides of vertebral bodies from base of skull to coccyx	In three sites anterior to spinal cord and close to major abdominal arteries	Close to or in walls of effectors

Q9.   c, a, d, b.

Q10. a, immediate synapse in trunk ganglion; b, T1; c, L2; d, C3; e, sacral; f, grey rami; g, spinal nerves; h, splanchnic; i, prevertebral; j, plexuses; k, abdomen; l, postganglionic; m, cannot; n, postganglionic.

Q11.

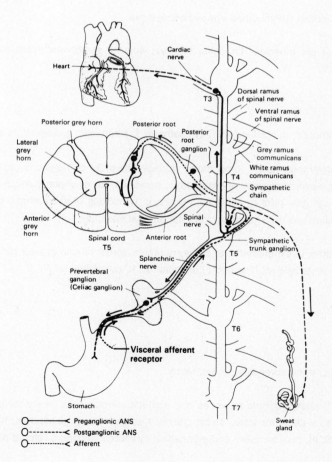

Q12. Cranial and sacral parasympathetic outflow.

Q13.

Cranial nerve		Name of Terminal Ganglion	Structures Innervated
Number	Name		
a. III	Oculomotor	Cillary	Iris and ciliary muscle of eye
b. VII	Facial	1. Pterygopalatine 2. Submandibular	1. Nasal mucosa, palate, pharynx, lacrimal gland 2. Submandibular and submaxillary salivary glands
c. IX	Glosso-pharyngeal	Otic	Parotid salivary gland
d. X	Vagus	Ganglia in cardiac and pulmonary plexuses and in abdominal plexuses	Thoracic and abdominal viscera

a, III; b, Oculomotor; c, Ciliary; d, VII; e, Facial; f, Nasal mucosa, palate, pharynx, lacrimal gland; g, Submandibular and submaxillary salivary glands; h, IX; i, Otic; j, Parotid salivary gland; k, X; I. Vagus; m, Thoracic and abdominal viscera.

Q14. Sa, Pb, Sc, Pd, Se, Sf, Sg, Sh, P and S for i, Sj.

Q15. The adrenal medulla. The glands function like modified sympathetic ganglia.

Q16. a, dual; b, sweat glands; arrector pili muscles, fat cells, kidneys, adrenal gland, and most blood vessels; c, lacrimal glands.

Q17. 1a, 2b, 1c, 1d, 1e.

Q18. a, cholinergic; b, adrenergic; c, adrenergic; d, cholinergic; e, sympathetic; f, adrenergic; g, adrenal; h, sympathetic.

Q19. a, acetylcholine; b, catechol-O-methyltransferase; c, monoamine oxidase (the order of b and c is not important); d, noradrenaline; e, sympathetic; f, greater divergence of sympathetic neurones, for example, through the extensive sympathetic trunk chain and through grey rami to all spinal nerves; g, mimicking of sympathetic responses via release of catecholamines (adrenaline and noradrenaline) from the adrenal medulla.

Q20. a, nicotinic; b, muscarinic; c, nicotinic; d, sympathetic; e, parasympathetic (order of your answer not important); f, muscarinic; g, postganglionic; h, postganglionic; i, smooth; j, muscarinic; k, acetylcholine.

Q21. No.

Q22. True.

Q23. a, alpha; b, effector; c, sympathetic; d, noradrenaline; e, excitatory.

Q24. a, P postganglionic neurones; b, S postganglionic neurones and somatic effector cells, acetylcholine, always; c, muscarinic; d, P; e, blood vessels, skeletal muscles, sweat glands; f sometimes; g, decreases; h, increases; i, ACh; j, nicotine; k, muscarinic; l, S; m, noradrenaline and adrenaline; n, catecholamine; o, alpha; p, excitatory; q, constrict; r, out of.

Q25. a, Noradrenaline; b, increase; c, adrenaline, d, beta; e, propranolol (refer to a pharmacology book for more information); f, decreases; g, decreased.

Q26. a, Beta$_2$; b, dilatation; c, easier; d, relaxation; e, decreases; f, constrict; g, high; h, blocker.

Q27. b, P↓ S↑; c, P– S↑; d, P↑ S↓; e, P↓ S↑; f, P↑ S↓; g, P– S↑; h, P– S↑; i, P– S↑; j, P↓ S↑.

Q28. Sympathetic – promotes the conversion of glycogen into glucose and the conversion of noncarbohydrates in the liver into glucose (gluconeogenesis); decreases bile secretion.
Parasympathetic – promotes glycogen synthesis; increases bile secretion.

Q29. Either somatic or visceral afferents.

Q30. Cardiac, respiratory, vasomotor, swallowing and vomiting.

Q31. c, j, a, e, f, g, d, b, h, i.

Q32. a, do not; subconscious.

Q33. Hypothalamus.

Q34. The posterior and lateral portion of the hypothalamus controls the sympathetic.
The anterior and medial portion of the hypothalamus controls the parasympathetic.

Q35. b, c, d, e,

Q36. a, e, f.

Q37. a, c, e, g.

Q38. a, b, e, f.

Q39. b.

Q40. e.

Q41. c.

Q42. d.

Overview and key terms

The endocrine system

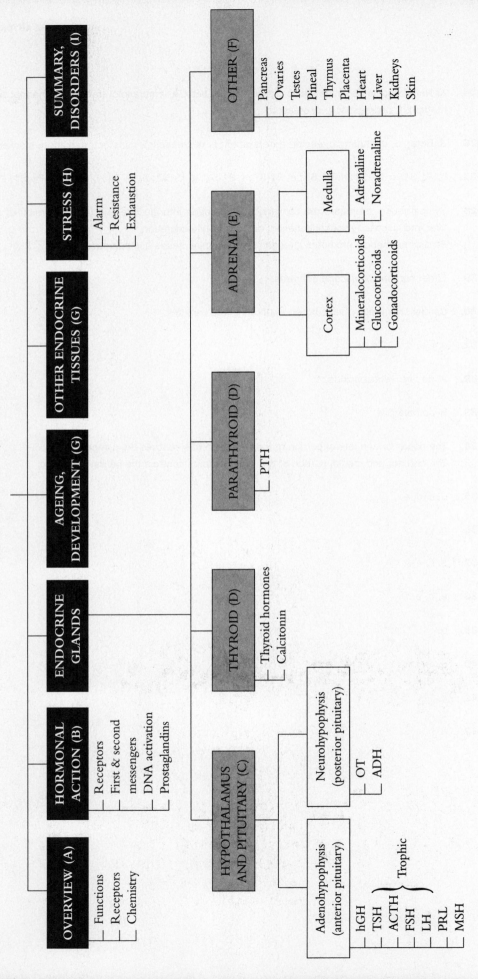

11. The Endocrine System

Learning outcomes

1. To list the components of the endocrine system.

2. To show an awareness of the relationship between the nervous system and the endocrine system.

3. To name seven main effects of hormones in the body.

4. To outline how hormones are transported in the blood and how they interact with target cell receptors.

5. To describe the structure and function of the main endocrine glands (anterior and posterior pituitary, thyroid, parathyroid, adrenals, ovaries, testes, pancreas, pineal and thymus).

6. To explain with appropriate examples the control of hormonal secretions via both negative and positive feedback mechanisms.

7. To discuss the signs and symptoms associated with under- or oversecretion of some of the endocrine glands.

8. To define the general adaptation syndrome (GAS).

Chapter 18

INTRODUCTION

The endocrine system consists of a series of glands referred to as endocrine glands. Their main role is to co-ordinate the functions of all body systems through producing secretions known as *hormones*. These secretions are directly poured into the bloodstream where they are carried to distant target cells and exert their effects. The hormones may be said to be *first messengers*. The overall function of the endocrine system is to maintain various homeostatic controls in the body.

The endocrine and the nervous system influence each other and can thus be referred to as a *neuroendocrine system*. The study here focuses mainly on endocrine functions, although you will meet a neuroendocrine example when you study the posterior lobe of the pituitary gland.

This study should assist you in understanding the structure and function of the main endocrine glands and hormones, and also their *receptors*. The last section will deal with the hormonal responses to stress.

THE ENDOCRINE SYSTEM

For questions 1, 2 and 4, see 📖 *Page 518*

Q1. **Giving an example of each, differentiate between an exocrine and an endocrine gland.**

_____

_____

_____

_____

Q2. **Compare the ways in which the nervous and endocrine systems exert control over the body. Write 'N' (nervous) or 'E' (endocrine) next to the descriptions that fit each system.**

_____ a. Sends messages to muscles, glands and neurones only.

_____ b. Sends messages to virtually any part of the body.

_____ c. Effects are generally faster and short-lived.

Q3. **Figure 11.1 shows some of the endocrine glands in the body and their anatomical position in relation to other organs. Label A–H and 1–10.**

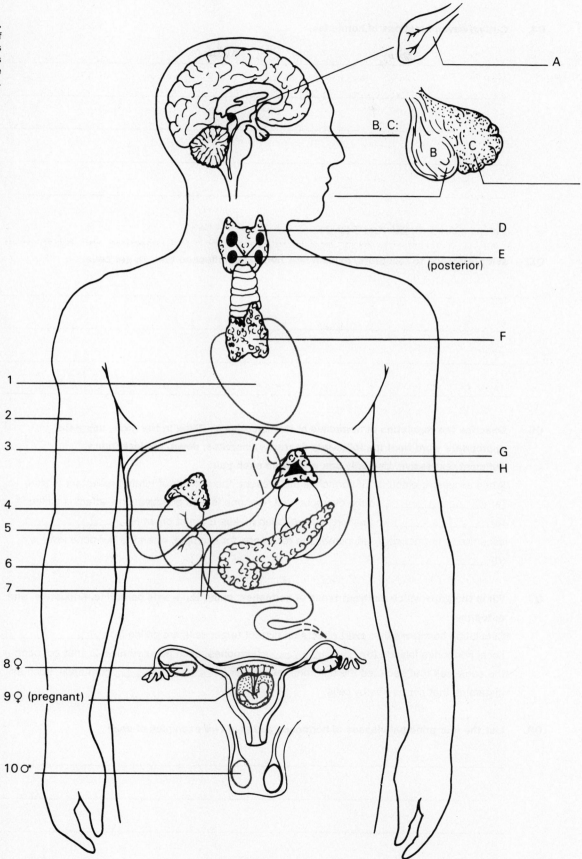

Figure 11.1.
Diagram of endocrine glands (A–H) and organs containing endocrine tissue (1–10).

Q4.   Outline seven functions of hormones.

_____

_____

_____

_____

_____

For questions 5–9, 📖 Page 519-21.

Q5.   With reference to receptors, explain how hormones influence their target cells.

_____

_____

_____

_____

Q6.   Describe the regulation of hormones in this exercise by filling in the gaps, using the appropriate word from the following: decrease/increase, down/up, less/more, deficient/excessive. Use only one word from each pair.

When excessive amounts of hormones are present, the number of related receptors is likely to (a) _____ , so the overabundant hormone is less effective. This effect is called (b) _____ -regulation. Up-regulation makes a target organ (c) _____ sensitive to hormones by an increase in receptors, for example, when the hormone level is (d) _____ .

Q7.   Fill in the gaps which contrast types of hormones, using the words paracrine, endocrine, and autocrine.

Circulating hormones that exert effects on distant target cells are called (a) _____ . Local hormones include (b) _____ hormones, such as interleukin-2, that act upon the same cell that secreted the hormone, as well as (c) _____ hormones, such as histamine that act on nearby cells.

Q8.   List the four principal classes of hormones and give two examples of each.

_____

_____

_____

_____

Q9.   Giving a rationale for your answer, explain why insulin, which is usually given to diabetic individuals, is administered by injection rather than by mouth.

_____

_____

Q10.   Study the mechanisms of hormone actions and their regulation (📖 _Pages 522–4_) and then complete the exercise below.

A hormone such as antidiuretic hormone (ADH), which is released from the (a) _____ , acts as the (b) _____ messenger, as it delivers its message to the (c) _____ cells, where it acts (in this case the kidney cells). ADH binds to receptors on the outer surface of the (d) _____ membrane, causing activation of (e) _____ proteins. Such activation increases the activity of the enzyme (f) _____ _____ , located on the (g) _____ surface of the plasma membrane. This enzyme catalyses conversion of (h) _____ to (i) _____ _____, which is known as the (j) _____ messenger. Cyclic AMP then activates one or more enzymes known as (k) _____ _____ to help transfer (l) _____ from ATP to a protein, usually an enzyme. The resulting chemical can then set off the target cell's response. In the case of ADH, this is an increase in permeability of kidney cells, with a resulting decrease in (m) _____ production.

The effects of cyclic AMP are (n) _____ -lived, as it is rapidly degraded by an enzyme called (o) _____ . A number of hormones are known to act by means of the cyclic AMP mechanism and the majority of them are (p) _____ soluble.

Q11.   Name two chemicals besides cyclic AMP that may act as second messengers. 📖 _Page 523_

_____

For questions 12 and 13, read the section on amplification of hormone effects and hormonal interactions, 📖 Page 524

Q12.   Explain briefly what is meant by amplification of hormone effects.

_____

_____

_____

Q13.   Briefly explain the antagonistic effect of hormonal interaction, giving appropriate examples.

_____

_____

_____

Q14.   Giving two examples of each, explain what you understand by the terms negative and positive feedback mechanisms in relation to hormonal regulation.

_____

_____

_____

_____

_____

Now that you have completed an overview of hormonal effects, their chemistry and mechanisms of action, you can proceed to study the hypothalamus and the pituitary gland and some of the target cells.

For questions 15–17, 📖 *Pages 525–6 & 531*

Q15.   On Figure 11.2, which shows the hypothalamus and the pituitary gland, identify the following: hypothalamus, infundibulum, pars intermedia, neurohypophysis, adenohypophysis and sphenoid bone.

Figure 11.2.
Diagram of the
hypothalamus and the
pituitary gland.

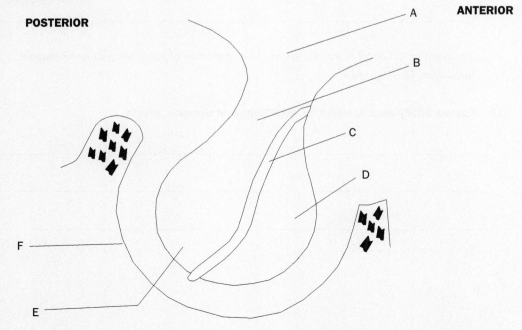

Q16.   Complete the exercise below, which gives an overview of the pituitary gland.

The pituitary gland is also known as the (a) _____ and is situated within the (b) _____ bone. It is connected to the (c) _____ by a stalk-like structure called the (d) _____ . The pituitary consists of two main lobes. The anterior lobe accounts for (e) _____ % of the gland. The posterior lobe is also referred to as the (f) _____ . The posterior lobe contains axons whose cell bodies lie in the paraventricular and (g) _____ nuclei. The cell bodies produce two hormones, which are known as ADH and (h) _____ .

The anterior pituitary gland is also known as the (i) _____ and it contains five principal types of pituitary cells, which secrete (j) _____ major hormones. The anterior pituitary gland is stimulated by releasing hormones and suppressing hormones also known as (k) _____ hormones from the (l) _____ .

Q17.   What are the functions of the three types of anterior pituitary cells mentioned below?

a. Lactotrophs.

_____

b. Somatotrophs.

_____

c. Gonadotrophs.

_____

Q18.   Define the term trophin or trophic hormones and give four examples.

_____

_____

_____

_____

Q19. **Complete the table below, listing the releasing → trophic → target hormone relationships. Fill in the name of a hormone next to each letter.** 📖 *Pages 525–31*

Hypothalamic hormone	Anterior pituitary hormone	Target hormone
GHRH (growth hormone releasing hormone)	a.	None
CRH (corticotrophin releasing hormone)	b.	c.
d.	TSH (thyrotrophin)	e.
GnRH (gonadotrophic releasing hormone)	FSH (follicle stimulating hormone)	f.

Q20. **Name the three main hypothalamic inhibiting hormones.**

_____

_____

_____

The most abundant anterior pituitary hormone is human growth hormone (hGH) which is secreted by the somatotrophs cells. **Study the functions of growth hormone and then complete the exercise below.** 📖 *Pages 528–30*

Q21. Growth hormone is also known as (a) _____ and its main function is to stimulate growth and maintain the size of (b) _____ and (c) _____ muscles. Human growth hormone stimulates protein synthesis by increasing the rate at which (d) _____ enter cells.

During fasting and starvation the effect of hGH is to stimulate (e) _____ catabolism to produce (f) _____ . hGH also influences carbohydrate metabolism. For example, it decreases (g) _____ uptake by cells, but accelerates the conversion of (h) _____ to glucose. Excess of hHG causes a rise in blood sugar and this is referred to as (i) _____ .

hGH from the anterior pituitary is controlled by two hormones from the (j) _____ . One stimulates the release of growth hormone and is called (k) _____ , whilst the other inhibits its secretion and is known as (l) _____ .

Q22. **Which condition is likely to occur as a result of hyposecretion of hGH during childhood?**

_____

Q23. Which condition is likely to occur as a result of hypersecretion of hGH in the adult?

_____

Now that you have grasped the facts about growth hormone, you can move on to study a second hormone from the anterior pituitary lobe, thyroid stimulating hormone and its effect on the thyroid gland.

THYROID STIMULATING HORMONE AND THE THYROID GLAND

Q24. Figure 11.3 is a schematic representation of the hypothalamus, the pituitary, the thyroid gland and the hormones they secrete. The numbers 1–4 represent the different hormonal secretions. Write the name of the hormones against each of the numbers.

Figure 11.3. Diagram of the hypothalamus, pituitary and thyroid gland, with one single follicle.

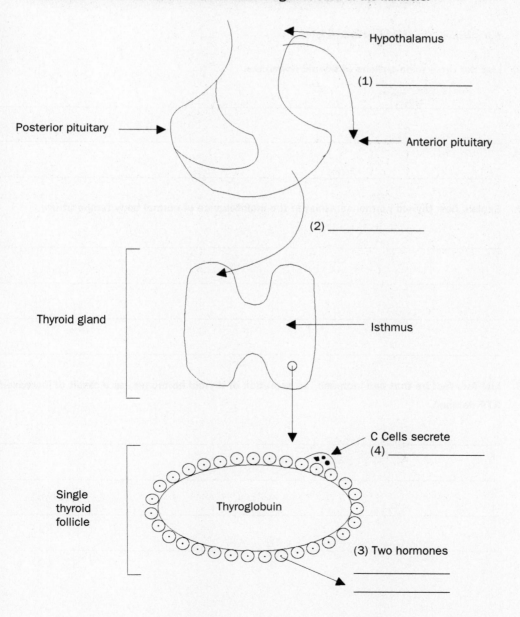

Hypothalamus

(1) _____

Posterior pituitary

Anterior pituitary

(2) _____

Thyroid gland

Isthmus

C Cells secrete
(4) _____

Single thyroid follicle

Thyroglobuin

(3) Two hormones

_____
_____

Q25. **Now that you have identified the various hormones that are important for the proper functioning of the thyroid gland, you can complete the exercise below.** 📖 *Pages 535–9*

The thyroid gland is located below the (a) _____ . It contains two lobes, which lie on either side of the (b) _____ . The thyroid is composed of two types of glandular cells, known as (c) _____ cells, which secrete **tri-iodothyronine** (T_3) and (d) _____ (T_4) and (e) _____ (cells) which produce (f) _____ (hormone that controls calcium metabolism).

In the thyroid follicular cells, the ion (g) _____ is highly concentrated and is the essential component of T_3 and T_4. The follicular cells also synthesise (h) _____ (a storage form of thyroid hormone), which is released in the lumen of the follicles and this is then referred to as (i) _____ . Since T_3 and T_4 are (j) _____ -soluble, they diffuse through the (k) _____ _____ to enter the blood. In the blood, T_3 and T_4 are transported as (l) _____ _____ _____ (TBG).

For questions 26–28, 📖 *Pages 537–8*

Q26. **List the three main actions of thyroid hormones.**

_____

_____

_____

Q27. **Explain how thyroid hormones assist in the maintenance of normal body temperature.**

_____

_____

_____

_____

Q28. **List four factors that can increase the secretion of thyroid hormones, as a result of increased ATP demand.**

_____

_____

_____

_____

Clinical application 📖 *Pages 538–9*

Over-secretion (hypersecretion) or under-secretion (hyposecretion) of thyroid hormones gives rise to conditions that require treatment. Hyposecretion gives rise to what can be referred to as **hypothyroidism,** whilst hypersecretion leads to **hyperthyroidism. When you have read the section on clinical application, complete the following exercise.**

Q29. Hyposecretion of thyroid hormones during fetal life or infancy results in (a) _____ and the affected individual exhibits (b) _____ , because the skeleton fails to grow and mature. Hyposecretion in the adult gives rise to the condition known as (c) _____ and the affected individual may have (d) _____ (a slow heart rate) and also

(e) _____ (low body temperature). Individuals suffering from hyposecretion of thyroid hormones will require oral thyroid hormones for the rest of their lives.

Hypersecretion of thyroid hormones leads to (f) _____ , the most common form of which gives rise to the condition known as (g) _____ _____ . A primary sign may be the (h) _____ of the thyroid gland, and the affected individual may also have a peculiar type of oedema behind the eyes, causing them to protrude, and this is called (i) _____ .

Although many thyroid disorders can cause enlargement of the thyroid gland, this can also occur when there is a lack of or inadequate (j) _____ in the diet. This results in a low level of thyroid hormones in the blood and because of the (k) _____ feedback mechanism, there is an increase in (l) _____ from the anterior lobe of the

(m) _____ gland.

Now that you have studied the thyroid gland, it is appropriate to discuss the location and functions of the **parathyroid** glands 📖 *Page 540. Please note that the parathyroid glands are not influenced by the pituitary gland.*

Q30. The parathyroid glands are situated on the posterior surfaces of the (a) _____ gland. They secrete (b) _____ , which increases the number and activity of

(c) _____ . This results in an increase in the amount of phosphates and

(d) _____ in the blood.

With respect to blood calcium level, **PTH** and (e) _____ are antagonistics. PTH also acts on the (f) _____ to promote the formation of the hormone

(g) _____ (also known as 1,25-dihydroxy cholecalciferol, which increases the rate of calcium, (h) _____ and magnesium absorption from the gastrointestinal tract.

Q31. In relation to blood calcium level, explain the relationship between PTH and calcitonin when:
a.   Blood calcium level falls.

_____

b.   Blood calcium level rises.

_____

Q32. An increase in parathormone can lead to (a) _____ (rise in blood calcium) whereas a decrease may give rise to (b) _____ (decrease in blood calcium). Decreased blood calcium results in an abnormal increase in nerve impulses to muscles, and the condition known as (c) _____ .

GONADOTROPHIN STIMULATING HORMONES (FOLLICLE STIMULATING HORMONE AND LUTEINIZING HORMONE) IN THE MALE AND THE FEMALE

The gonadotroph cells of the anterior pituitary produce **two** major hormones that regulate the functions of the gonads (ovaries and testes): follicle stimulating hormone (FSH) and luteinizing hormone (LH).

By working on a series of exercises, you will become familiar with the functions of these hormones.

For questions 33–34, 📖 *Pages 530 and 553 and for specific detail* 📖 *Pages 949–52*

FSH and LH in females

Q33. FSH release from the anterior pituitary is controlled by (a) _____ _____ _____ from the hypothalamus. FSH stimulates the ovaries and causes the development of the (b) _____ follicles. It also stimulates follicular cells to secrete (c) _____ . (d) _____ together with FSH brings about the process of (e) _____ . Following ovulation, (f) _____ promotes the formation of (g) _____ _____ and the secretion of (h) _____ preparing the (i) _____ for implantation of a fertilised ovum. Both (j) _____ and (k) _____ regulate the (l) _____ cycle. FSH secretion is inhibited by (m) _____ .

Q34. **Which hormone causes dilatation of the uterine cervix towards the end of pregnancy?**

_____

FSH and LH in males

For question 35, 📖 *Page 530 and for more detail* 📖 *Pages 925–6, Figure 28.3*

Q35. In males, FSH acts on the (a) _____ tubules in the (b) _____ to promote the development of (c) _____ . LH acts on specialised cells known as cells of (d) _____ (also known as interstitial cells) to secrete (e) _____ .

PROLACTIN, OXYTOCIN AND ANTIDIURETIC HORMONE

It is appropriate to move on to the hormones prolactin, oxytocin and antidiuretic hormone, now that you have studied the two major gonadotrophins.

For questions 36–39, 📖 Pages 531–5

Q36. **Describe the functions of the posterior pituitary hormones by labelling Figure 11.4. Write your answers on the lines provided, using the list of terms provided.**

Figure 11.4.
Posterior pituitary
hormones.

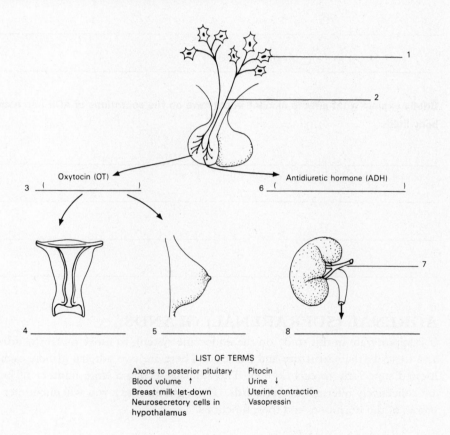

LIST OF TERMS

Axons to posterior pituitary	Pitocin
Blood volume ↑	Urine ↓
Breast milk let-down	Uterine contraction
Neurosecretory cells in hypothalamus	Vasopressin

Q37. Milk secretion and ejection are referred to as (a) _____ . Milk is produced by the hormone (b) _____ after the mammary glands have been primed by various hormones. PRL (prolactin) secretion is regulated by both the (c) _____ _____ _____ from the (d) _____ , which inhibits release of PRL, and the (e) _____ _____ _____ which raises the level of PRL, for example during pregnancy. The release of PRL from the (f) _____ lobe of the (g) _____ is controlled by the suckling reflex on the nipples by the infant.

Oxytocin has two target tissues, the (h) _____ and the (i) _____ . Oxytocin is released via a (j) _____ feedback mechanism from the (k) _____ lobe of the pituitary. The neurosecretory cells for oxytocin are situated in the (l) _____ in the hypothalamus.

Q38. If you were to drink a large amount of a sugary solution, explain what effects this would have on your body with regard to ADH and the homeostasis of body fluids. Give the rationale for your answer.

_____

_____

_____

_____

Q39. Briefly explain what effects alcohol would have on the secretions of ADH and homeostasis of body fluids.

_____

_____

_____

_____

ADRENAL (SUPRARENAL) GLANDS

It is appropriate in this study on the endocrine system, to move on to the **adrenal glands** and to study their structure and function. There are two adrenal glands, each of which is located superiorly to each kidney. The adrenals secrete a large number of hormones that are collectively referred to as **steroids.** Through this study, you will encounter the different names of the hormones and their functions.

Q40. Figure 11.5 shows the relationship between the hypothalamus, the anterior pituitary gland and the adrenal cortex. Number 1 refers to the hormone from the hypothalamus which stimulates the anterior lobe to release hormone number 2, which eventually stimulates the cortex to release its three main groups of hormones (numbers 5, 6 and 7). Write on the diagram the names of all the hormones involved. 📖 _Pages 531–5 & 542–8_

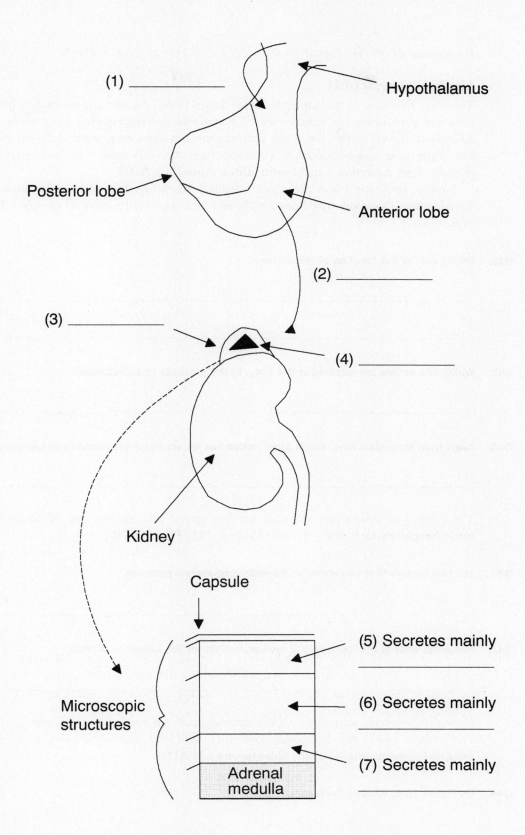

Figure 11.5.
The relationship between the hypothalamus, the anterior pituitary and the adrenal gland.

Hypothalamus

(1) _____

Posterior lobe

Anterior lobe

(2) _____

(3) _____

(4) _____

Kidney

Capsule

Microscopic structures

(5) Secretes mainly
_____

(6) Secretes mainly
_____

(7) Secretes mainly
_____

Adrenal medulla

For questions 41–45, 📖 *Pages 544–5*

Mineralocorticoids

The main functions of the mineralocorticoids are those of water and electrolyte homeostasis and particularly the concentration of **sodium** and **potassium.** One of the main mineralocorticoids is the hormone **aldosterone.** In regulating water and electrolytes, **blood pressure** is also maintained. Four important chemicals assist in the control of blood pressure. They are **renin, angiotensin, aldosterone**, and **ADH** .

Now to understand how these four chemicals work together, you will be directed to complete some exercises (questions 39-43) and then you will be asked to complete Figure 11.6.

Q41. **Briefly outline the function of aldosterone.**

_____

_____

Q42. **Which two anions are retained in the body, in the presence of aldosterone?**

_____

Q43. **Apart from potassium ions, which other cation has its excretion promoted by aldosterone?**

_____

The control of aldosterone secretion involves several mechanisms, one of which is the **renin–angiotensin** pathway (refer to 📖 *Page 545, Figure 18.20*).

Q44. **List two factors that can activate the renin–angiotensin pathway.**

_____

Q45. **Name the cells in the kidneys that are responsible for the secretion of renin.**

_____

Now that you have some ideas of the renin–angiotensin system, you can refer to Figure 11.6, which shows the hormonal control of fluid and electrolyte balance and blood pressure by **renin, angiotensin, aldosterone** and **ADH.**

Q46. **On Figure 11.6, identify the numbers 1–8.**

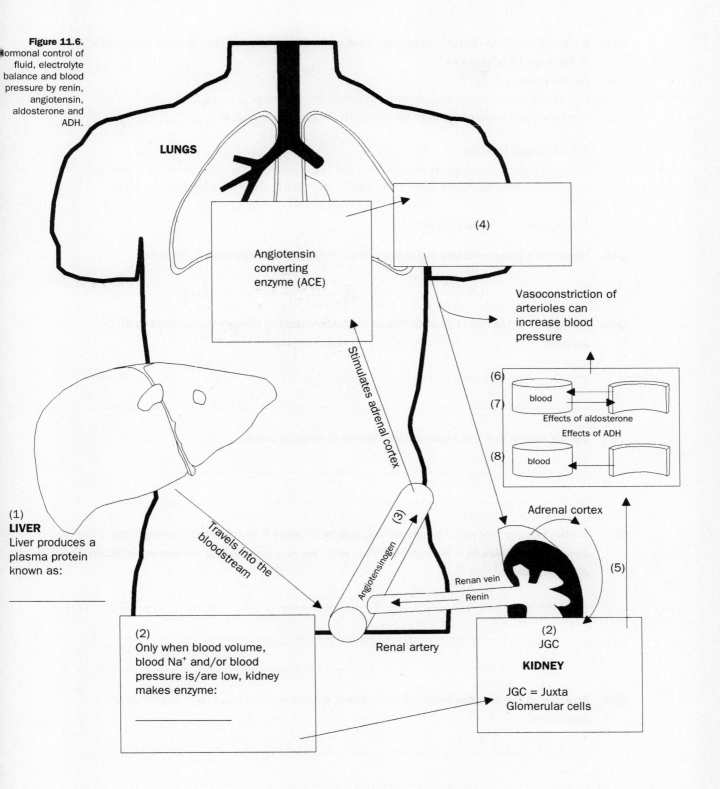

Figure 11.6.
Hormonal control of fluid, electrolyte balance and blood pressure by renin, angiotensin, aldosterone and ADH.

LUNGS

Angiotensin converting enzyme (ACE)

(4)

Vasoconstriction of arterioles can increase blood pressure

(6)

(7)

blood

Effects of aldosterone

Effects of ADH

(8)

blood

Stimulates adrenal cortex

Adrenal cortex

(1)

LIVER
Liver produces a plasma protein known as:

_____

Travels into the bloodstream

Angiotensinogen

(3)

Renan vein

Renin

Renal artery

(5)

(2)
Only when blood volume, blood Na$^+$ and/or blood pressure is/are low, kidney makes enzyme:

_____

(2)
JGC

KIDNEY

JGC = Juxta Glomerular cells

Q47.   A clinical challenge. Determine whether each of the following conditions is likely to increase or decrease blood pressure.

a.   Excessive renin production: _____ .

b.   Use of angiotensin converting enzyme (ACE) inhibitor medication: _____ .

c.   Aldosteronism (for example, due to a tumour of the zona glomerulosa): _____ .

Glucocorticoids

The glucocorticoids regulate metabolism and resistance to stress. The exercises below will only concentrate on metabolism, stress will be dealt with as the final topic in this chapter.

For questions 48–53, 📖 *Pages 545–7*

Q48.   Name three glucocorticoids and indicate the one that is most abundant in the body.

_____

Q49.   Briefly outline the role of glucocorticoids in gluconeogenesis through the catabolism of proteins.

_____

_____

Q50.   List six factors that can stimulate the release of glucocorticoids.

_____

_____

Q51.   Explain why the process of wound healing may be retarded if an individual is taking large amounts of steroids for a medical condition. Hint: you may assume that the steroids contain glucocorticoids.

_____

_____

_____

Q52.   Referring to the negative feedback mechanism, explain how the blood level of cortisol is maintained.

_____

_____

_____

_____

_____

Q53. When there is a high blood level of ACTH as a result of a disease such as Cushing's syndrome, explain why the skin of the affected individuals becomes darker.

_____

_____

Having gained some knowledge on the functions of the **mineralocorticoids** and **glucocorticoids,** you can now study the last group of hormones from the adrenal cortex which are called the **gonadocorticoids.**

For question 54, 📖 *Page 547*

Q54. Name two hormones that are gonadocorticoids.

_____

Now that you have completed the study on the adrenal cortex, you can move on to review the **medulla.** Please note that the hormones produced by the medulla **epinephrine** and **norepinephrine** are also known as **adrenaline** and **noradrenaline,** respectively. In the United Kingdom adrenaline and noradrenaline are the preferred names.

Q55. What is the name for the hormone-producing cells in the medulla?

_____

Q56. Which of the hormones secreted by the medulla accounts for 80% of the gland's secretion?

_____

Q57. Why are adrenaline and noradrenaline referred to as sympathomimetic?

_____

_____

Q58. Name the chemical group to which adrenaline and noradrenaline belong.

_____

OTHER ENDOCRINE GLANDS: PANCREAS AND PINEAL GLAND 📖 *Pages 549–54*

You have already met some of the functions of the pancreas when you studied the digestive system. Here, you will be introduced mainly to the endocrine functions and hence the hormones that control carbohydrate metabolism.

Q59.   What is the name of the endocrine tissues found in the pancreas?

_____

Q60.   Name the four types of islet cells.

_____

Q61.   Complete the exercise below, which relates to glucagon.

_____

Glucagon is produced by (a) _____ cells and it increases blood sugar in two ways. Firstly, it stimulates the breakdown of (b) _____ to glucose, a process known as (c) _____ . Secondly, it stimulates the conversion of amino acids and other compounds to (d) _____ . This process is called (e) _____ .

Control of glucagon secretion is determined by the effect of blood (f) _____ level directly on the pancreas. When blood glucose is low, then a (g) _____ level of glucagon will be produced. This will raise the level of blood sugar.

Q62.   Complete the exercise below, which relates to insulin.

Insulin is secreted by the (a) _____ cells of the islets of Langerhans. Its main action is to (b) _____ the level of blood glucose. For example, it converts glucose to glycogen, a process known as (c) _____ .

Insulin secretion is regulated by the blood (d) _____ level. When blood glucose level is (e) _____ , insulin secretion is increased, whereas when blood sugar level is low, insulin level is (f) _____ .

Q63.   Contrast type I and type II diabetes mellitus by writing I or II next to the related descriptions.

☐   a. Also known as maturity-onset diabetes mellitus.

☐   b. The more common type of diabetes mellitus.

☐   c. Related to insensitivity of body cells to insulin, rather than to absolute insulin deficiency.

☐   d. Also known as insulin-dependent diabetes mellitus.

☐   e. More likely to lead to serious complications such as ketoacidosis.

Q64. List three or more factors that increase insulin secretion.

_____

_____

_____

Q65. Define the following terms: hypoglycaemia, hyperglycaemia, and glycosuria.

_____

_____

_____

Q66. Explain why polydipsia and polyuria occur in individuals suffering from diabetes mellitus. Please note that this is likely to occur when the diabetes is not well controlled.

_____

_____

PINEAL GLAND

Q67. Where is the pineal gland situated?

_____

Q68. Which hormone is secreted by the pineal gland?

_____

Q69. Outline why bright light therapy is used in the treatment of seasonal affective disorder.

_____

_____

Eicosanoids

Under 'chemistry of hormones' 📖 *Page 520*, you met the term 'eicosanoids'. Through working on question 70, you will understand the roles of the eicosanoids in both normal and altered physiology.

Q70.   Briefly outline the functions of the following: leukotrienes, prostaglandins and thromboxane.

_____

_____

_____

_____

STRESS AND HOMEOSTASIS

The last section to be considered in this study concerns **stress** and **homeostasis**. To be able to understand the physiology of stress, you really need to have an overview of the functions of the **hypothalamus,** the **pituitary gland**, the **thyroid**, **adrenal cortex** and the **medulla.**

For the study on stress, 📖 _Pages 556–60_

Q71.   Define and give two examples of stressors.

_____

_____

Q72.   Complete the exercise below, which summarises the body's response to stress.

The part of the brain that senses stress and initiates the response is the (a) _____ .
It responds by two main mechanisms. First is the (b) _____ reaction involving the
adrenal (c) _____ and the sympathetic division of the (d) _____ nervous
system. Second is the (e) _____ reaction. Playing key roles in this response are
three anterior pituitary hormones: (f) _____ , which is controlled by thyrotrophin
releasing hormone, (g) _____ , which is controlled by corticotrophin releasing
hormone and (h) _____ , which is controlled by growth hormone releasing hormone.
These three hormones and the appropriate target hormones activate the adrenal
(i) _____ to secrete its hormones.

**Q73.   By completing the exercise below, you will have described the events that characterise the
first (or alarm) stage of response to stress.**

The alarm reaction is sometimes called the (a) _____ response. During this stage
blood glucose (b) _____ (increases? decreases?) by a number of hormonal
mechanisms, including those of the adrenal medulla hormones (c) _____ and
(d) _____ . Glucose must be available for cells to have energy for the stress
response.

Oxygen must also be available to tissues; the respiratory system (e) _____
(increases? decreases?) its activity. Heart rate and blood pressure (f) _____

(increase? decrease?). Blood is shunted to vital tissues such as the (g) _____ ,
(h) _____ , and (i) _____ , and is directed away from reservoir organs
such as the (j) _____ , (k) _____ , and (l) _____ .

Nonessential activities such as digestion (m) _____ (increase? decrease?).
Sweating (n) _____ (increases? decreases?) in order to control body temperature
and eliminate wastes.

Q74. **When you have answered this question, you should understand the functions of four important hormones in the resistance stage. Describe the effects of each of the following hormones in the resistance stage:**

a.   Glucocorticoids

_____

b.   Thyroxine

_____

c.   Human growth hormone

_____

d.   Mineralocorticoids

_____

_____

Q75. **When the resistance stage fails to combat the stressor, the body moves into (a) _____ . Explain how this is related to:**

b.   Loss of potassium.

_____

c.   Depletion of glucocorticoids.

_____

d.   Weakening of organs.

_____

Congratulate yourself, you have now completed the endocrine system. Well done. Now you could check your progress by working on the Checkpoints Exercise which follows.

CHECKPOINTS EXERCISE

Q76. **Match the terms with the descriptions of hormones.**

| 1. Steroid 2. Eicosanoids 3. Peptides/protein 4. Biogenic amines |

☐ a. Chains of 3 to about 200 amino acid residues that may form glycoproteins; most hormones are in this category.

☐ b. Related to cholesterol; include hormones from the adrenal cortex, ovary and testis.

☐ c. Chemically, the simplest hormones; examples include thyroid hormones (T3 and T4) and catecholamines (adrenaline and noradrenaline).

☐ d. Derived from a 20-carbon-atom fatty acid; examples are prostaglandins and leukotrienes.

Q77. **Complete the following exercise about growth hormone.**

Hypersecretion of GH leads to (a) _____, whereas deficiency causes pituitary (b) _____ . Excess hGH after closure of epiphyseal plates causes (c) _____, characterised by bones in three areas: face, (d) _____, and (e) _____.

Q78. **Complete the following exercise which relates to posterior pituitary hormones.**

The time period from the start of a baby's suckling at the breast to the delivery of milk to the baby is about (a) _____ . Although afferent impulses (from the breast to the hypothalamus) require only a fraction of a second, passage of the oxytocin through the (b) _____ to the breasts requires about (c) _____ seconds.

If your body becomes dehydrated, for example through excessive sweating, your ADH is likely to (d) _____ (increase? decrease?). This will therefore tend to (e) _____ (increase? decrease?) urine production.

The effects of diuretic medications are (f) _____ (similar? opposite?) to ADH. In other words, diuretics will (g) _____ (increase? decrease?) urine production and thus will (h) _____ (increase? decrease?) blood volume and blood pressure. Too much diuretic may lead to (i) _____ and therefore (j) _____ (a low blood volume).

Inadequate ADH production, as occurs in diabetes (k) _____ results in large daily volumes of urine. Unlike the urine produced in diabetes mellitus, the urine does not contain (l) _____ .

Alcohol (m) _____ (its effect on ADH secretion) ADH secretion, which contributes to the (n) _____ (increase? decrease?) of urine production after alcohol intake.

Q79. **This question indicates the contrast between growth hormone and thyroid hormone functions. Fill in either the word catabolism or anabolism.**

Like growth hormone, thyroid hormone increases protein (a) _____ . Unlike hGH, thyroid hormone increases most aspects of carbohydrate (b) _____ .

Q80. **When you have completed this exercise, you should understand the effects of glucorticoids in metabolism and resistance to stress.**

These hormones promote (a) _____ (catabolism? anabolism?) of proteins. In this respect their effects are (b) _____ (similar? opposite?) to those of both growth hormone and thyroid hormone. However, glucocorticoids may stimulate conversion of amino acids and fats to glucose, a process known as (c) _____ . In this way glucocorticoids, like hGH (d) _____ (increase? decrease?) blood glucose levels. In times of stress, both glucocorticoids and hGH production are increased. By raising blood glucose levels, these hormones make energy available to cells most vital for a response to stress. During stress, glucocorticoids also act to (e) _____ (increase? decrease?) blood pressure and to (f) _____ (enhance? limit?) the inflammatory process.

Q81. **Aspirin is widely used in medicine. Its main function is to inhibit the synthesis of an important chemical substance in the body.**

a. Name the chemical substance.

_____

b. List **three** therapeutic effects of aspirin.

_____

_____

_____

Q82. **Test your understanding of these hormones by writing the name of the correct hormone after each of the following descriptions.**

a. Stimulates release of growth hormone: _____ .

b. Stimulates testes to produce testosterone: _____ .

c. Promotes protein anabolism, especially of bones and muscles: _____ .

d. Trophic hormone for thyroxin: _____ .

e. Stimulates development of ova in females and spermatozoa in males: _____ .

f. Present in bloodstream of nonpregnant women to prevent lactation: _____ .

g. Stimulates the ovary to release the ovum and change the follicle cells into corpus luteum: _____ .

h. Stimulates uterine contractions and also breast milk let-down: _____ .

i. Inhibited by MIH: _____ .

j. Stimulates kidney tubules to produce a small volume of concentrated urine: _____ .

k. Target hormone of ACTH: _____ .

l. Increases blood calcium: _____ .

m. Decreases blood calcium and phosphate: _____ .

n. Contains iodine as an important component: _____ .

o. Raises blood glucose level (three answers): _____ , _____ and _____ .

p. Lowers blood glucose level: _____ .

q. Serves anti-inflammatory functions: _____ .

r. Mimics many effects of sympathetic nerves: _____ .

Q83.   Match the disorder with the hormonal imbalance.

> **1. Acromegaly 2. Addison's disease 3. Cretinism 4. Diabetes insipidus 5. Diabetes mellitus.
> 6. Grave's disease. 7. Myxoedema 8. Tetany 9. Phaeochromocytoma 10. Pituitary dwarfism
> 11. Simple goitre**

☐ a. Deficiency of hGH in child; slow bone growth.

☐ b. Excess of hGH in adult; enlargement of hands, feet and jawbones.

☐ c. Deficiency of ADH; production of enormous quantities of 'insipid' urine.

☐ d. Deficiency of effective insulin; hyperglycaemia and glycosuria.

☐ e. Deficiency of thyroxin in child; short stature and mental retardation.

☐ f. Deficiency of thyroxin in adult; oedematous facial tissues, lethargy.

☐ g. Excess of thyroxin; protruding eyes, 'nervousness' and weight loss.

☐ h. Deficiency of thyroxin due to lack of iodine; most common reason for enlarged thyroid gland.

☐ i. Result of deficiency of PTH; decreased calcium in blood and fluids around muscles resulting in abnormal muscle contraction.

☐ j. Deficiency of adrenocorticoids; increased K^+ and decreased Na^+ resulting in low blood pressure and dehydration.

☐ k. Tumour of adrenal medulla causing sympathetic-type responses, such as increased pulse and blood pressure, hyperglycaemia and sweating.

Q84.   Arrange the answers in the correct sequence.

1.   Steps in action of TSH upon a target cell:

a. Adenylate cyclase breaks down ATP.

b. TSH attaches to receptor site.

c. Cyclic AMP is produced.

d. Protein kinase is activated to cause the specific effect mediated by TSH, namely, stimulation of thyroid hormone.

e. G-protein is activated.

2.   Steps in renin–angiotensin mechanism to increase blood pressure:

a. Angiotensin I is converted to angiotensin II .

b. Renin converts angiotensinogen, a plasma protein, to angiotensin I.

c. Angiotensin II causes vasoconstriction and stimulates aldosterone production, which causes water conservation and raises blood pressure.

d. Low blood pressure or low blood Na^+ level causes secretion of the enzyme renin from cells in kidneys.

Q85.   All of these compounds are synthesised in the hypothalamus except:

a. ADH

b. GHRH

c. CT

d. PIH

e. Oxytocin.

Q86. Choose the false statement about endocrine glands.

a. They secrete chemicals called hormones.

b. Their secretions enter extracellular spaces and then pass into blood.

c. Sweat and sebaceous glands are endocrine glands.

d. Endocrine glands are ductless.

Q87. All of the following hormones are secreted by the anterior pituitary except:

a. ACTH

b. FSH

c. Prolactin

d. Oxytocin

e. hGH.

Q88. Choose the false statement about the anterior pituitary.

a. It secretes at least seven hormones.

b. It develops from mesoderm.

c. It secretes trophic hormones.

d. It is stimulated by releasing factors from the hypothalamus.

e. It is also known as the adenohypophysis.

Q89. Choose the false statement.

a. Both ADH and aldosterone tend to lead to retention of water and increase blood pressure.

b. PTH activates osteoclasts, leading to bone destruction.

c. Tetany is a sign of hypocalcaemia.

d. ADH and OT pass from the hypothalamus to the posterior pituitary via pituitary portal veins.

PATIENT SCENARIO

Maureen Sylvester, a 21-year-old university student, is admitted for a subtotal thyroidectomy. She was diagnosed as suffering from **thyrotoxicosis** two years ago. She has been treated medically by her general practitioner mainly with the drug, carbimazole (Neo-Mercazole) and propranolol.

On admission, Maureen appears very nervous and anxious. Further nursing assessment indicates that she dislikes the warm weather, and does not like to be in a warm environment. She also reports that she always feels warm. She has lost weight, although she has an increased appetite and she is always hungry. She sometimes suffers from bouts of diarrhoea. She states that at times she feels that her heart is 'racing'.

Nursing observations indicate that her blood pressure is 120/80 mmHg, pulse is 140/minute and regular, and respiration is 24/minute and regular.

Q90.   In physiological terms, briefly explain why Maureen should feel warm.

_____

_____

_____

Q91.   What can the nurse do to assist Maureen in settling in the rather warm ward environment?

_____

_____

_____

_____

_____

Q92.   What is the likely physiological explanation for Maureen's palpitation and diarrhoea?

_____

_____

_____

_____

Q93.   Discuss the nursing observations that Maureen would require immediately on return to the ward from theatre. Give the rationale for your answer.

_____

_____

_____

_____

A few hours following surgery, whilst you are caring for Maureen, you notice that she has slight hoarseness.

Q94.   What may be the possible reason for Maureen's hoarseness?

_____

_____

_____

_____

_____

Maureen is to be monitored for blood serum calcium level for the next few days following surgery.

Q95. Explain the reason why the calcium level is being monitored.

_____

_____

_____

_____

_____

Q96. Outline the actions of carbimazole and propranolol that Maureen has been prescribed.

_____

_____

_____

_____

_____

Q97. Maureen was advised by her general practitioner to stop taking her carbimazole two weeks prior to surgery. Explain the rationale for this advice.

_____

_____

Q98. Briefly outline any possible long-term complications, following surgery.

_____

_____

_____

QUESTIONS FOR DISCUSSION

1.   Discuss the nursing management of Maureen until she is discharged home three days post-operatively.

2.   What specific advice should you give to Maureen to ensure that she remains in good health?

SOME FACTS ABOUT THYROTOXICOSIS

Hyperthyroidism is also called **thyrotoxicosis.** It is a very common endocrine disorder affecting both men and women, although the incidence is higher for women. It results from excessive secretion of thyroxine (T_4) or tri-iodothyronine (T_3). The most common causes are toxic diffuse goitre (Grave's disease) and toxic nodular goitre. Grave's disease is caused by antibodies (thyroid stimulating immunoglobulins) that abnormally stimulate thyroid hormones. Thyroid stimulating immunoglobulins, are also referred to as long-acting thyroid stimulators. It would also appear that the thyroid gland no longer responds in the normal way to thyroid stimulating hormone and indeed it may regulate itself. There is increased metabolic rate and this may have serious effects on the heart. Thyroxine also has a direct effect on the heart.

Patients with Grave's disease usually have a goitre (swelling of the thyroid gland), most of the signs associated with hyperthyroidism and also an abnormal protrusion of the eyes which is called **exophthalmos.** Exophthalmos may give rise to **ptosis** (drooping of the eyelids) and also irritation of the eyes (because of the protrusion of the eyes, the eyelids fail to cover the eyes and they remain exposed) leading to conjunctivitis.

An important sign of Grave's disease, as a result of increased blood flow, is a noise (referred to as a bruit) which can be heard with a stethoscope placed over the thyroid gland. Most of the symptoms in thyrotoxicosis are the result of sympathetic nervous stimulation.

Diagnostic tests

Thyroid functions can be assessed through many tests, of which the following are common: measurement of serum T_4 and T_3 concentrations, radioactive iodine uptake, thyroid scan, thyroid ultrasound, thyroid antibody test and thyroid stimulating immunoglobulins.

Overview of treatment

If patients do not respond to medications, surgery is usually the next option. Part of the thyroid may be removed, but in hyperthyroidism, a subtotal thyroidectomy may be performed. In this operation, as much as five-sixths of the gland is removed.

In well-planned surgery with no complications, patients can be discharged home on the fourth of fifth day following surgery. The wound incision is usually held together by means of clips. These are used, as they minimise scar formation. Due to the vascularity of the blood supply to the neck, the wound heals very quickly and the clips can be removed 72 hours following surgery.

The wound may be drained by one or two sealed vacuum drainage bottles, but they are usually removed 24 hours after surgery, if there is no drainage.

Specific nursing observations and care will be discussed in the answer section.

Answers to questions

Q1. An exocrine gland pours its secretion directly into a duct, whilst an endocrine organ pours its secretion directly into the bloodstream. Because of this difference, endocrine disorders usually affect many body systems. Exocrine secretions are localised and if there is dysfunction, the effects will mainly be localised. An example of an endocrine gland is the thyroid. An example of an exocrine gland is the gastric glands.

Q2. Na, Eb, Nc.

Q3. A, pinneal; B, posterior pituitary; C, anterior pituitary; D, thyroid; E, parathyroid; F, thymus; G, andrenal cortex; H, adrenal medulla.

1, heart; 2, skin; 3, liver; 4, kidney; 5, stomach; 6, pancreas; 7, intestine; 8, ovary; 9, placenta; 10, testis.

Q4. 1. Regulate the chemical composition and volume of body fluids.
2. Regulate metabolism and energy balance.
3. Control muscle contractions and secretions of glands.
4. Maintain homeostasis despite the effects of various stressors.
5. Play a role in the immune system.
6. Control growth and development.
7. Important for all reproductive processes.

Q5. Hormones bind and interact with their specific receptors present only on target cells. There are mainly two types of hormonal receptors, those that are found in the plasma membrane and those that are found in the cytosol (cytosolic receptors). Steroids interact for example with cytosolic receptors, whilst adrenaline interacts with membrane-bound receptors.

Q6. a, decrease; b, down; c, more; d, deficient.

Q7. a, Endocrine; b, Autocrine; c, paracrine.

Q8. *Steroids* – examples oestrogen and testosterone.
Biogenic amines – examples thyroxine and noradrenaline.
Peptides and proteins – examples oxytocin and insulin.
Eicosanoids – examples prostaglandins and leukotrienes.

Q9. Because it is a protein, and if given by mouth it would be broken down by pepsin.

Q10. a, Hypothalamus; b, first; c, target; d, plasma; e, G; f, adenylate cyclase; g, inner; h, ATP; i, cyclic AMP; j, second; k, protein kinases; l, phosphate. m. urine; n, short; o, phosphodiesterase; p, water.

Q11. Calcium ions and cyclic guanosine monophosphate.

Q12. Amplification of hormone effects indicates that a very low concentration of a hormone can cause a chain of reactions to occur (referred to as a cascade system). Each step of the cascade amplifies the next. For example, a single molecule of a hormone such as adrenaline could bind to its receptor, and in so doing activate a hundred G proteins. Each G protein can then activate an adenylate cyclase molecule. This can then produce many hundreds of cyclic AMP molecules.

Q13. The effect of one hormone on a target cell is opposed by another hormone. An example is **insulin** which lowers the blood sugar level and **glucagon**, which raises it.

Q14. Negative feedback can be explained in terms of a system in which there is an input and output with a control centre. There is usually a fine tuning between the input and output (homeostasis). Thus, if for example the input is increased, the control centre will sense this and will therefore reduce the production level, until a normal level is achieved. Similarly, if there is a decrease in output, the control centre senses this and triggers an increase in input. In terms of most endocrine secretions, the hypothalamus may be regarded as the control centre. To illustrate the negative feedback, let us use the hormone **thyroxine** which is produced by the thyroid gland. This hormone circulates in the bloodstream and is maintained at an 'acceptable' level. The production of thyroxine is controlled by **thyrotrophin stimulating hormone** from the anterior pituitary gland, and this gland itself is controlled by the hypothalamus (**thyrotrophin releasing hormone**). The thyroxine is the stimulus to the hypothalamus, so that when the thyroxine level is high, the hypothalamus reduces the secretion of releasing hormone and hence the level of thyrotrophin stimulating hormone. Therefore, the level of thyroxine is regulated. Conversely, when the level of thyroxine is low, the reverse occurs.

Two examples of hormones regulated by negative feedback are thyroxine and cortisol.

Positive feedback mechanisms operate differently from negative feedback. Rather than decreasing the output when the hormone level is high, more of the hormone is produced. An example of positive feedback is oxytocin.

Q15. A, hypothalamus; B, infundibulum; C, pars intermedia; D, adenohypophysis; E, neurohypophysis; F, sphenoid bone.

Q16. a, Hypophysis; b, sphenoid; c, hypothalamus; d, infundibulum; e, 75; f. neurohypophysis; g, supraoptic; h, oxytocin; i, adenohypophysis; j, seven; k. releasing; l, hypothalamus.

Q17.
a. Lactotrophs secrete prolactin.
b. Somatotrophs secrete human growth hormone.
c. Gonadotrophs secrete follicle stimulating hormone and luteinizing hormone.

Q18. A trophin is a hormone that influences another endocrine gland. Examples are thyrotrophin stimulating hormone, ACTH, follicle stimulating hormone and luteinizing hormone. ◻ *Page 525.*

Q19. a, hGH (human growth hormone); b, ACTH (corticotropin); c, cortisol; d, TRH (thyrotropin releasing hormone); e, thyroxine; f, oestrogen.

Q20. Growth hormone inhibiting hormone, prolactin inhibiting hormone and MSH inhibiting hormone.

Q21. a, Somatotrophin; b, bones; c, skeletal; d, amino acids; e, fat; f, ATP; g, glucagon; h, glycogen; i, hyperglycaemia; j, hypothalamus; k, growth hormone releasing hormone; l, growth hormone inhibiting hormone or somatostatin.

Q22. Pituitary dwarfism.

Q23. Acromegaly.

Q24. 1. Thyrotrophin releasing hormone.
2. Thyroid stimulating hormone.
3. Thyroxine and tri-iodothyronine.
4. Calcitonin.

Q25. a, Larynx; b, trachea; c, follicular; d, thyroxine; e, parafollicular cells or clear cells; f. calcitonin; g, iodide; h, thyroglobulin; i, colloid; j, lipid; k. plasma membrane; l, thyroxine binding globulin.

Q26. 1. Regulate oxygen use and basal metabolic rate.
2. Regulate cellular metabolism.
3. Regulate growth and development.

Q27. Thyroid hormones control the rate at which oxygen in the cells is used to produce ATP. As the cells use more oxygen to produce ATP, more heat is given off, and therefore the body temperature rises. This is referred to as the calorigenic effect of thyroid hormones and plays a role in the maintenance of normal body temperature.

Q28. 1. Stimulation of protein synthesis.
2. Increase in lypolysis.
3. Enhancement of cholesterol excretion in bile.
4. Stimulation of the synthesis of the enzyme sodium, potassium adenosine triphosphatase.

Q29. a, Cretinism; b, dwarfism; c, myxoedema; d, bradycardia; e, hypothermia; f, thyrotoxicosis; g, Grave's disease; h, swelling; i, exophthalmos; j, iodine; k, negative; l, thyroid stimulating hormone; m, pituitary.

Q30. a, Thyroid; b, parathormone; c, osteoclasts; d, calcium; e, calcitonin; f. kidneys; g, calcitriol; h, phosphate.

Q31. a. When blood calcium level falls, more PTH is released and less calcitonin is released.
b. When blood calcium level rises, less PTH is released, but more calcitonin is secreted.

Q32. a, Hypercalcaemia; b, hypocalcaemia; c, tetany.

Q33. a, gonadotrophin releasing hormone; b, graafian follicle; c, oestrogen; d. luteinizing hormone; e, ovulation; f, luteinizing hormone ; g, corpus luteum; h, progesterone; i, uterus; j, FSH; k, LH; l, menstrual; m, a high level of oestrogen.

Q34. Oxytocin.

Q35. a, Seminiferous; b, testes; c, cells of Sertoli; d, Leydig; e, testosterone.

Q36. 1, neurosecretory cells in hypothalamus; 2, axons to posterior pituitary; 3, pitocin; 4, uterine contraction; 5, breast milk let-down; 6, vasopressin; 7, blood volume ↑ (by increased reabsorption of water from urine in kidneys); 8, unrine ↓.

Q37. a, Lactation; b, prolactin; c, prolactin inhibiting hormone; d, hypothalamus; e, prolactin releasing hormone; f, anterior; g, pituitary; h, uterus; i, breast; j, positive; k, posterior; l, paraventricular

Q38. Osmolality (increase in concentration of solutes) of blood will increase and therefore the osmoreceptors in the hypothalamus will be stimulated. These cells are sensitive to a decrease or increase in osmolality. Increase in osmolality causes the release of ADH, which will therefore increase the permeability of the kidney tubules, and more fluids will be absorbed. This will restore the balance of body fluids. Short-term physiological changes will include increase in thirst and also possibly an increase in the volume of urine passed (as a result of osmodiuresis). Glucose could also appear in the urine, if it greatly exceeds the renal threshold.

Q39. Alcohol inhibits the secretion of ADH and therefore more fluid is lost in the urine. This could lead to dehydration. Fortunately, in a healthy individual, the thirst mechanism comes into play and the person drinks more fluid, and water homeostasis is restored. One assumes that the person drinks nonalcoholic fluids before he is completely drunk.

Q40. 1. Corticotrophin releasing hormone.
2. Adrenocorticotrophic hormone.
3. Cortex.
4. Medulla.
5. Mineralocorticoids.
6. Glucocorticoids.
7. Gonadocorticoids.

Q41. Aldosterone promotes the reabsorption of sodium and decreases the reabsorption of potassium from the renal tubules. It also promote the excretion of hydrogen ions in the urine.

Q42. Chloride and bicarbonate ions.

Q43. Hydrogen ion.

Q44. Decrease in blood volume from dehydration, and haemorrhage.

Q45. Juxtaglomerular cells.

Q46. 1. Angiotensinogen.
2. Renin.
3. Angiotensin I.
4. Angiotensin II.
5. Aldosterone.
6. Sodium and water.
7. Potassium and hydrogen ions.
8. Water.

Q47. a, Increase;
b, Decrease;
c, Increase.

Q48. Cortisol, corticosterone and cortisone. Cortisol is the most abundant.

Q49. Proteins are broken down, and amino acids are removed and transported to the liver. Amino acids can then be converted to glucose.

Q50. Fasting, fright, bleeding, infection, high altitude and temperature extremes.

Q51. Since glucocorticoids are anti-inflammatory compounds, they inhibit the inflammatory response ($\square\!\!\!\square$ *Page 546*). They reduce the number of mast cells, blood capillary permeability and phagocytic actions. They also interfere with connective tissue regeneration and this therefore slows down wound healing.

Q52. Cortisol is secreted by the adrenal cortex. When the level of cortisol is elevated, the blood reaching the hypothalamus acts as the stimulus and reduces the secretion of corticotrophin releasing hormone. This also reduces the level of ACTH by the anterior pituitary and hence the level of cortisol by the cortex. Conversely, when the level of cortisol is low, the stimulus to the hypothalamus causes an increase in corticotrophin releasing hormone. This also causes an increase in ACTH, which stimulates the cortex to secrete more cortisol. This explains the negative feedback mechanism, for when CRF is suppressed, ACTH is also reduced and hence the level of cortisol is reduced, and vice versa.

Q53. At high concentration ACTH mimics the skin darkening effects of melanocyte stimulating hormone. This results in excessive skin pigmentation.

Q54. Oestrogen and androgen.

Q55. Chromaffin cells.

Q56. Adrenaline.

Q57. This is because they produce effects that are similar to those brought about by the sympathetic division of the autonomic nervous system.

Q58. Catecholamines.

Q59. Islets of Langerhans.

Q60. Alpha, beta, delta and F-cells.

Q61. a, Alpha; b, glycogen; c, glycogenolysis; d, glucose; e, gluconeogenesis; f, glucose; g, high.

Q62. a, Beta; b, decrease; c, glycogenesis; d, glucose; e, high; f, decreased.

Q63. II a. II b. II c. I d. I e.

Q64. Rise in blood glucose level – Increased blood levels of certain amino acids can also stimulate insulin secretion; human growth hormone and adrenocorticotrophic hormone can also stimulate insulin release.

Q65. Hypoglycaemia is a low level of blood glucose. Hyperglycaemia is a high level of blood glucose, such as that which is normally found in a diabetic individual. Glycosuria is the presence of glucose in the urine. This again occurs in diabetics. Glucose can also sometimes appear in the urine of otherwise healthy individuals, but this happens when the glucose renal threshold is surpassed. It can for example occur in a child who has consumed large amounts of carbohydrates.

Q66. These are explained in chapter 16, under the patient scenario.

Q67. It is situated in the brain and is attached to the roof of the third ventricle.

Q68. Melatonin.

Q69. It is believed that seasonal affective disorder arises when day-length is short and thus stimulates overproduction of melatonin. Bright light therapy inhibits melatonin secretion, since the latter is produced during darkness. Reducing the level of melatonin is believed to give relief to sufferers of seasonal affective disorder.

Q70. Leukotrienes stimulate chemotaxis of white blood cells, which are important in the inflammatory process.

Prostaglandins act in a paracrine or autocrine fashion in most tissues of the body. They can alter smooth muscle contraction and therefore they can induce labour. They can also alter secretion, blood flow and platelet function. They play a role in inflammation. They can promote fever and they can also intensify pain. For more information, 📖 *Page 556.*

Thromboxanes can constrict blood vessels and promote platelet aggregation.

Q71. Any stimulus that produces a stress response is called a stressor. Two examples are heat and cold. 📖 *Page 556.*

Q72. a, Hypothalamus; b, alarm; c, cortex; d, autonomic ; e, resistance; f, thyroid stimulating hormone; g, ACTH; h, growth hormone; i, cortex.

Q73. a, Fight or flight; b, increases; c, adrenaline; d, noradrenaline; e, increases; f, increase; g, skeletal muscles; h, heart; i, brain; j, spleen; k, gastrointestinal tract; l, skin. m. decrease; n, increases.

Please note that some of your answers may not be in the same order, but do not worry, as long as you have obtained the right responses.

Q74. a. Glucocorticoids – Stimulate gluconeogenesis, therefore producing glucose from noncarbohydrate sources. They also reduce inflammation.
b. Thyroxine – Stimulates the production of ATP from glucose.
c. Human growth hormone – Stimulates the catabolism of fats and the conversion of glycogen to glucose.
d. Mineralocorticoids – Hormones such as aldosterone acts to conserve sodium and to eliminate hydrogen ions. Conservation of sodium also increases water retention, which therefore maintains the blood pressure and also brings about homeostasis of water balance. Elimination of hydrogen ions prevents acidosis.

Q75. a. Exhaustion.
b. Loss of potassium – This occurs because of increased aldosterone activity. Potassium is excreted in exchange for the sodium which is reabsorbed.
c. Depletion of glucocorticoids – The cortex no longer responds to the stressor and therefore there is less secretion of glucocorticoids.
d. Weakening of organs – This is because cells lack nutrients such as glucose and therefore are depleted of ATP. This may affect enzyme functions. The loss of potassium from the cells will also affect water homeostasis. The sodium–potassium pump is also affected and there is disruption of electrolytes balance.

Q76. 3a, 1b, 4c, 2d.

Q77. a, Giantism; b, dwarfism; c, acromegaly; d, hands; e, feet.

Q78. a, 30–60 seconds; b, bloodstream; c, 30–40; d, increase; e, decrease; f. opposite; g, increase; h, decrease; i, dehydration; j, hypovolaemia; k, insipidus; l, glucose; m, inhibits; n, increase.

Q79. a, Anabolism; b, catabolism.

Q80. a, Catabolism; b, opposite; c, gluconeogenesis; d, increase; e, increase; f, limit.

Q81.   a. Prostaglandin.

b. It is an antipyretic (reduces body temperature), it is an anti-inflammatory medication and it is also an analgesic.

Q82.   a. Growth hormone releasing hormone.

b. Luteinizing hormone.

c. Human growth hormone and also testosterone.

d. Thyroid stimulating hormone.

e. Follicle stimulating hormone.

f. Prolactin inhibiting hormone.

g. Luteinizing hormone.

h. Oxytocin.

i. Melanocyte stimulating hormone.

j. Antidiuretic hormone.

k. Glucocorticoids.

l. Parathormone.

m. Calcitonin.

n. Thyroid hormone.

o. Glucagon, glucocorticoids, noradrenaline, adrenaline and growth hormone (any three hormones are acceptable). Please also note that the order of your answer is not important.

p. Insulin.

q. Adrenocorticoid.

r. Adrenaline and noradrenaline.

Q83.   10a, 1b, 4c, 5d, 3e, 7f, 6g, 11h, 8i, 2j, 9k.

Q84.   1. b, e, a, c, d.

2. d, b, a, c.

Q85.   c.

Q86.   c.

Q87.   d.

Q88.   b.

Q89.   d.

Q90.   Due to the increased thyroxine secretion, there is an increase in metabolic rate. There is an increase in ATP production. Therefore, a large amount of heat is generated and this increases body temperature, which explains why Maureen feels warm.

Q91.   If it is possible, Maureen should be nursed in a single cubicle and preferably one where there is a window. She should then be able to control her own environment with regard to reducing the heat. The nurse should provide a fan, which will also assist with heat regulation. Maureen could be encouraged to drink plenty of fluids, so as to maintain water homeostasis. Maureen can be instructed to take regular showers or baths, which could also help in controlling body temperature.

Q92.   Palpitation: Maureen's palpitation is obviously a result of increased heart rate (tachycardia). This occurs because thyroxine directly stimulates the heart and therefore increases sympathetic activity. This is why many patients with thyrotoxicosis are treated with beta-blocker medication, which reduces sympathetic activity and therefore reduces heart rate. For further information on beta-blockers, refer to the answer to Q7

Diarrhoea: This occurs because of increased peristaltic activity of the intestines. It is due to over-activity of the sympathetic nervous system. This is rather like the 'intestinal hurry' that you may have experienced when you are over-anxious or stressed, for example when you are attending an interview or when taking an examination.

Q93.   Nursing observations: Since the surgery is in the neck region, it is vital that breathing is monitored, as possible complications may occur, such as haemorrhage, swelling as a result of haematoma (collection of blood in the tissues), or oedema in the vicinity of the vocal cords and the larynx.

On return to the ward, every step should be taken to ensure that, when Maureen is placed in bed, she is well supported with pillows, so that the neck is not extended. This will keep the airway patent and assist with breathing. The nurse should monitor breathing, so as to detect early signs of cyanosis (bluish tinge of the skin which indicates poor oxygenation).

Haematoma/swelling: N.B. It is vital that essential equipment is at the bedside, e.g. clip remover, which may be needed for example if the patient has a choking sensation, or difficulty in breathing as a result of haematoma.

The nurse should check the dressing frequently, for any excessive bleeding. Record and monitor blood pressure, pulse rate and respiration in accordance with the agreed regime. Report any deviations from baseline observations. Ensure that oxygen equipment is available, should this be required. Check the amount of drainage, taking note of the time of the observation.

Monitoring of pain: Pain is an important factor in any type of surgery, but following thyroidectomy, due to the extension of the neck during the surgical procedure, the patient may have severe pain which could affect breathing; but it may also cause difficulty in swallowing and coughing. Pain should be regularly assessed and monitored and analgesia given as prescribed.

Q94.   Laryngeal damage: Maureen may be hoarse, or may speak with a weak voice or may show signs of stridor. This may be due to laryngeal nerve damage (some degree of hoarseness is quite normal immediately following surgery) and would require careful monitoring as breathing could be affected, especially if there is also oedema at the site of the vocal cords and larynx. It is wise, at an early stage, for the nurse not to give any specific explanation with regard to the hoarseness which could be in contradiction with the surgeon's view. It could well be that the hoarseness may be permanent.

Q95.   Tetany (this is due to hypocalcaemia, a low blood calcium level): It is important for the nurse to realise that when the thyroid has been removed, the parathyroid glands might also have been removed in the process, since they are embedded in the posterior wall of the thyroid.

Although signs of tetany are not usually seen immediately following surgery, it could occur. The nurse should observe for signs of tetany which are manifested on account of nerve excitability. They are **carpopedal spasm** (unusual spasm of the hands and feet), **paraesthesia** (pins and needles around the mouth, hands and feet), **Trousseau's and Chvostek's signs.** The nurse may detect Trousseau's sign when recording the blood pressure. This is because the inflated cuff obliterates the blood flow to the upper arm and because of the lack of calcium there is muscle spasm. Trousseau's sign can be purposely elicited by the use of an inflated cuff. Chvostek's sign can also be elicited by gently tapping the facial nerve – the muscle of the face goes into spasm. Should tetany be detected, the emergency management is usually by the administration of calcium gluconate or other calcium preparation intravenously.

Q96.   Carbimazole: This drug is used to establish euthyroid (normal function of the thyroid). It is an antithyroid agent and its main action is to prevent uptake of iodine by the thyroid gland and thus it blocks the synthesis of thyroxine and tri-iodothyronine. Due to the reduction of hormone by the thyroid, and as a result of the negative feedback mechanism, there is an increase in thyrotrophin and this causes marked enlargement of the gland (hyperplasia) with vascularisation.

The side effects may be as follows: paraesthesia, headache, vertigo, skin rash, nausea, vomiting and dyspepsia. Serious side effects are thrombocytopenia, leukopenia and agranulocytosis.

The patient should be warned to report sore throat, fever and rashes (these are likely to occur in the first few months of treatment).

Propranolol: This drug is a nonselective beta-blocker of both cardiac (beta$_1$) and beta$_2$ adrenoreceptors and competes with adrenaline and noradrenaline for available beta receptor sites. The main action is to reduce the heart rate, myocardial irritability and force of contraction, depressing the automaticity of the sinus node (pacemaker). The prescribed dose is usually 10–40mg three to four times daily.

The side effects may be as follows: giddiness, weakness, drowsiness, insomnia, vivid dreams, visual hallucinations, profound bradycardia, various arrhythmias, dry eyes, nausea, vomiting, constipation and flatulence. More serious side effects are agranulocytosis, hypoglycaemia, and bronchospasm.

Patients should be advised to take the medication before meals and at bedtime. It is believed that if the medication is taken on a full stomach, this might interfere with absorption. The patient should also be instructed to take their radial pulse rate before each dose and to report any change, such as a slower pulse rate, to the general practitioner. Patients should also take alcohol in moderation.

Q97. As explained above, the drug causes vascularisation and if it is not stopped prior to surgery, it could increase the risk of haemorrhage, thus putting the patient at risk.

Q98. Complications: Possible complications are as follows: hypothyroidism, tetany, hoarseness of the voice and recurrence of thyroidism.

Hypothyroidism is perhaps the commonest complication and it can occur as a result of a severe reduction in the activity of the thyroid gland. If this should happen, the patient will require thyroid hormone replacement, which can be given as long acting thyroxine (can be taken orally).

The reasons for the other complications have all been explained above.

Overview and key terms

Cardiovascular system (1)

HEART

BLOOD VESSELS

BLOOD

DISORDERS

STRUCTURE
- Layers
- Conducting system
- Coronary arteries

FUNCTION
- Cardiac output
- Peripheral resistance
- Control of BP
- Hormones

Blood vessels:
- Arteries
- Arterioles
- Vasoconstriction
- Vasodilatation
- Capillaries

Blood:
- Clotting
- Fibrinolysis

Disorders:
- Atheroma
- Atherosclerosis
- Coronary thrombosis
- Myocardial infarction
- Angina pectoris
- Shock and B.P.
- Electrocardiogram
- arrhythmias
- Thrombolysis

12. The Cardiovascular System (1): Heart Blood Vessels and Blood

Learning outcomes

1. To understand the structure and function of the heart and blood vessels, and blood clotting.

2. To relate this knowledge of structure and function to an understanding of the nature of coronary artery disease.

3. To identify the common patient problems in myocardial infarction.

4. To provide a physiological rationale for these problems.

5. To provide a rationale for the principles of care and treatment following a myocardial infarction.

INTRODUCTION

This chapter is concerned with the heart, blood vessels and blood, and the way in which the structure and function of these relate to a common cardio-vascular condition.

The first part of the chapter is concerned with questions that deal with normal anatomy and physiology. This provides the basis for the next section and the patient scenario – a man who has coronary artery disease. This condition is explained and the relevant problems and aspects of care and treatment are approached through the use of questions.

THE HEART ▦ *Chapter 20.*

Figure 12.1.
Diagram of a frontal section of the heart.

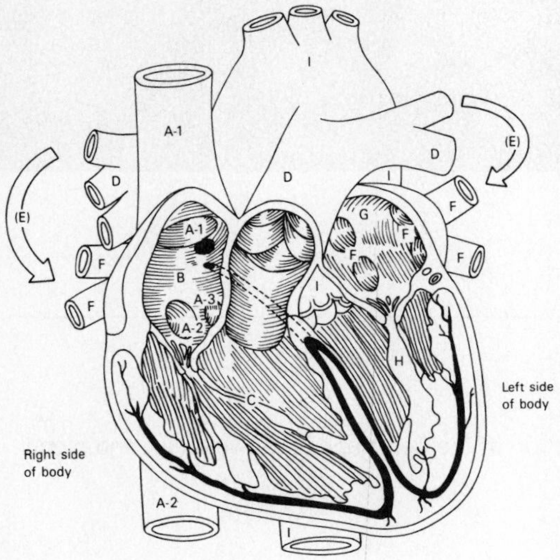

A–1 _____

A–2 _____

A–3 _____

B _____

C _____

D _____

E _____

F _____

G _____

H _____

I _____

Q1. **Refer to Figure 12.1 to complete the following exercise.**

a. Identify all structures with letters (A–I) by writing labels on lines A–I.

b. Draw arrows on Figure 12.1 to indicate direction of blood flow.

c. Colour red the chambers of the heart and vessels that contain highly oxygenated blood; colour blue the regions in which blood is low in oxygen and high in carbon dioxide.

d. On Figure 12.1, label the four valves that control blood flow through the heart.

Q2. **Add the labels (1–6) to Figure 12.2. Colour right and left coronary arteries.**

Q3. **Check your understanding of heart structure and the pathway of blood through the heart by selecting terms that fit the descriptions below. Not all answers need be used.**

---

1. Atria 2. Pulmonary vein 3. Chordae tendineae 4. Septum 5. Pulmonary artery
6. Ventricles 7. Papillary muscles

☐ a. Thin-walled chambers that receive blood from veins.

☐ b. Blood vessel that carries blood that is rich in oxygen from lungs to left atrium.

c. Wall separating right side from left side of the heart.

d. Strong tendons that anchor atrioventricular valves to ventricular muscle.

e. Sites of most of the myocardium.

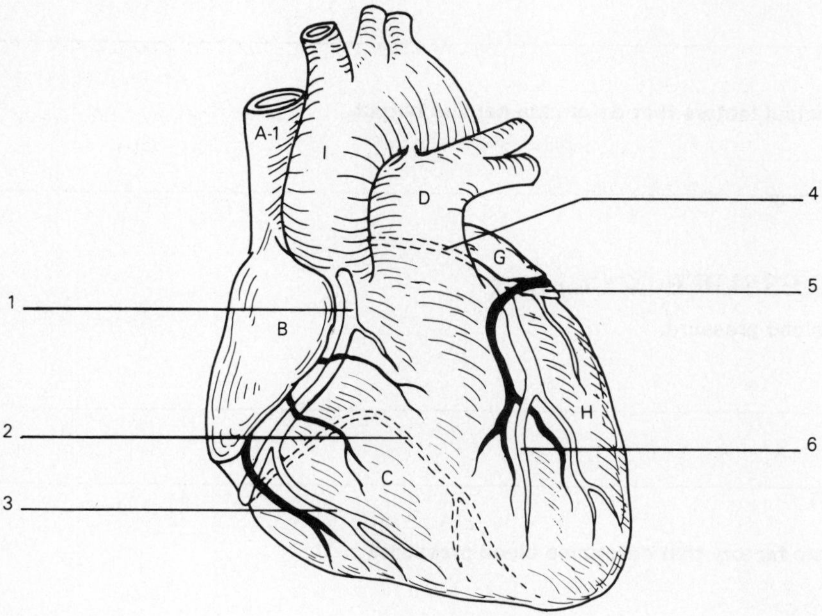

Figure 12.2.
nterior view of the
heart.

Label

Anterior interventricular branch

Circumflex branch

Left coronary artery

Marginal branch

Right coronary artery

Posterior interventricular branch

Colour:

◯ Left coronary artery and branches

◯ Right coronary artery and branches

Q4.   List the four main elements of the conduction system of the heart.

_____

_____

_____

_____

Q5.   Briefly describe how the cardiac impulse spreads across the heart.

_____

_____

Q6.   Define the term 'cardiac output' and give its average value.

_____

_____

Q7.   Give the two principal factors that determine cardiac output.

_____

BLOOD PRESSURE 📖 *Chapter 21.*

Q8.   Define the term blood pressure.

_____

_____

Q9.   What are the three factors that determine blood pressure?

_____

_____

_____

Q10.   Briefly describe the term total peripheral resistance. What are the structures that define this?

_____

_____

Q11.   What structure controls the heart rate? Where is it situated?

_____

Q12.   Name the two inputs to the cardiovascular centre and give a brief description of the action of each.

_____

_____

_____

_____

Q13. Higher centres also have an effect on the cardiovascular centre. Give an example of this.

_____

Q14. Briefly describe the effects of the two hormones, adrenaline and noradrenaline, on blood flow in the body.

_____

_____

_____

Q15. If these two hormones raise cardiac output and peripheral resistance, what is the effect on blood pressure?

_____

Q16. Name the two nerves that connect the cardiovascular centre with the heart, and state their effect on the heart's action.

_____

_____

Q17. If the heart rate increases, what will be the effect of this on the following?

a. Cardiac output.

_____

b. Blood pressure.

_____

Q18. If cardiac output rises, then blood pressure can remain unchanged, in which of the following cases?
a. Peripheral resistance rises.
b. Peripheral resistance falls.
c. Blood volume rises.

VASCULAR SYSTEM 📖 *Pages 624–9.*

Q19.   **What are the names of the three layers of an artery?**

_____

Q20.   **What is the special feature of blood in the arteries?**

_____

Q21.   **Generally in what direction – in relation to the heart – do arteries carry blood?**

_____

Q22.   **Arterioles are small arteries that can determine total peripheral resistance** (📖 *Page 631*). **What are the names of the two movements that determine this property?**

_____

Q23.   **If vasoconstriction occurs and cardiac output remains unchanged, what will be the effect on blood pressure?**

_____

Q24.   **What will be the effect of vasodilatation on rising blood pressure?**

_____

Q25.   **Where is the location of the control centre for vasoconstriction and vasodilatation?** 📖 *Pages 637–8.*

_____

Q26.   **What is the primary function of capillaries?**

_____

_____

Q27.   **What are the two major differences between arteries and veins?**

_____

_____

BLOOD CLOTTING 📖 *Pages 579–85.*

Q28. **What are the three basic mechanisms of haemostasis?**

_____

Q29. **Briefly describe the stages of coagulation.**

_____

_____

Q30. **What is fibrinolysis?**

_____

Q31. **What is the action of plasmin?**

_____

CHECKPOINTS EXERCISE

Q32. **Imagine that your blood pressure is slightly lower than your body needs right now. Do this exercise to see how your body is likely to respond to increase your blood pressure.**

Refer to Figure 12.3 and fill in box 1 to describe types of receptors that trigger changes in blood pressure: (a) _____-receptors and (b) _____-receptors. Baroreceptors are sensitive to changes in (c) _____, and chemoceptors are activated by chemicals such as (d) _____. These receptors are located in three locations: (e) _____ ____, _____, and _____.

Nerve messages from the carotid sinuses travel to the brain via cranial nerve (f) _____, whereas messages from the aorta and right atrium travel by cranial nerve (g) _____. Write in these cranial nerve on Figure 12.3.

This **input** reaches the cardiovascular centre located within the (h) _____ of the brain. Fill in box 3 in Figure 12.3 to indicate this region of the brain. This centre receives input from other parts of the brain also. Note three of these brain parts in box 2: (i) _____, _____ and _____.

Consider the cardiovascular centre as comparable to the control centre of an automobile. The centre has an accelerator portion (like an accelerator pedal) and an inhibitor portion (like the (j) _____ of a car). When baroreceptors report that blood pressure is too low (as if the car is running too slowly), the (k) _____ (cardiostimulatory? cardio-inhibitory?) centre must be activated; in the car analogy, you would (l) _____ (step on the accelerator? step on the brake?). At the same time, the cardio-inhibitory centre must be deactivated. Continuing with the car analogy, what response do you make? (m) _____. What is the outcome for the car/heart? (n) _____.

In addition, a vasomotor portion of the cardiovascular centre responds to lower blood pressure by (o) _____ (stimulating? inhibiting?) the smooth muscle of blood vessels, resulting in (p) _____ (vasoconstriction? vasodilatation?). This helps to increase blood pressure by (q) _____ -creasing systemic vascular resistance.

Summarise nervous **output** to effectors from the cardiovascular centre by writing in box 4 in Figure 12.3 the three factors that are altered: (r) _____ _____ _____. The result of this output is an attempt to restore homeostasis by (s) _____-creasing blood pressure.

Overall, Figure 12.3 demonstrates (t) _____ (positive? negative?) feedback mechanisms for regulating blood pressure, since a decrease in blood pressure initiates factors to increase blood pressure.

Figure 12.3.
Factors regulating blood pressure.

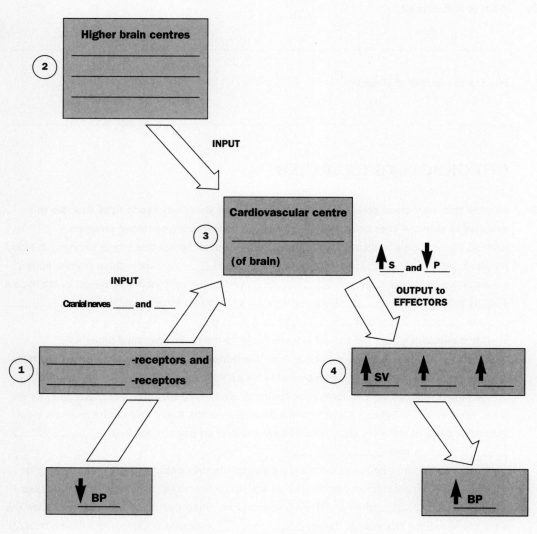

Q33. What properties of arterioles are important in the regulation of blood pressure?

Q34. **a. Vasodilatation tends to** _____ **blood pressure.**

  b. Vasoconstriction tends to _____ **blood pressure.**

Q35. **Following clot formation, clots undergo two changes. Summarise these.**

First, clot (a) _____ , or syneresis occurs. Figure 12.4 shows the next step: clot dissolution, or (b) _____. An inactive enzyme (F on the figure) is activated to G, which dissolves clots. Label F: (c) _____, and G: (d) _____ on the figure. Clot dissolution is activated by chemicals produced within the body, for example, from damaged blood vessels, and also by (e) _____.

Figure 12.4.
Summary of steps in clot dissolution.

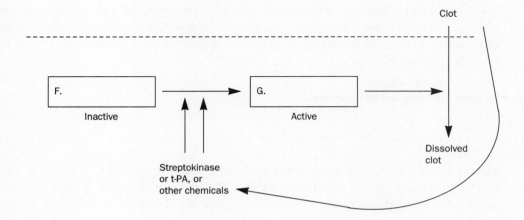

PATIENT SCENARIO

Mr William Brown is a 65-year-old former train driver. He has felt unwell at home; he has chest pain which radiates to his left shoulder. This has been preceded by indigestion-type pains in the previous few days. Also, he appears pale and his blood pressure is low.

Mr Brown lives with his wife in a small terraced house. Their grown-up children (two) live away from home.

Mrs Brown summoned the general practitioner, Dr Cole, who suspected a **myocardial infarction**. He arranged for Mr Brown to be conveyed immediately to hospital by ambulance.

Myocardial infarction

The term **myocardial infarction** (MI) means that part of the heart muscle (myo = muscle, cardia = heart) has died (infarction). This has happened because one of the coronary arteries – or its branches – has become damaged and blocked by a blood clot. This arterial damage is known as **atheroma**. The next section will discuss the nature of this – and relate it to normal arterial anatomy.

Atheroma and atherosclerosis

Mr Brown suffers from damage to the coronary arteries and this is the result of the disease process known as **atheroma**. The term **atherosclerosis** is used synonymously, whilst the term **arteriosclerosis** is a general label that is applied to any sort of arterial disease — including atheroma.

Atheroma is characterised by an accumulation of cholesterol (and fat) on the otherwise smooth lining of blood vessels. As the condition spreads, so fibrous tissue may form and the wall of the artery can become ulcerated and weakened. This deposit of atheroma narrows the internal diameter of the blood vessel and as a result the blood supply (in the case of arteries and arterioles) to the tissues is reduced. The atheroma also provides a site on which blood can clot.

This blood clot is known as a **thrombus**, hence the term **thrombosis**, meaning the formation of a blood clot. Thrombosis has been termed one of the greatest killers in the world today. In Western countries the processes of atheroma and thrombosis account for 40–50% of all deaths.

Q36. How many coronary arteries are there?

These normally supply the heart muscle with blood. Under the effects of atheroma they can become narrowed and lose their elasticity. The effect of this is to deprive the heart muscle of blood; this occurs in the first instance when the coronary arteries are called upon to dilate and supply more blood. This would happen during exercise, when the heart is speeding up so that oxygenated blood can be supplied to the skeletal muscles.

As a result, the heart muscle is now **ischaemic** — deprived of its full quota of blood. This gives rise to a characteristic chest pain that can radiate to the left shoulder and arm, and is known as **angina pectoris.**

Mr Brown's problems

Without blood, the area of myocardium will not recover and it will now be replaced by a scar (📖 *Page 121*). This scar will not have the same properties as heart muscle, so the heart will now lose some of its strength and be functionally weakened; as a result, chronic heart failure may occur at some point in the future.

In the meantime, Mr Brown is likely to suffer from some characteristic problems. It is an important nursing function to be able to recognise these when they are occurring (actual problems) and when they **may** occur (potential problems).

Q37. What is the name for pain that is felt at a site that is distant from the site of damage, e.g. left shoulder/arm pain resulting from myocardial infarction?

Q38. What treatment would Mr Brown receive for this pain?

Q39. **What do you think Mr Brown's mental state will be on admission to hospital?**

_____

_____

Q40. **How is his mental state likely to affect his condition?**

_____

_____

_____

Q41. **How can Mr Brown's anxiety be lessened?**

_____

_____

_____

_____

The following questions are based on 📖 _Pages 608–11 and 635–8._

Q42. **Mr Brown has low blood pressure. Explain why this is occurring.**

_____

_____

_____

Q43. **What is the normal homeostatic response that will occur as a result of Mr Brown's low blood pressure?**

_____

_____

_____

Q44. What observations – other than a rapid pulse and blood pressure measurement – will tell you that Mr Brown is in shock?

_____

_____

_____

_____

_____

Figure 12.5 is a summary of the body's responses in cardiogenic shock.

Figure 12.5.
A summary of the body's responses in cardiogenic shock.

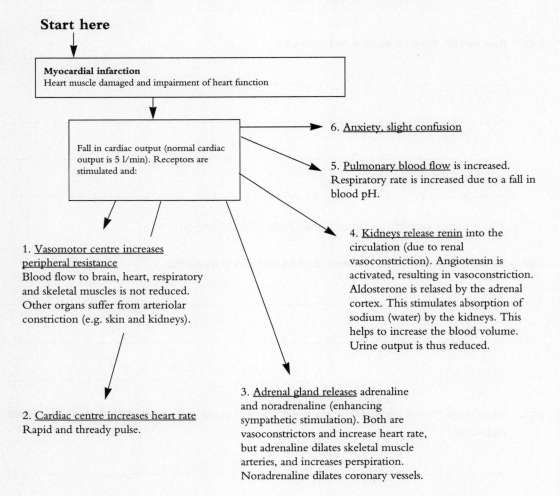

Start here

Myocardial infarction
Heart muscle damaged and impairment of heart function

Fall in cardiac output (normal cardiac output is 5 l/min). Receptors are stimulated and:

6. <u>Anxiety, slight confusion</u>

5. <u>Pulmonary blood flow</u> is increased. Respiratory rate is increased due to a fall in blood pH.

4. <u>Kidneys release renin</u> into the circulation (due to renal vasoconstriction). Angiotensin is activated, resulting in vasoconstriction. Aldosterone is relased by the adrenal cortex. This stimulates absorption of sodium (water) by the kidneys. This helps to increase the blood volume. Urine output is thus reduced.

1. <u>Vasomotor centre increases peripheral resistance</u>
Blood flow to brain, heart, respiratory and skeletal muscles is not reduced. Other organs suffer from arteriolar constriction (e.g. skin and kidneys).

2. <u>Cardiac centre increases heart rate</u>
Rapid and thready pulse.

3. <u>Adrenal gland releases</u> adrenaline and noradrenaline (enhancing sympathetic stimulation). Both are vasoconstrictors and increase heart rate, but adrenaline dilates skeletal muscle arteries, and increases perspiration. Noradrenaline dilates coronary vessels.

Q45. If Mr Brown's heart should stop working, how would this be recognised and treated?

_____

_____

_____

_____

Q46. One way in which Mr Brown's condition can be continuously monitored is by recording his electrocardiogram (ECG) (📖 *Page 604*) on a small screen, like a TV. What would this display look like if Mr Brown should have a cardiac arrest?

_____

_____

Q47. What is thrombolytic therapy? And why may Mr Brown receive it?

_____

_____

_____

Q48. What are the dangers of giving Mr Brown thrombolytic therapy?

_____

_____

Q49. What health promotion advice should Mr Brown be given prior to his discharge?

_____

_____

_____

_____

In the long term Mr Brown may require surgery to replace his damaged coronary arteries – a coronary artery bypass graft. Alternatively, he may go on to develop a complication such as congestive cardiac failure – which will form the subject of the next chapter. In addition, there are some other cardiovascular problems that Mr Brown may encounter. These will also be dealt with in the following chapter.

QUESTIONS FOR DISCUSSION

1. How are Mr Brown's other activities of daily living likely to be affected by his problems and treatment? Draw up a list of problems.

2. What is the effect of cardiac arrest on acid–base balance? How can this be counteracted?

3. What are the common drugs – and side effects – that are used for treating cardiac-related pain?

4. What are the effects of atheroma on other sites in the body?

5. What form of treatment is given for other arrhythmias, such as atrial fibrillation and extrasystoles?

6. What are the homeostatic mechanisms that are triggered by low blood pressure and are designed to improve blood flow (and pressure) to the kidney? Briefly describe them.

Answers to questions

Q1.

a. A-1, superior vena cava; A-2, inferior vena cava; A-3, coronary sinus; B, right atrium; C, right ventricle; D, pulmonary trunk and arteries; E, vessels in lungs; F, pulmonary vein; G, left atrium; H, left ventricle; I, aorta.

b. See figure opposite.

c. See 📖 *Page 595, Figure 20.3.*

d. See figure opposite.

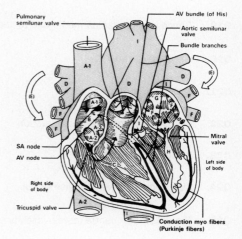

Q2. See 📖 *Page 600, Figure 20.5.*

Q3. 1a, 2b, 4c, 3d, 6e.

Q4. Sinoatrial node
Atrioventricular node
Bundle of His
Conduction myofibres (Purkinje fibres)

Q5. From the sinoatrial node across the atria and down the atrioventricular node – and across the ventricles.

Q6. The amount of blood pumped out by the heart in 1 minute. The average value of cardiac output is approximately 5 litres/minute.

Q7. Heart rate and stroke volume.

Q8. The pressure exerted by blood on the wall of a blood vessel. For clinical purposes this is the brachial artery in the upper arm.

Q9. Cardiac output, total peripheral resistance and blood volume.

Q10. All the vascular resistance offered by the blood vessels, mostly in the arterioles.

Q11. Cardiovascular centre, situated in the medulla oblongata.

Q12. Baroreceptors monitor blood pressure in the carotid sinus and aorta, and send messages to the cardiovascular centre and act to regulate blood pressure. Chemoreceptors in the same region monitor O_2 and acid levels in the blood. A fall in O_2 or a rise in acid levels will lead to vasoconstriction and an increase in blood pressure.

Q13. Anxiety or fear will increase heart rate.

Q14. The two hormones increase cardiac output and vasodilatation of cardiac and muscle arteries, and cause vasoconstriction of skin and abdominal vessels. Thus, blood flow to heart and muscles will increase, and flow to skin and abdomen will decrease.

Q15. Blood pressure will rise.

Q16. The vagus nerve slows the heart down, and the sympathetic nerves speed the heart up.

Q17. a. Rises
b. Rises

Q18. b.

Q19. Tunica interna, tunica media and tunica externa.

Q20. It is oxygenated.

Q21. Away from the heart.

Q22. Vasoconstriction and vasodilatation.

Q23. Blood pressure will rise.

Q24. Blood pressure will stabilise or fall.

Q25. The vasomotor centre (cardiovascular centre) in the medulla oblongata.

Q26. To allow the passage of oxygen and nutrients from the blood into the tissues, and to allow carbon dioxide and waste to travel in the opposite direction.

Q27. Veins have valves and also have a much thinner muscle coat.

Q28. Vascular spasm, platelet plug formation and coagulation (clotting).

Q29. 1. Formation of prothrombinase
2. Conversion of prothrombin to thrombin
3. Conversion of fibrinogen to fibrin. Fibrin forms the clot.

Q30. Dissolution of a clot.

Q31. It dissolves blood clots.

Q32. a, Baro; b, chemo; c, blood pressure; d, H^+, CO_2, and O_2; e, carotid arteries, aorta, and right atrium; f, IX; g, X; h, medulla; i, cerebral cortex, limbic system, and hypothalamus; j, brakes; k, cardiostimulatory; l, step on the accelerator; m, take your foot off the accelerator; n, car goes faster/heart beats faster and with greater force of contraction; o, stimulating; p, vasoconstriction; q, in; r, ↑ stroke volume (SV), ↑ heart rate (HR), and ↑ systemic vascular resistance (SVR); s, in; t, negative.

Q33. Vasoconstriction and vasodilatation.

Q34. a. Lower
b. Raise

Q35. a, Retraction; b, fibrinolysis; c, plasminogen; d, plasmin; e, thrombin.

Q36. Two.

Q37. This is known as referred pain (📖 *Pages 448–9*), and occurs because the brain interprets the pain as coming from the receptors at the distal end of the nerve, which are in the shoulder and arm (see 📖 *Page 449, Figure 15.2*). In the days preceding an MI patients often complain about indigestion-type pains, however.

Q38. A strong analgesic (pain killing) drug, such as diamorphine (heroin).

Q39. He is likely to be extremely anxious.

Q40. Research has shown that anxiety increases pain, and lowering anxiety can help to lessen the need for analgesic drugs. Also, anxiety produces sympathetic stimulation (📖 *Pages 557–9*). In addition, adrenaline and noradrenaline will be released by the adrenal glands (📖 *Pages 548–9*). The net effect of these two hormones, and the sympathetic stimulation, is that the heart rate will increase. This will add stress to an already weakened heart muscle, but it will also help to maintain Mr Brown's blood pressure – at a time when it is falling, because of the damaged heart muscle.

Q41. By providing him with information and reassurance about his hospitalisation, care and treatment. This can help prevent him from worrying and becoming more anxious, with the consequences as discussed above. It is hoped that his homeostasis (📖 *Page 10*) will be restored. Talking to Mr Brown about such matters, as well as about his home and family, are of fundamental importance in his psychological care. In this way, one can have a desirable **psychosomatic** effect on the patient (*psych* = mind; *soma* = body).

Additionally, the secondary effect of strong analgesics, such as diamorphine, is to allay anxiety and promote sedation and rest. Rest is important if his heart is to recover from this damage. Unfortunately, diamorphine also tends to make people feel nauseous and a drug such as Stemetil, is usually given to counteract this.

Q42. Part of his heart muscle is dead, so the capability of the heart is reduced and the volume of blood that the heart can pump is reduced. This is known as the cardiac output and is a vital part of maintaining blood pressure (📖 *Pages 608–10*). In shock, the systolic blood pressure is often reduced to below 90mmHg, but there is no decrease in blood volume – as there might be in other types of shock that are associated with haemorrhage. The main problem with Mr Brown is that the 'pump' has been damaged. Hence, the term cardiogenic shock is used (cardio = heart, genesis = birth of).

Q43. The cardiovascular centre, in the medulla oblongata, will stimulate an increase in heart rate and vasoconstriction (as will the hormones mentioned in question 40). (📖 *Pages 636–7*).
This will increase cardiac output and peripheral resistance and hence blood pressure; remember that:

Blood pressure = cardiac output x peripheral resistance.

This increase in pressure will help to keep his tissues supplied with oxygen – particularly the heart muscle itself and the brain. It is estimated that 20% of all patients who suffer a myocardial infarction die at the time because the remaining healthy heart muscle is unable to maintain cardiac output. The remaining 80% maintain a cardiac output (blood pressure) of varying degrees.

Q44. Mr Brown will appear pale and cold to touch. This is because the blood vessels in his skin are constricted (vasoconstriction). This is a part of the homeostatic response to a fall in blood pressure, which results in blood being diverted away from 'non-essential' organs such as the skin and abdominal viscera and towards essential organs such as the heart and brain. If the blood supply to the brain remains low, then the cells will not function properly and an indication of this will be that Mr Brown becomes confused and perhaps incoherent, and progresses into semiconsciousness. These are important signs that can be gauged by talking to him, and they will reveal whether his condition is improving, or not.

The kidneys rapidly lose their blood supply once blood pressure starts to fall. The immediate consequence of this will be a reduction in renal function and urine output. Therefore, this is another important observation. Should urine volume fall, then this could indicate the onset of renal failure. (The kidneys have a characteristic homeostatic response when their blood supply is reduced.) *See 📖 Pages 877–8 for further details of this.*

Q45. When the heart stops beating (cardiac arrest), the following signs occur:

Loss of consciousness.
No pulse or blood pressure.
Cessation of respiration.
Dilatation of the pupils.

Within 3–4 minutes the brain cells will undergo irreversible damage and Mr Brown will die. Hence, hospitals have a recognised emergency procedure for dealing with cardiac arrest. Help is summoned and **cardiopulmonary resuscitation** is commenced. The heart is massaged by compressing the lower one-third of the sternum and this squeezes the heart between the sternum and the vertebral column, ensuring cardiac output.

At the same time, the lungs are ventilated by mouth-to-mouth breathing or by using mechanical aids. Hence oxygen is supplied to the lungs – and bloodstream – and ultimately the brain. Drugs such as adrenaline can be given to try and stimulate the heart into action.

Q46. The ECG might display a straight line:

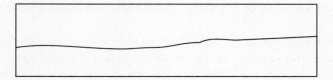

This is known as **asystole**, which literally means absence of contraction. Alternatively, it might display ventricular fibrillation:

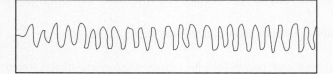

Here, there is no co-ordinated activity and so no ventricular contraction – and thus no cardiac output. The trace is produced because the heart muscle is quivering in a completely unco-ordinated manner.

These two examples are disturbances of rhythm (**arrhythmias**). There are others, which are less serious but may be the precursors of serious states such as cardiac arrest. Hence, it is an important skill for nurses and doctors to be able to recognise these and act upon them.

The ECG is also a very useful way of monitoring the success of the cardiopulmonary resuscitation procedure, in addition to feeling for the patient's pulse and observing the pupils.

Q47. Thrombolysis means the breakdown (lysis) of a blood clot (thrombus). The therapeutic substances (streptokinase and tissue plasminogen activator) are naturally present in the body (📖 *Page 582)* and activate plasminogen into plasmin.

Plasmin will then dissolve blood clots, such as the one which is blocking Mr Brown's coronary circulation. This will then allow oxygenated blood to flow through and reach the heart muscle. If this is done soon enough, then the heart muscle may not die (and be replaced by scar tissue) but undergo recovery. In the long term, Mr Brown will then make a better recovery and have little chance of developing chronic heart failure.

Q48. These thrombolytic substances may dissolve other blood clots in his body, for example, at shaving sites, intra-muscular injection sites or around intravenous cannulas. Thus, these sites need to be carefully observed for any haemorrhage.

Q49. He should be advised about the importance of gentle exercise. The aim is not to do too much, whilst at the same time not becoming housebound. Most physicians advise a return to sexual intercourse within a week or two – unless chest pain is experienced. He may also be advised to stop smoking, lose weight and/or readjust his diet to eat less cholesterol/saturated fat. This may require professional help from dietitians or Weight Watchers (*see* 📖 *Pages 612–13).*

Overview and key terms

Cardiovascular system (2)

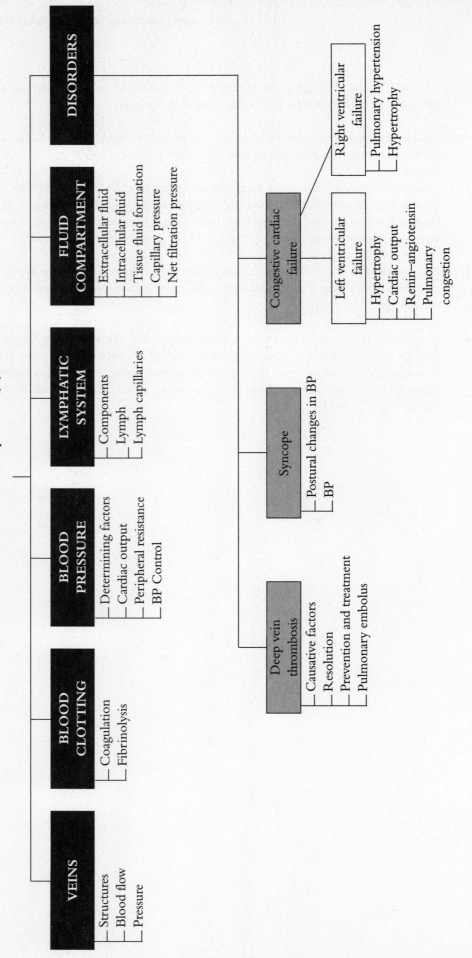

15. The Cardiovascular System (2): Veins, Blood Clotting, Lymphatics and Fluid Balance

Learning outcomes

1. To understand the main components of the venous system and blood flow.

2. To relate this to the complications of deep vein thrombosis and pulmonary embolus.

3. To understand the control of blood pressure and how this relates to fainting (syncope).

4. To describe the main components of fluid compartments and tissue fluid formation.

5. To describe the circulatory and fluid compartment changes that arise in left ventricular failure and congestive cardiac failure.

6. To understand how right ventricular failure (cor pulmonale) may be caused.

Chapters 19, 21, 22, 27

INTRODUCTION

This chapter extends and builds on the cardiovascular (1) chapter, which dealt with the chief components of the circulation (heart, blood and vessels), and related these to Mr Brown, who had a myocardial infarction.

The present chapter will deal mainly with other problems that Mr Brown may develop, both in the short and long term. These are related to the venous system, blood clotting, the regulation of blood pressure, the lymphatic system and the distribution of water and electrolytes in the body. The questions in the first part of this chapter will provide the basis from which these topics can be explored.

VEINS 📖 *Pages 624–32*

Q1. **Refer to Figure 13.1 and complete this exercise on blood vessels.**

a. Label vessels 1–7. Note that numbers are arranged in sequence of the pathway of blood flow. Use the following labels.

Aorta and other large arteries	Small artery
Arteriole	Small vein
Capillary	Venule
Inferior vena cava	

b. Colour the vessels according to colour code ovals.

c. The human circulatory system is called a(n) (open? closed?) system. State the significance of this fact.

_____

_____

Q2. **Complete this exercise about the structure of veins.**

Veins have (a) _____ (thicker? thinner?) walls than arteries. This structural feature relates to the fact that the pressure in veins is (b) _____ (more? less?) than in arteries. The pressure difference is demonstrated when a vein is cut. Blood leaves a cut vein in (c) _____ (rapid spurts? an even flow?).

Q3. **When a person is at rest, what percentage of the blood volume is in the veins?**

_____

Q4. **What is the average blood pressure in the small and large veins?**

_____

Figure 13.1.
Diagram of blood
vessels of the
human body.

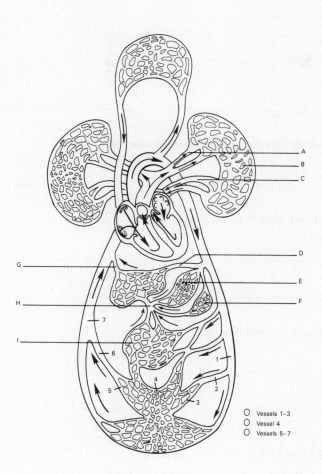

BLOOD CLOTTING 📖 *Pages 579–83.*

Q5.   **Briefly describe the three stages of blood clotting.**

_____

_____

_____

Q6.   **What type of feedback is involved in the process of clot formation?**

_____

_____

_____

_____

_____

_____

_____

Q7.   Name the two major factors that can cause intravascular clotting:

_____

Q8.   What is fibrinolysis and what is its purpose?

_____

_____

Q9.   What is the function of an anticoagulant?

_____

_____

BLOOD PRESSURE 📖 *Pages 630–44.*

Q10.   What are the two factors that determine blood pressure?

_____

Q11.   Which structure controls heart rate?

_____

Q12.   Which sets of nerves control heart rate, and what is their function?

_____

_____

Q13.   What other factors can increase heart rate?

_____

_____

Q14.   If blood pressure starts to fall, name the three mechanisms by which it can be restored.

_____

THE LYMPHATIC SYSTEM ◫ *Pages 683–9*

Q15.   List the components of the lymphatic system.

_____

_____

Q16.   Briefly describe the structure and location of the lymphatic capillaries.

_____

_____

Q17.   Briefly describe the formation and flow of lymph.

_____

_____

Q18.   The lymphatic system does not have a separate heart for pumping lymph. Describe two principal factors that are responsible for return of lymph from the entire body to major blood vessels in the neck. (Note that these same factors also facilitate venous return.)

_____

_____

FLUID COMPARTMENTS ◫ *Pages 905–6*

Q19.   What are the names of the two major fluid compartments in the body?

_____

Q20.   a. About 66% of body fluids are (inside? outside?) cells. _____ .

b. Check your understanding of fluid compartments by circling all fluids that are considered extracelluar fluids (ECF).

Blood plasma.

Aqueous humour and vitreous humour of the eyes.

Endolymph and perilymph.

Fluid within liver cells.

Fluid immediately surrounding liver cells.

Lymph.

Pericardial fluid.

Synovial fluid.

Cerebrospinal fluid (CSF).

You will need to refer to 📖 Pages 632–5 to answer these questions.

Q21.   Describe the types of fluid in the body and their relationships to homeostasis by completing these statements and Figure 13.2.

Figure 13.2.
Diagram of body
fluids.

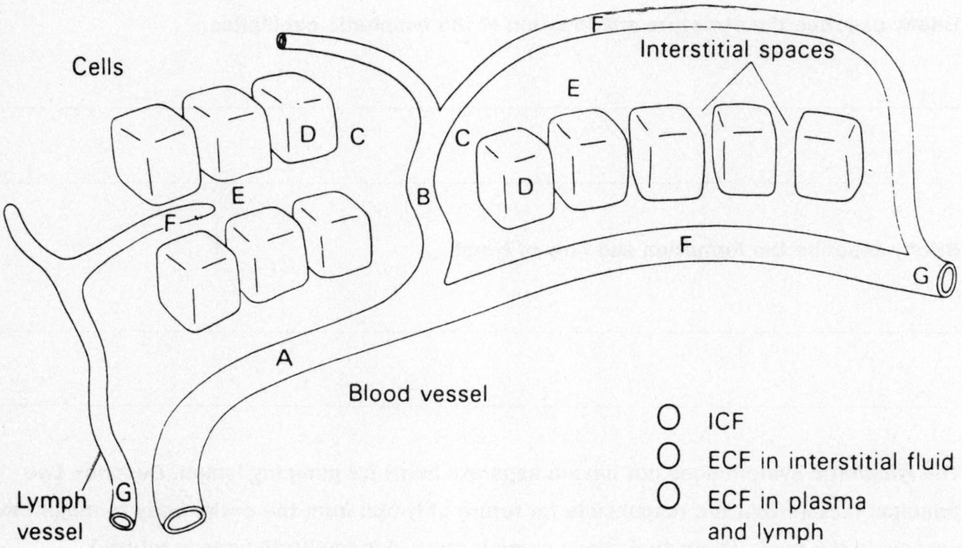

Q21 continued:

Fluid inside cells is known as (a) _____ fluid (ICF). Colour areas containing this type of fluid yellow.

Fluid in spaces between cells is called (b) _____. It surrounds and bathes cells and is one form of (c) _____ (intracellular? extracelluar?) fluid. Colour the spaces containing this fluid light green.

Another form of extracellular fluid is located in (d) _____ vessels and (e) _____ vessels. Colour these areas dark green. The body's 'internal environment' (that is, surrounding the cells) is (f) _____ -cellular fluid (ECF) (all green areas in your figure). Maintaining ECF in relative constancy is known as (g) _____.

Q22.   Refer again to Figure 13.2. Show the pattern of circulation of body fluids by drawing arrows connecting letters in the figure in alphabetical order (A → B → C →, etc.). Now fill in the blanks below describing this lettered pathway: A (arteries and arterioles) → B (blood capillaries) → C (_____) → D (_____) → E (_____) → F (_____) → G (_____).

Q23.   Interstitial fluid (tissue fluid) is formed because (a) _____ pressure exceeds (b) _____ pressure at the (c) _____ of the capillary.

Q24. Fluid is returned at the (a) _____ of the capillary because (b) _____ pressure is less than (c) _____ pressure.

Q25. Briefly describe what is meant by net filtration pressure (NFP).

_____

_____

CHECKPOINTS EXERCISE

Q26. Is pressure higher or lower in veins, in comparison to arteries?

_____

Q27. Inspiration (breathing in) causes the diaphragm to lower, and thus increases pressure inside the abdomen. What is the likely effect of this on blood flow in the inferior vena cava?

_____

_____

Q28. Many leg veins run through and close to muscles. What will be the effect on these veins of muscular activity?

_____

_____

Q29. From which fluid compartment do lymph capillaries drain?

_____

Q30. Where is lymph returned to?

_____

Q31. What is the driving force for the passage of water and electrolytes from the circulatory system into the tissue spaces?

_____

Q32. Fluid will not remain in the tissues because _____ _____ _____ effectively 'sucks' it back into the circulation.

PATIENT SCENARIO

Chapter 12 described Mr Brown's illness and examined some aspects of his care and treatment. The remainder of this chapter will deal with some other problems – related to the circulatory and lymphatic system – that he may develop. These are the problems of blood clots forming in the leg veins – known as **deep vein thrombosis**, **postural hypotension** which means a fall in blood pressure – with consequent dizziness – when a person stands upright, and finally, a long-term complication of heart muscle damage, known as **congestive cardiac failure**. Once again, the emphasis will be on explaining these in relation to normal anatomy and physiology.

THE CARDIOVASCULAR SYSTEM AND THE PROBLEMS OF BEDREST

Whilst bedrest is part of the treatment for Mr Brown's condition, it is not without its problems. Sitting in bed can lead to damage in several systems of the body. For example, blood clots can form in the legs, chest infections can occur, muscle weakness may develop and psychological depression may arise.

The following section, however, will be concerned with those problems that are related to the cardiovascular system. These are the formation of blood clots in the legs, and the loss of normal blood pressure-regulating mechanisms.

Deep vein thrombosis

A deep vein thrombosis (DVT) is a complication of bedrest. It is a blood clot that usually occurs in a vein in the calf region (the 'deep' veins, 📖 *Page 669, Figure 21.29*). The patient experiences pain and slight swelling at the site. Upon examination, the doctor will try to elicit **Homans' sign**; this is calf pain that is experienced when the foot is flexed towards the lower leg. In addition, there may be a slight rise in body temperature (pyrexia). The causes of a DVT are explored further below.

Poor blood flow

Lying in bed leads to a sluggish blood flow because of inactivity. This is particularly marked in the leg veins, as they are channelling blood – at low pressure – from the feet up to the abdomen, and subsequently the heart. The additional pressure of the calf resting on the bed will further slow the blood flow.

The following questions are based on 📖 Pages 630–5.

Q33.   What is the normal pressure within the veins?

Normally the venous system is a low-pressure circulation which returns blood to the heart. Additionally, the leg veins are also working against the pull of gravity for most of an individual's life.

Q34. **Explain the two mechanisms that help to return the blood flow from the lower limbs to the heart.**

_____

_____

_____

These two mechanisms are, of course operating at a minimal level when someone is confined to bed. Those patients with broken limbs will thus be particularly prone to DVT formation because of the additional necessity of keeping them immobile whilst healing takes place.

Increased platelet and clotting activity

This occurs particularly after surgical operations or episodes of trauma that involve broken bones and tissue damage.

Q35. **What is the first step in blood clotting?** 📖 _Page 579._

_____

The patient is then in a **hypercoaguable** state, and so will readily form blood clots. Hence, a DVT is usually – but not exclusively – regarded as a complication in patients who are recovering from surgery.

Vascular disease

As previously discussed, Mr Brown has atherosclerosis. This damage to the vessel wall can predispose to blood clot formation, because of the loss of the normally smooth lining of the blood vessel, although atherosclerosis is typically associated with arterial, and not venous, problems.

Additionally, any period of cardiac failure shock (📖 _Page 641_) will lead to a reduced blood flow, and thus predispose Mr Brown to blood clot formation.

Other factors

Taking the contraceptive pill is something that predisposes the recipients to forming blood clots. Also, dehydration will thicken the blood, and once again may lead to clot formation. Thickening of the blood also occurs in **polycythaemia**, a condition in which there is a proliferation of red blood cells.

However, Mr Brown is mostly predisposed to a DVT because of the inactivity of being in bed, arterial disease and the fact that he has already formed a thrombus – albeit in his coronary arteries.

Q36. **If part of this blood clot (DVT) should break off, in which direction would the blood flow carry it?**

_____

_____

_____

Q37. What will happen to the clot once it enters the pulmonary circulation? What effect will this have on Mr Brown?

_____

_____

_____

_____

_____

Q38. What will happen to this blood clot?

_____

_____

_____

_____

Q39. From a knowledge of the causes, how is it possible to prevent Mr Brown from forming a DVT?

_____

_____

_____

_____

Q40. Following a few days of bedrest, Mr Brown is allowed to get out of bed and sit in an armchair. Whilst doing this, he starts to feel dizzy. Why is this?

_____

_____

_____

_____

_____

Q41.   What actions would you take if Mr Brown felt dizzy?

_____

_____

_____

CONGESTIVE CARDIAC FAILURE

In the previous chapter, it was seen that the nature of Mr Brown's condition was essentially that of a damaged heart muscle, arising from a blockage in its blood supply. The damaged heart muscle will not, however, regenerate itself. It will be replaced by scar tissue (📖 *Page 122*) which, functionally, does not have the properties of cardiac muscle. This means that, despite a good recovery, Mr Brown's heart will always have a weakness. This may, in the years to come, lead to the heart being unable to cope with bodily demands. This is known as chronic heart failure – or **congestive cardiac failure**.

Chronic heart failure – terminology and definitions

Books and lecturers tend to take different approaches to the classification and subdivisions of this condition. This can be confusing for the student. Therefore, it is worthwhile, at the outset, to try to discern the reasoning behind these different approaches.

The condition is divided into three connected topics (some authors only use the first two).

Left heart failure

This is sometimes just called left ventricle failure (LVF). This is the most common type, and results from conditions, like myocardial infarction and high blood pressure, that impose a burden primarily on the left side of the heart.

However, because the two sides of the heart are connected via the lungs, the flow of blood from the right side of the heart (📖 *Page 672, Figure 21.31*) is soon affected. This is known as right heart failure.

Right heart failure

This, then, occurs as a **secondary** result of the failure of the left side of the heart. However, right sided failure can occur **primarily** from lung disease which imposes a strain on the right heart (📖 *Page 672, Figure 21.31*). This condition is called **cor pulmonale**.

Some authors maintain that because both sides of the heart are connected, it is artificial, and an over-simplification, to talk of left and right sided failure.

Congestive cardiac failure

This term is used when both right and left sided heart failure are present. Shock and cardiac arrest, as discussed in the previous chapter, are forms of **acute** heart failure. In the long term, however, Mr Brown's heart may develop chronic heart failure. The following questions should help you to differentiate between the different forms of chronic heart failure and to understand the underlying physiology and how this logically leads to the nature of care and treatment.

Q42. As Mr Brown's heart starts to weaken, so the cardiac output will start to fall. What will be the homeostatic response to this?

_____

_____

_____

Q43. What are the likely effects on Mr Brown's body of a diminished cardiac output?

_____

_____

_____

The other effect of a reduced blood flow is that the homeostatic mechanism (📖 *Page 10*) known as the renin-angiotensin system comes into play.

The following questions relate to 📖 Pages 544–5.

Q44. What is renin and what is its action?

_____

Q45. What is the trigger for the release of renin?

_____

Q46. What are the two effects of angiotensin?

_____

_____

Q47. What is the action of aldosterone?

_____

Q48. What is reabsorbed – along with sodium – by the kidney tubules?

_____

Q49. What is the effect on the body of the kidneys reabsorbing extra Na and water from the glomerular filtrate?

_____

_____

_____

Q50. The other effect of a reduced cardiac output is that 'up-stream' there will be a reduced blood flow. What changes will occur as a result of this?

_____

_____

Q51. What will be the effect as blood pressure inside the pulmonary capillaries exceeds the colloid osmotic pressure?

_____

_____

_____

Q52. What is the homeostatic response as Mr Brown's blood CO_2 level rises?

_____

_____

_____

Q53. What is the effect of left ventricular failure, and pulmonary congestion, on the right ventricle?

_____

_____

_____

_____

Q54. What is the effect on the net filtration pressure (NFP), at the venous end of the capillary, if pressure within the vein starts to rise?

_____

_____

_____

_____

PULMONARY HEART DISEASE

So far it has been seen that Mr Brown may first develop left ventricular failure as a result of his myocardial infarction. This can then lead to a strain on the right ventricle – and subsequent failure. This is then known as **congestive cardiac failure**. However, right ventricular failure can also occur directly as a result of lung disease. This usually begins with blood gas changes.

Q55. In severe lung disease, such as chronic bronchitis, there is retention of CO_2 and a lowering of blood O_2 because of impaired gas exchange. What will be the effect of these changes on blood pressure, particularly in the lungs?

_____

_____

_____

_____

QUESTIONS FOR DISCUSSION

1. Contrast and compare the three classifications of chronic heart failure, and relate this to normal structure and function.

2. What are the likely effects of systemic venous congestion on abdominal organs such as the stomach and liver? What problems will this cause for Mr Brown?

3. Postural hypotension (fainting) can also occur as a side effect of taking medication for high blood pressure. Find three examples of this medication, and in relation to normal anatomy and physiology explain how they can cause postural hypotension. What other effects may ensue from this?

4. Using a nursing model, devise a care plan for Mr Brown, assuming that he has developed congestive cardiac failure.

5. Some methods of DVT prevention are claimed to be better than others. Discuss the relative merits of each method.

Answers to questions

Q1. a. 1. Aorta
2. Small artery
3. Arteriole
4. Capillary
5. Venule
6. Small vein
7. Inferior vena cava

b. See 📖 *Page 647, Figure 21.19.*

c. Closed; blood is carried from the heart within a closed system of tubes which contributes to haemodynamics. For example, large arteries convert stored energy into kinetic energy of blood, so that blood continues to move on through smaller vessels.

Q2. a, Thinner; b, less; c, an even flow.

Q3. 60%.

Q4. Approximately 5–8 mmHg.

Q5. 1. Formation of prothrombinase.
2. Conversion of prothrombin to thrombin.
3. Conversion of fibrinogen to fibrin.

Q6. Positive feedback.

Q7. Roughed endothelial surface, and slow blood flow.

Q8. The dissolution (dissolving) of a blood clot. This is a natural mechanism, which operates to prevent blood clots from forming within the vascular system. Fibrinolysis is also the mechanism by which blood clots, formed from trauma and tissue damage in other parts of the body are dissolved.

Q9. It prevents blood clotting, and so stops a blood clot from spreading.

Q10. Cardiac output, and peripheral resistance.

Q11. Cardiovascular centre in the medulla oblongata.

Q12.   Vagus nerve, decreases heart rate; and sympathetic nerves, increase heart rate.

Q13.   Adrenaline, noradrenaline, thyroxine and body temperature rise.

Q14.   Increasing heart rate, stroke volume or vasoconstriction.

Q15.   Lymph, lymph vessels and lymph organs (such as tonsils, spleen and lymph nodes).

Q16.   Slightly larger than blood capillaries and found in tissues throughout the body (except nervous system, spleen and bone marrow).

Q17.   Lymph is fluid derived from tissue fluid spaces, which is then returned via lymphatic vessels to the circulatory system. 📖 *Pages 684–5.*

Q18.   Skeletal muscle contraction and respiratory movements squeeze lymphatics, which contain valves that direct the flow of lymph.

Q19.   Extracelluar fluid, and intracellular fluid.

Q20.   a. Inside
            b. All answers except fluid within liver cells.

Q21.   a, Intracellular; b, interstitial (or intercellular or tissue) fluid; c, extracelluar; d, blood; e, lymph; f, extra; g, homeostasis.

Q22.   C, (interstitial, intercellular fluid) → D (intracellular fluid) → E (interstitial, intercellular fluid) → F (blood or lymph capillaries) → G (venules and veins or lymph vessels).

Q23.   a, Blood; b, colloid osmotic; c, arterial end.

Q24.   a, Venous end; b, blood; c, colloid osmotic.

Q25.   The pressure that forces fluid out of a capillary. 📖 *Page 633, Figure 21.10.*

Q26.   Lower.

Q27.   Blood flow – venous return to the heart – will be squeezed, and thus assisted on its journey to the heart.

Q28.   The veins will be squeezed and thus blood flow will be assisted. This is the so-called 'muscle pump effect'.

Q29.   Interstitial fluid (extracelluar compartment).

Q30.   The circulatory system.

Q31.   Blood pressure.

Q32.   Colloid osmotic pressure.

Q33.   16 mmHg (average).

Q34. 1. The muscle pump effect of the leg muscles squeezing the veins (see Figure 13.5).
2. The respiratory pump. Breathing in increases abdominal pressure, by lowering the diaphragm. This squeezes blood up the inferior vena cava (see Figure 13.4).

Q35. Platelet activation.

Q36. Blood flow in the veins is towards the direction of the heart, so the blood clot would pass up the femoral and iliac veins, towards the inferior vena cava and into the right side of the heart (📖 *Page 664*) and then into the pulmonary circulation. Finally, it will pass into a vessel that has a smaller diameter than itself; then it will become stuck.

Q37. The effect of this will be to stop the flow of blood to an area of the lung. The larger the vessel that is blocked, the larger the area of tissue damage (see Figure 13.3).

   When this happens – usually a sudden event – Mr Brown will experience various symptoms, and the severity of these will depend upon the size of lung tissue that is damaged. With a small embolus, Mr Brown will just experience some breathlessness and chest pain, and will possibly cough up some blood.

   On the other hand, a large embolus may block the circulation – from the heart – and stop the heart pumping (cardiac arrest). This is a feared complication, amongst surgeons, and undoubtedly was one of the factors that gave rise to the well-known phrase: 'The operation was a success, but the patient died'.

Figure 13.3.
The effects of an embolus (thrombus) lodging in the lungs (pulmonary embolus).

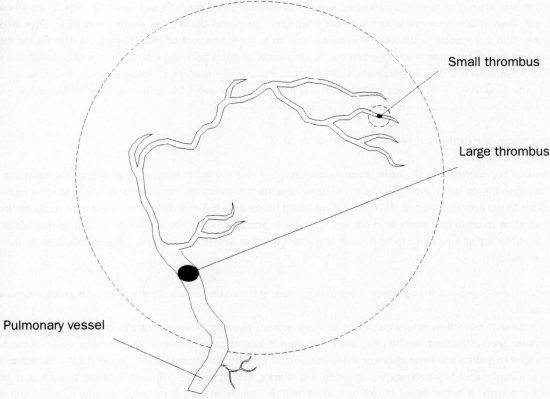

Small thrombus

Large thrombus

Pulmonary vessel

-------------- Area of tissue damage

Q38. Plasmin *(📖 Page 582)* will dissolve the blood clot (fibrinolysis). However, this will not prevent another blood clot from forming, and if the conditions (bedrest, lack of movement, arterial disease) exist for the formation of a first clot, then there are good reasons why a second one should form. For this reason, Mr Brown will be prescribed an **anticoagulant** (e.g heparin) that will prevent his blood from clotting – and thus stop a second clot from forming. But note that drugs such as heparin are not fibrinolytic – they will not dissolve the blood clot in the lungs.

Q39. Heparin can be given. Some surgeons routinely give this to patients undergoing major surgery. In addition, special stockings can be worn by the patient. These are called TED (Thrombo embolic deterrent) stockings and they act by compressing the ankle more than the thigh – this helps push blood up the leg. Thus they aid venous flow and return. Remember that blood pressure in the veins is quite low *(📖 Page 631, Figure 21.9)* and so the flow is quite sluggish.

Also, Mr Brown should not be allowed to become dehydrated. It is an important aspect of his nursing care to ensure that he receives sufficient fluid intake, and to monitor this by keeping an accurate fluid balance chart.

Probably one of the most important aspects of prevention is to allow Mr Brown up and out of bed. This will bring into play the muscle pump *(📖 Page 634, Figure 21.11)* and this will immediately improve blood flow in the leg veins. Uncrossing the legs, whilst in bed, will at least relieve compression on the calf, which may cause a DVT.

The trend to early mobilisation over the last few decades – both after surgery as well as following myocardial infarction – has undoubtedly been prompted by the above reasons. With the increasing use of day surgery, one would expect to see a further trend in the reduction of DVT formation.

Q40. Mr Brown is starting to feel faint (syncope), and this is because blood tends to sink down the legs as he stands upright. Thus, the venous return to the heart is reduced. The Frank–Starling law of the heart *(📖 Page 609)* ensures that if the return to the heart is reduced, then so is the cardiac output *(📖 Page 636)*. This means that the blood flow to the brain is reduced and this is what leads to dizziness – and ultimately loss of consciousness.

The reason that this does not normally happen is that whenever we assume a vertical position, the cardiovascular centre *(📖 Page 636)* speeds up the heart and produces vasoconstriction of the leg veins. Thus cardiac output and peripheral resistance are increased, and so is blood pressure.

Blood pressure = cardiac output x peripheral resistance

This does not happen with Mr Brown, because his period of rest has led to his cardiovascular centre becoming a bit sluggish ('if you don't use it, you lose it'). Thus, when he stands up, his blood pressure starts to fall – and he may fall to the floor in a faint. In doing this he will effect his treatment, because in assuming a horizontal position, he will allow blood to flow easily from his legs to his heart and then brain. The only danger is that he may break a bone and/or suffer a head injury as a result of the fall! And this sometimes happens when people faint for 'emotional' reasons.

Q41. Lay him down again and then proceed more slowly, allowing his cardiovascular centre to accommodate his movements.

If a person who is feeling faint cannot be laid flat, perhaps because they are on a crowded train, then there are two other approaches that can be used to try and prevent loss of consciousness. Blood flow to the brain can be increased by putting the head between the knees and/or by using the muscle pump (Figure 13.5). The effect of this can be enhanced by alternately contracting and relaxing the leg muscles. This will increase blood flow to the heart and brain. It is something taught to soldiers and policemen who are sometimes required to stand still for long periods of time. Taking deep breaths (the respiratory pump, Figure 13.4) will also aid venous return.

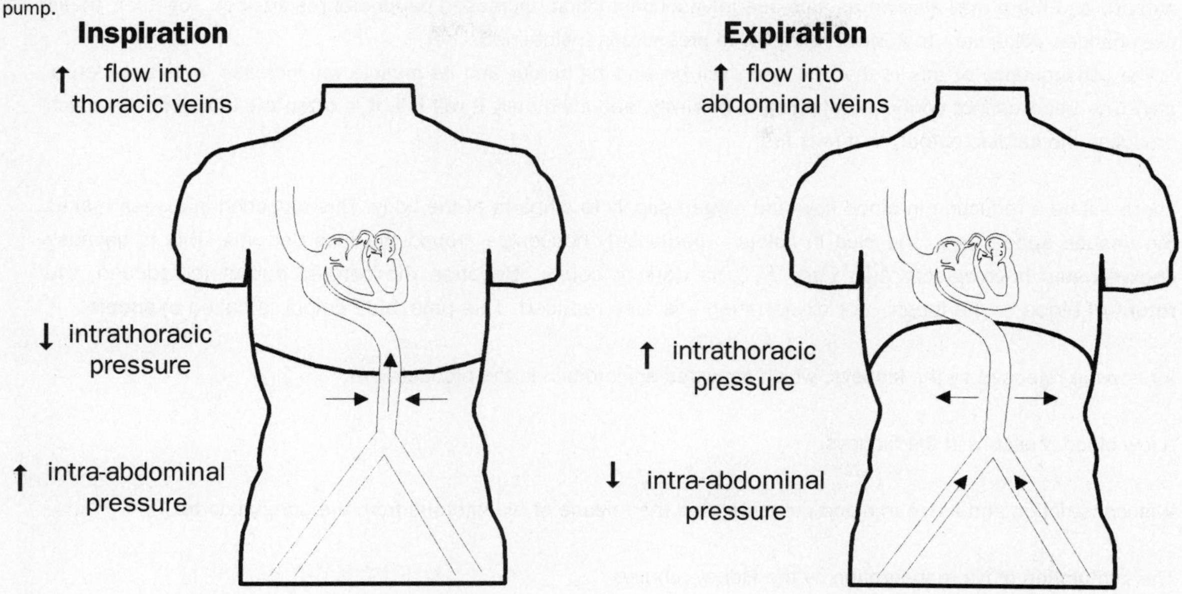

Figure 13.4.
The respiratory
pump.

Inspiration

↑ flow into
thoracic veins

↓ intrathoracic
pressure

↑ intra-abdominal
pressure

Expiration

↑ flow into
abdominal veins

↑ intrathoracic
pressure

↓ intra-abdominal
pressure

Figure 13.5.
The skeletal muscle
pump.

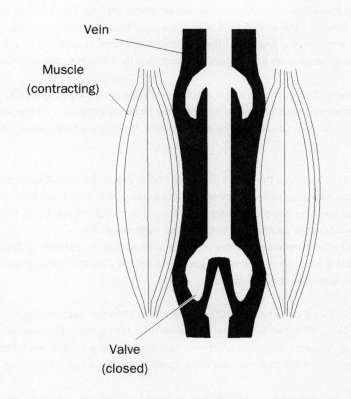

Vein

Muscle
(contracting)

Valve
(closed)

Q42. The baroreceptors will prompt the cardiovascular centre *(▢▢ Pages 636–40)* to increase the heart rate (cardiac output), and there may also be an increase in vasoconstriction (increased peripheral resistance). Together, these two changes will ensure that Mr Brown's blood pressure is maintained.

   The consequence of this is that the heart will be working harder and its muscle will increase in size (hypertrophy). The heart cannot continue enlarging in this way, and eventually it will fail. It is often the left ventricle, which produces the cardiac output, that fails first.

Q43. There will be a reduction in blood flow and oxygen supply to all parts of the body. This reduction in oxygen makes the tissues appear pale and blue in colour – particularly noticeable around the face and lips. This is because deoxygenated haemoglobin *(▢▢ Page 570)* is dark in colour. Because the cardiac output is reduced, the return of blood to the lungs – for oxygenation – is also reduced. This pale/blue colour is called **cyanosis**.

Q44. An enzyme released by the kidneys, which activates angiotensin in the bloodstream.

Q45. A low blood pressure in the kidneys.

Q46. Vasoconstriction and a rise in blood pressure; and the release of aldosterone from the adrenal cortex.

Q47. The stimulation of Na reabsorption by the kidney tubules.

Q48. Water

Q49. Blood volume will start to rise *(▢▢ Page 630)*. Coupled with vasoconstriction, this means that blood pressure will rise. Hence, this is another homeostatic response to a fall in cardiac output (BP). Unfortunately, the increase in blood volume is only an appropriate response in someone whose blood pressure is low because of blood loss (Mr Brown's BP is low because of failure of the 'pump' – the heart). The effect of this extra volume is to place extra strain on the heart, and this will probably worsen the degree of heart failure. This problem can be treated by giving Mr Brown drugs that will expel the excess fluid from the body. These work by increasing urine production and some of them oppose the action of aldosterone. They are called **diuretics**. In addition, he will be given a drug called **digoxin**, which will strengthen and steady the heart's action, and thus improve cardiac output.

Q50. Up-stream of the left ventricle is the left atrium and the pulmonary circulation *(▢▢ Page 647, Figure 21.19)*. The pressure inside these structures will start to rise as blood flow becomes congested, in the same way that the pressure inside a hose pipe rises if one squeezes the end. If visible, the lungs would appear rather swollen and bulging.

Q51. Fluid will be forced from the capillaries into the alveoli *(▢▢ Page 633, Figure 21.10)*. If fluid collects in the alveoli then this will slow down gas exchange between the alveoli and the capillary. This is because diffusion distance *(▢▢ Page 745)* is increased when fluid is present. Also this means that oxygen uptake into the capillary will be reduced and CO_2 will not move from the capillaries into the alveoli quite so quickly.

   In its severest form this is called **pulmonary oedema** (oedema is an abnormal collection of fluid in the tissues). This state can be life-threatening because of reduced O_2 uptake. In addition, breathing would become difficult and some of the fluid would be coughed up as watery sputum.

Q52. Chemoreceptors *(▢▢ Page 735)* will detect a rising CO_2 level and stimulate the respiratory centre to increase the rate and depth of breathing. Thus, Mr Brown will appear as though he is having difficulty breathing (**dyspnoea**).

   This dyspnoea can occur in nocturnal attacks (paroxysmal nocturnal dyspnoea) because, when lying flat, fluid that has collected in the lower half of the body can now move upwards into the lungs. This will have an immediate effect on gas exchange.

   As mentioned earlier, the use of digoxin to improve cardiac output will prevent pulmonary congestion and the ensuing problems of CO_2 retention, O_2 lack and difficulty with breathing.

Figure 13.6 provides a summary of the effects on the body of left heart (ventricle) failure.

Figure 13.6.
A summary of the
effects on the body
of left heart failure.

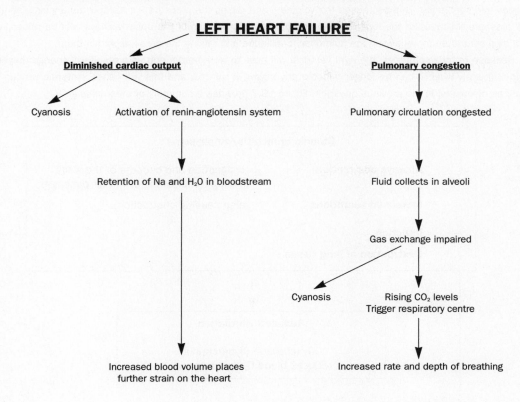

LEFT HEART FAILURE

Diminished cardiac output

Cyanosis   Activation of renin-angiotensin system

Retention of Na and H_2O in bloodstream

Increased blood volume places
further strain on the heart

Pulmonary congestion

Pulmonary circulation congested

Fluid collects in alveoli

Gas exchange impaired

Cyanosis   Rising CO_2 levels
Trigger respiratory centre

Increased rate and depth of breathing

Q53. The right ventricle is trying to pump blood into an already congested pulmonary circulation. The right ventricle, like the left, will now start to enlarge (hypertrophy) as it works harder. When this is no longer possible, it will fail.

The effect of this will be to cause congestion in those structures that are draining blood into the right side of the heart. The superior vena cava drains blood from those structures above the level of the heart (📖 *Page 661, Figure 21.25*) whilst the inferior vena cava drains all the structures below the level of the heart. The abdominal organs and lower limbs will thus become congested with blood, and pressure within their veins will rise.

Q54. Net filtration pressure will rise and have a positive value. (📖 *Page 633, Figure 21.10).* This means that there will be no reabsorption of fluid at the venous end of the capillary; and coupled with fluid formed in the tissues at the arterial end, this will mean an overall increase in fluid within the tissues, the condition known as **oedema**.

The fluid will collect, under gravity, in the sacral region in patients who are in bed. It can be detected by pressing gently with the thumb. If this leaves a small hollow in the skin, then that is a sign of oedema. If Mr Brown is up and about, then the fluid will collect in his ankles. It will also collect around the abdominal organs such as the stomach, and impair their function, which may lead to loss of appetite.

Excess fluid in the circulation will cause veins, which normally have a low pressure to bulge (📖 *Page 631, Figure 21.9),* and this may be observed in Mr Brown's neck as the jugular veins (📖 *Page 661, Figure 21.25)* became more pronounced.

Digoxin and diuretics will prevent oedema forming and promote its removal.

Q55. Blood pressure in the pulmonary circulation will rise and this will put a strain on the right ventricle as it attempts to keep pumping blood into a circulation which now has an increased pressure. (Imagine trying to blow more air into an already over-inflated balloon.)

The pressure in the pulmonary circulation is further raised because the lung disease leads to destruction of alveoli and capillaries. This decreases the volume – and raises the pressure – in the pulmonary circulation. Alveolar pressure, because of the lung disease and blockage by sputum of the upper airways, will be raised, and this will also contribute to squeezing the pulmonary capillaries and raising the pressure within them.

Because of these changes, the right ventricle will have to work harder and as a result will change (**hypertrophy**) and ultimately when it can no longer become any bigger, it will fail, and this will cause systemic venous congestion, as discussed in the previous question. Figure 13.7 provides a summary of these changes.

Figure 13.7.
A summary of right heart failure and its causation by lung disease (cor pulmonale).

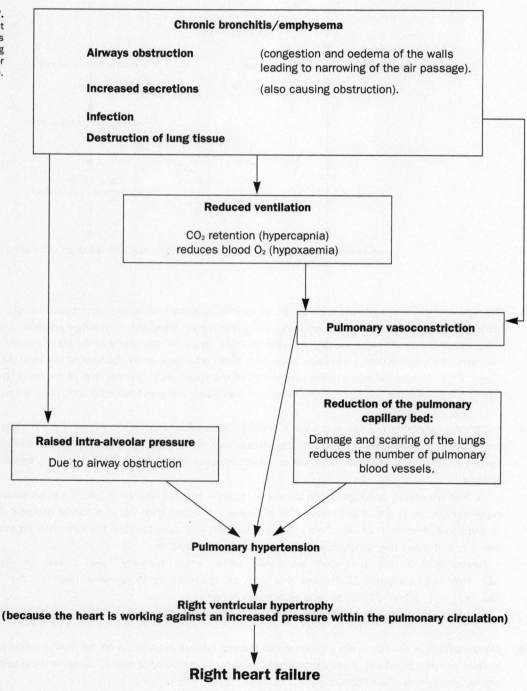

Chronic bronchitis/emphysema

Airways obstruction (congestion and oedema of the walls leading to narrowing of the air passage).

Increased secretions (also causing obstruction).

Infection

Destruction of lung tissue

Reduced ventilation

CO_2 retention (hypercapnia)
reduces blood O_2 (hypoxaemia)

Pulmonary vasoconstriction

Reduction of the pulmonary capillary bed:

Damage and scarring of the lungs reduces the number of pulmonary blood vessels.

Raised intra-alveolar pressure

Due to airway obstruction

Pulmonary hypertension

Right ventricular hypertrophy
(because the heart is working against an increased pressure within the pulmonary circulation)

Right heart failure

Overview and key terms
Lymphatic system and immunity

LYMPHATIC SYSTEM

- **ORGANISATION (A)**
  - Lymphatic vessels
  - Lymph circulation
- **LYMPHATIC TISSUE (B)**
  - Nodes
  - Tonsils
  - Spleen
  - Thymus
- **DEVELOPMENT (C)**

RESISTANCE TO DISEASE

- **NONSPECIFIC RESISTANCE (D)**
  - Skin, mucosa
    - Mechanical factors
    - Chemical factors
  - NK cells
  - Antimicrobial substances
    - Transferrins
    - Interferon
    - Complement
    - Properdin
  - Phagocytosis
    - Chemotaxis
    - Opsonisation
    - Adherence
    - Ingestion
    - Killing
  - Inflammation
    - Pain, redness, swelling, heat
    - Stages
  - Fever
- **IMMUNITY: SPECIFIC RESISTANCE (E)**
  - Antigens
    - Immunogenicity
    - Reactivity
    - MHC antigens
    - APCs
  - Cytokines
    - Interleukins
    - Interferons
    - Lymphotoxin
    - Perforin
  - Cell-mediated immunity (CMI)
    - T cells
      - cytotoxic (T_C)
      - helper (T_H)
      - 3 others
  - Antibody-mediated immunity (AMI)
    - B cells
    - Plasma cells
    - Antibodies
      - Ig
  - Active
  - Passive

AGEING AND IMMUNITY (F)

DISORDERS (G)

- Cancer
- AIDS
- Autoimmune
- Hypersensitivity
  - allergy
  - tissue rejection

14. The Lymphatic System, Nonspecific Resistance to Disease, and Immunity

Learning outcomes

1. To describe the components and functions of the lymphatic system.

2. To discuss how oedema develops.

3. To discuss the roles of the skin and mucous membranes, antimicrobial substances, phagocytosis, inflammations and fever in nonspecific resistance to disease.

4. To define immunity and describe how T cells and B cells are produced.

5. To explain the relationship between an antigen (Ag) and an antibody (Ab).

6. To describe the roles of antigen presenting cells, T cells and B cells in cell-mediated and antibody-mediated immunity.

7. To outline how self-tolerance occurs.

8. To show an awareness in the possible effect of ageing on the immune system.

9. To outline some of the clinical symptoms in acquired immune deficiency syndrome and hypersensitivity reactions.

10. To describe altered physiology in tissue rejection following transplantation.

Chapter 22

INTRODUCTION

The chapter on immunology should help you to understand how the immune system of the body operates and also why an immunisation programme is beneficial to mankind. As health care professionals, you will be expected to give sound advice to clients on all aspects of immunity and it is therefore imperative that you are conversant with the relevant materials on the immune system.

A major component of the immune system is the lymphatic system, the one which plays an important role in specific resistance to disease (immunity), through the production of antibodies and various types of T cells. It is also important to consider the role of the body in nonspecific resistance to disease, which is provided by a variety of structures and mechanisms such as the skin, mucus and white blood cells. The lymphatic system also assists in the regulation of body fluids by returning proteins and fluids to blood vessels.

To maximise your learning on this topic, you will need to refer to 📖 *Chapter 22*, which covers the lymphatic system, and nonspecific and specific resistance to disease. You will first be introduced to the structure and functions of the lymphatic system, before moving on to immunity.

LYMPHATIC SYSTEM

For questions 1–6 see 📖 *Pages 683–7*

Q1. Identify the vessels that form the lymphatic system and outline how they assist in draining lymph fluid back to the heart.

_____

_____

_____

_____

Q2. List two functions of the lymphatic system, other than the draining of lymph fluid.

_____

Q3. Lymphatic vessels drain, from tissue spaces, (a) _____ that are too large to pass readily into blood capillaries. They also transport (b) _____ from the gastrointestinal tract to the bloodstream. The defensive functions of the lymphatic system are carried out largely by white blood cells known as (c) _____ (B or T) lymphocytes, which destroy foreign substances directly, whereas B lymphocytes lead to the production of (d) _____ .

Q4. **Briefly differentiate between a lymph node and a lymphatic nodule.**

_____

_____

_____

Q5. **Label A–E on Figure 14.1, which shows the structure of a lymph node.**

A – Vessels for entrance of lymph into node.

B – Site of B lymphocyte proliferation into antibody-secreting plasma cells.

C – Vessels for exit of lymph out of node.

D – Channels for flow of lymph in the cortex of the node.

E – Dense strands of lymphocytes, macrophages and plasma cells.

Figure 14.1.
ructure of a lymph
node.

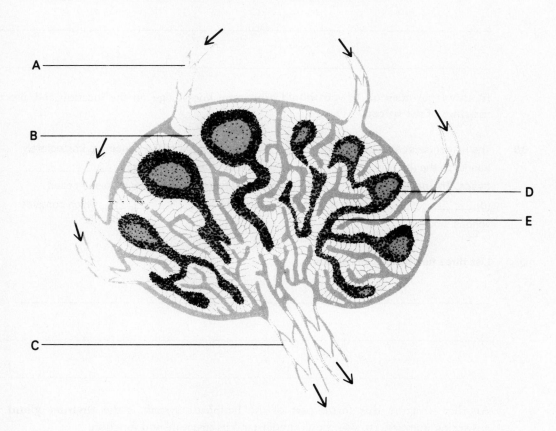

Q6. **Describe the structure of a lymph node making reference to its function. You may find** 📖 *Page 688, Figure 22.5,* **very useful in answering this question.**

_____

_____

_____

_____

Q7. **Outline how T cells and B cells are produced in the body.**

_____

_____

_____

In answering question 8, you should gain some knowledge on the location and also the structure of the **spleen**.

Q8. The spleen is located in the (a) _____ quadrant of the abdomen, immediately inferior to the (b) _____ . It consists of a large mass of (c) _____ tissue. The parenchyma of the spleen consists of two different types of tissue called (d) _____, which is lymphatic tissue and (e) _____ which contains venous sinuses.

Q9. **List three functions of the spleen.**

_____

_____

_____

Another structure that forms part of the lymphatic system is the **thymus gland**. In answering question 10, you should understand its structure and function.

Q10. The thymus gland is located in the superior (a) _____ , posterior to the (b) _____ bone and between the (c) _____ . Its size is relatively (d) _____ in childhood. The thymus gland contains a medulla surrounded by a (e) _____ . Within the cortex are densely packed (f) _____ . The thymus is the site of maturation of (g) _____ throughout life.

NONSPECIFIC RESISTANCE TO DISEASE

Your body is constantly bombarded by various **pathogens**, and many other components that can produce diseases, yet if you maintain a healthy life style, it is rare that your body will become infected; or, to put it in another way, you are unlikely to succumb to many infections in your lifetime. So, how does the body achieve this? Your answer to question 11 will demonstrate this to you.

Q11. **Giving the rationale for your answer, briefly discuss the role of the body in nonspecific resistance to disease.**

_____

_____

_____

_____

Q12. **Match the following conditions or factors with the nonspecific resistance that is lost in each case.**

> **1. Cleansing of oral mucosa 2. Cleansing of vaginal mucosa 3. Flushing of microbes from urinary tract 4. Lacrimal fluid with lysozyme 5. Respiratory mucosa with cilia 6. Closely packed layers of keratinized cells 7. HCl production – pH 1 or 2 8. Sebum production**

- [ ] a. Long-term smoking.
- [ ] b. Excessive dryness of the skin.
- [ ] c. Use of anticholinergic medications that decrease salivation.
- [ ] d. Vaginal atrophy related to normal ageing.
- [ ] e. Dry eyes related to decreased production of tears, as in ageing.
- [ ] f. Decreased urinary output, as in prostatic hypertrophy.
- [ ] g. Skin wound.
- [ ] h. Partial gastrectomy (removal of part of the stomach).

Q13. **When you have completed questions 13 and 14 below, you should have gained some more knowledge on nonspecific defences in the body.** 📖 _Pages 693–4_

Interferons (IFNs) are proteins produced by cells infected with (a) ——————————.

Alpha interferon (alpha-IFN) is classified as type (b) —————————— interferon. This substance has been used in the treatment of individuals with an associated virus disorder giving rise to (c) _____ _____.

NK cells, or (d) _____ _____ cells, are a type of (e) _____.

Type II (gamma) IFNs stimulate the (f) _____ activity of these cells. NK cells are less functional in patients with (g) _____ and some forms of (h) _____.

Q14. Two types of white blood cells are involved in phagocytosis, of which the most numerous are the

(a) _____ followed by the (b) _____ . Other leukocytes, known as

(c) _____ , travel to infection sites and develop into highly phagocytic

(d) _____ cells. Macrophages form part of the reticuloendothelial, or

(e) _____ _____ system.

Q15. Outline the roles of the complement system with reference to C3, histamine, opsonisation and membrane attack complex. 📖 *Pages 693–4.*

_____

_____

_____

_____

Q16. Select the number in the box that best fits each description of a phase of inflammation.

1. Vasodilatation and increased capillary permeability 2. Phagocytic migration 3. Repair

☐   a. Brings defensive substances to the injured site and helps remove toxic wastes.

☐   b. Histamine, prostaglandins, kinins, leukotrienes and complement enhance this process.

☐   c. Causes redness, warmth and swelling of inflammation.

☐   d. Localises and traps invading organisms.

☐   e. Occurs within an hour after initiation of inflammation; involves margination, diapedesis, chemotaxis and leukocytosis.

☐   f. White blood cell and debris formation that may lead to abscess or ulcer.

Q17 Identify the chemicals in the box that fit the descriptions below.

1. Complement 2. Histamine 3. Interferon 4. Kinins 5. Prostaglandins 6. Leukocytosis-promoting factor 7. Leukotrienes 8. Transferrins

☐   a. Produced by damaged or inflamed tissues; aspirin and ibuprofen neutralise these pain-inducing chemicals.

☐   b. Produced by mast cells and basophils (two answers).

☐   c. Stimulates increase in production of neutrophils.

☐   d. Induces vasodilatation, permeability, chemotaxis and irritation of nerve endings (pain).

☐   e. Neutrophils are attracted by these chemicals present in the inflamed area (two answers).

☐   f. Proteins that inhibit bacterial growth by depriving micro-organisms of iron.

☐ g. Group of 20 serum proteins that stimulate release of histamine and also make bacteria 'tastier' to phagocytes by opsonisation.

☐ h. Made by some leukocytes and fibroblasts; stimulates cells near an invading virus to produce antiviral proteins that interfere with survival of the virus.

SPECIFIC RESISTANCE TO DISEASE (IMMUNITY) 📖 *Pages 697–712*

Now that you have completed the exercises on the lymphatic system and nonspecific resistance to disease, you can concentrate on specific resistance to disease. You will discover some of the factors that can influence the immune system.

To assist you with this part of the study, you will be presented with a patient scenario after you have been introduced to some important components of the immune system.

Q18. **Name the two types of immune response.**

_____

Q19. **This exercise will introduce you to the cells that carry out immune responses.**

The two categories of cells that carry out immune responses are (a) _____ and antigen presenting cells. The former cells originate mainly from the (b) _____ cells of the (c) _____ _____ and also from (d) _____ nodes.

Some immature lymphocytes migrate to the thymus and become (e) _____ cells. In the thymus, these cells develop immunocompetence, meaning that they have the ability to (f) _____ (more explanations are wanted here). Some T cells become CD4$^+$ cells and others become (g) _____ cells, based on the type of (h) _____ in their plasma membranes.

B cells mature into immune cells in the (i) _____ _____ .

Q20. **Contrast two types of immunity by writing AMI before descriptions of antibody-mediated immunity and CMI before those describing cell-mediated immunity.**

☐ a. Especially effective against micro-organisms that enter cells, such as viruses and parasites.

☐ b. Especially effective against bacteria present in extracellular fluids.

☐ c. Involves plasma cells (derived from B cells) that produce antibodies.

☐ d. Utilises killer T cells (derived from CD8$^+$ T cells) that directly attack the antigen.

☐ e. Facilitated by helper T (CD4$^+$) cells.

It is an appropriate stage in your study to consolidate your understanding of an antigen and an antibody. In working on question 21, you should become familiar with the term antigen.

Q21.   Complete the exercise below on antigens.

An antigen is defined as 'any chemical substance which, when introduced into the body, is recognised as (a) _____'. In general, they are (b) _____. When attached to a lipid, they are referred to as (c) _____ and when attached to a carbohydrate are called (d) _____ .

Antigens have **two** important properties. One is the ability to provoke an immune response and therefore the production of antibodies, and this is known as (e) _____. The second is the ability of the antigen to react specifically with the produced antibodies or cells, and this is referred to as (f) _____. An antigen that has both of the properties mentioned above is called (g) _____.

A partial antigen is known as a (h) _____. It has reactivity but not (i) _____. For example, the drug penicillin can evoke an immune response, but only if it is able to combine with (j) _____ in the body. Individuals who have this particular protein are said to be (k) _____ to penicillin.

The specific portions of antigen that can trigger immune responses are called antigenic determinants or (l) _____.

MAJOR HISTOCOMPATIBILITY COMPLEX (MHC) ANTIGENS 📖 *Pages 701–2*

To fully understand how an antigen triggers an immune response, i.e the production of antibodies, and also how T cells recognise foreign invaders in the body, it is essential to appreciate the role of the MHC antigens in these processes.

What are the MHC complex antigens ?

In simple terms, the MHC is a **chromosomal** region that codes for the synthesis of **self antigens** that are used by the specific immune system for the recognition of **self.** Usually, **immune responses** are only directed against **nonself antigens.** If this mechanism fails and the body is not able to recognise self antigens, an **autoimmune response** can occur and this gives rise to the so-called **autoimmune disorders.** An example of an autoimmune disorder is **rheumatoid arthritis**.

In humans, the gene cluster that contains the MHC is located on **chromosome number 6** and is called the **HLA** (human leukocyte antigen complex).

Question 22 refers to MHC antigens.

Q22.   Briefly differentiate between the two types of MHC antigens.

_____

_____

_____

_____

Q23. Define the term exogenous antigen.

_____

Q24. Name three types of antigen presenting cells.

_____

Q25. Place in correct sequence the statements below, which describe the steps that APCs or other body cells take to initiate an immune response to invading antigens.

a. Binding of peptide fragment to MHC-II.

b. Exocytosis and insertion of antigen fragment MHC-II into APC plasma membrane.

c. Fusion of vesicles of peptide fragments with MHC-II.

d. Partial digestion of antigen into peptide fragments.

e. Phagocytosis or endocytosis of antigen.

f. Presentation of antigen to T cell in lymphatic tissue.

_____ _____ _____ _____ _____ _____

CYTOKINES 📖 *Pages 702–3*

Lymphocytes and APCs secrete chemicals known as **cytokines.** These play different roles in immune responses.

Q26. Give the specific names for cytokines that are released by the lymphocytes and those that are released by monocytes or macrophages.

_____

Q27. Match the name of each of the cytokines from the list with the description that best fits.

1. Gamma interferon 2. Interleukin-2 3. Monokine 4. Macrophage migration inhibiting factor 5. Interleukin-4

☐ a. General name for a cytokine made by a monocyte.

☐ b. Made by activated helper T cells; stimulates B cells, leading to IgE production.

☐ c. Known as T cell growth factor, it is made by helper T cells; needed for almost all immune responses; causes proliferation of cytotoxic T cells (as well as B cells) and activates NK cells.

☐ d. Formerly called macrophage activating factor, stimulates phagocytosis in macrophages and neutrophils; enhances AMI and CMI responses.

☐ e. Prevents macrophages from leaving the site of infection.

ANTIBODIES

At this stage in your study, it is appropriate to look at the important molecules of the immune respose, **the antibodies**. 📖 *Pages 702–5.*

To fully understand the structure of an antibody, you will be introduced to a diagram showing an antibody and you will be asked to complete an exercise.

Q28. **Figure 14.2 shows a schematic structure of an antibody molecule. Label the parts indicated (A–I) which refer to variable light chain, constant light chain, constant heavy chain, variable heavy chain, antigen binding site, hinge region, disulphide bonds, carbohydrates and Fc region or 'fragment crystallisable'.**

Figure 14.2.
Diagram of an
antibody molecule.

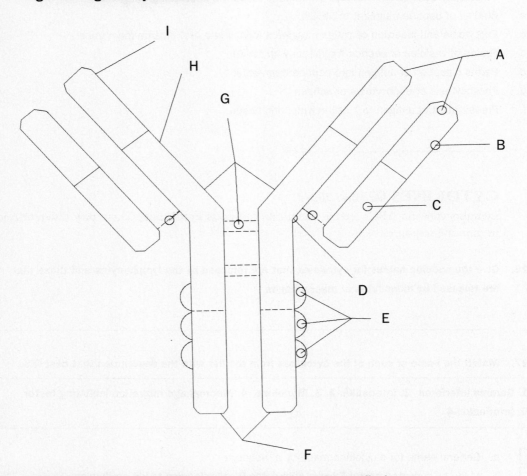

Q29. **Complete this exercise, which refers to the structure of an antibody.**

Chemically all antibodies are composed of glycoproteins, which are also known as
(a) _____ . They consist of (b) _____ (how many?) polypeptide chains.
The two heavy chains contain about (c) _____ amino acids; light chains contain
more than (d) _____ amino acids.

(e) _____ portions are diverse for different antibodies since these serve as
binding sites for different antigens. (f) _____ portions are identical for all antibodies
within the same class.

Since most antibodies have two antigen binding sites, they are said to be (g) _____ .
There are basically (h) _____ different classes of antibodies. The presence of

(i) _____ (which type?) antibodies indicates a recent infection, since they are the first ones to appear and are relatively short-lived.

Q30. **When you have answered this question, you will understand the different classes of immunoglobulin (Ig). Write the name of the related class of Ig next to each description.**

_____ a.   The first antibodies to be secreted after initial exposure to antigen, they are short-lived; destroy invading micro-organisms by agglutination and lysis.

_____ b.   The only type of Ig to cross the placenta, it provides specific resistance to newborns. Also significantly enhances phagocytosis and neutralisation of toxins in persons of all ages, since it is the most abundant type of antibody.

_____ c.   Found in secretions such as mucus, saliva, and tears, so protects against oral, vaginal, and respiratory infections.

_____ d.   Located on mast and basophil cells and involved in allergic reactions, for example, to certain foods, pollen, or bee venom.

_____ e.   Activates B cells to produce antibodies.

T LYMPHOCYTES

To fully understand how antibodies are produced in response to antigens, it is essential to recognise the roles of **T cells**. Question 31 should assist you in understanding the functions of T cells.

Q31. **Match the T cells from the list with descriptions of their roles.**

1. Delayed-type hypersensitivity cells 2. Memory T cells 3. Suppressor T cells
4. Cytotoxic T cells 5. Helper T cells

☐ a. Cells that may produce chemicals that inhibit production of B cells and T cells.

☐ b. Mediate allergic responses by secreting cytokines (such as gamma-IFN) that activate macrophages.

☐ c. Called T8 cells since developed from cells with CD8 protein; to become cytolytic, must be co-stimulated by IL-2 from T_H cells.

☐ d. Called T4 cells since developed from cells with CD4 protein; activated by APCs and co-stimulated by IL-I and IL-2; produce IL-2.

☐ e. Programmed to recognise the original invader; can initiate dramatic responses to reappearance of the intruder.

For question 32, see 📖 *Page 708*

Q32. **Describe the steps in antibody-mediated immunity, using the following key terms: activation of B cells, follicular dendritic cells, antigen-MHC-II, co-stimulation, plasma cells, four or five days, memory B cells, antibodies with identical structure to original antigen receptors, complement enzymes activated.**

_____

_____

_____

_____

IMMUNOLOGICAL MEMORY AND IMMUNISATIONS

So far you should have grasped that for the body to produce antibodies, it should be able to recognise specific antigens. The **B cells** produce **plasma cells** which produce antibodies and at the same time also give rise to **memory cells**. The memory cells play a vital role should the body encounter the same antigen at some time in the future. The **booster** dose of a vaccine can cause rapid proliferation of memory cells into plasma cells and hence a rise in antibodies.

When you have completed questions 33 and 34, you should understand the principles of immunisation.

Q33. **Complete this exercise on immunisations.**

Once a specific antigen has initiated an immune response, either by infection or by vaccination, the person produces some long-lived B and T cells called (a) _____. The level of antibody rises (b) _____ (slowly? rapidly?) after the initial immunisation. This level measured in the serum is known as the antibody (c) _____ . The antibody to rise first is (d) _____ and this is followed by (e) _____ .

Upon subsequent exposure to the same antigen, such as during another infection or by a (f) _____ dose of vaccine, memory cells provide a more intense response. Antibodies produced by this (g) _____ (primary? secondary?) response, also known as immunological memory, have a (h) _____ affinity for the antigen compared to antibodies produced in the (i) _____ response.

Q34. **Identify the types of immunity shown by the individuals below, by selecting from the answers in the box.**

1. Artificial active immunity 2. Artificial passive immunity 3. Natural active immunity **4. Natural passive immunity**

☐ a. Jim received tetanus immunoglobulins following a rusty nail injury which he sustained 10 days ago. He presented to the Accident and Emergency Department with a very serious wound infection.

☐ b. A one month old baby who is breastfed.

☐ c. A three month old baby who receives her scheduled MMR (measles–mumps–rubella) immunisation.

☐ d. An individual who has recovered from chickenpox.

Now that you have completed the section on immunity, you may find the following notes very interesting.

NOTES ON SOME ASPECTS OF IMMUNISATION

Immunisation is the method by which individuals in a population are protected from the harmful effects of bacteria and viruses (i.e specific infectious diseases) and this is achieved mainly through vaccination.

Vaccination is a way of increasing the body's resistance to diseases caused by harmful bacteria and viruses through introducing into the body a controlled amount of treated bacteria or viruses or their toxins in the form of a **vaccine.** The introduction of the vaccine into the body is known as **inoculation.** Vaccines are of two forms:

(a)   Live vaccines.

(b)   Killed vaccines.

Live vaccines

Live vaccines contain live micro-organisms that have been treated chemically and are in what is referred to as an **attenuated** form. These attenuated organisms stimulate the immune system of the body into producing antibodies. These antibodies may give lifelong immunity. Examples of live vaccines are: poliomyelitis (oral polio vaccine), measles, rubella, mumps and BCG.

Killed vaccines

Killed vaccines contain the inactivated organisms or their products. They also stimulate the body to produce its own antibodies. Examples of killed vaccines containing the inactivated organisms are: whooping cough, typhoid and inactivated poliomyelitis (IPV).

Killed vaccines containing inactivated products usually derived from toxins are: tetanus and diptheria. The chemically treated toxins are known as **toxoids**. The toxins are inactivated by formaldehyde.

Some vaccines contain **adjuvants**. These are substances that enhance the antibody response. Examples of adjuvants are aluminium phosphate and aluminium hydroxide.

Human normal immunoglobins (HNIG)

HNIG is derived from the pooled plasma of donors and contains antibodies to viruses which are currently prevalent in the general population. Immunosuppressed children exposed to measles, for example, can receive protection from **HNIG**.

Specific immunoglobins

Specific immunoglobulins are obtained from the pooled blood of convalescent patients, or those recently immunised with the relevant vaccine. It may be used for tetanus or hepatitis B. Both HNIG and specific immunoglobulin can only protect the body for a few weeks.

Recent advances

In 1988 combined **measles, mumps and rubella** (MMR) vaccine was introduced in the UK for young children. It is hoped that through this immunisation programme, the risk of rubella infection to nonimmune pregnant women will be reduced or even removed.

From October 1992, immunisation against **haemophilus influenzae type B** (HIB) became available. It is offered with the routine DPT immunisations of two, three and four months. It will also be made available to all other children under four years of age.

HIB bacteria can be a common cause of bacterial meningitis in children under five years. Other infections which can occur are epiglottitis, osteomyelitis, septic arthritis, cellulitis and septicaemia.

Immunisation procedures

(1) Observe safety aspects as for any medication to be administered.
(2) Cleaning of skin with Mediswabs containing alcohol only.
(3) Route of administration:

(a) By mouth – example, oral polio (OPV).
(b) Subcutaneous and intramuscular injection.

All vaccines, with the exception of BCG and OPV, must be given by intramuscular or deep subcutaneous injection.

Injection sites

In infants, the anterolateral aspect of the thigh or upper arm should be used. If the buttock is used, the injection should be given into the upper outer quadrant.

BCG injection is always given intradermally. A needle, size 25G, should be used. Refer to Tables 14.1 and 14.2, which give more detail about immunisation.

Table 14.1. Route of vaccine administration

Vaccine	Route of administration	Dose	Needle size
OPV	Oral	3 drops	Nil
IPV	Deep subcutaneous or intramuscular	0.5ml	23G
D/T/P and D/T	Deep subcutaneous or intramuscular	0.5ml	23G
Measles, mumps and rubella	Deep subcutaneous or intramuscular	0.5ml	23G
Typhoid	Deep subcutaneous or intramuscular	0.5ml	23G
BCG	Intradermal Infants	0.1ml 0.05ml	25G
Rabies	Deep subcutaneous or intramuscular Intradermal	1.0ml 0.1ml	23G 25G
Anthrax	Deep subcutaneous or intramuscular	0.5ml	23G
Hepatitis B	Deep subcutaneous or intramuscular	0.5ml	23G
HIB	Deep subcutaneous or intramuscular	0.5ml	23G

Table 14.2. Schedule for routine immunisation

Vaccine	Age	Notes
D/T/P and Polio, plus HIB	1st dose, 2 months; 2nd dose, 3 months; 3rd dose, 4 months	Primary course
Measles, mumps and Rubella (MMR)	12–18 months	Can be given at any age over 12 months
Booster D/T and Polio	4–5 years	
Rubella	10–14 years	Girls only
BCG	10–14 years	Interval of 3 weeks between BCG and rubella
Booster tetanus and polio	15–18 years	

Children should therefore have received the following vaccines:

By 6 months	–	3 doses of D/T/P and polio, or D/T and polio
By 18 months	–	measles/mumps/rubella
By school entry	–	4th D/T and polio; measles/mumps/rubella if missed earlier
Between 10 and 14 years	–	BCG, rubella for girls
Before leaving school	–	5th polio and tetanus

Adults should receive the following vaccines:

Women sero-negative for rubella	–	rubella
Previously unimmunised individuals	–	polio, tetanus
Individuals in high risk groups	–	hepatitis B, influenza

Conditions that do not contraindicate vaccinations

(a) Asthma, eczema, hay fever or 'snuffles'.

(b) Treatment with antibiotics or locally acting (e.g topical or inhaled) steroids.

(c) Child being breast fed.

(d) History of jaundice after birth.

(e) Under a certain weight.

(f) Over the age given in immunisation schedule.

(g) Previous history of pertussis, measles, rubella or mumps infection.

(h) Prematurity: immunisation should not be postponed.

(i) Stable neurological conditions, such as cerebral palsy and Down's syndrome.

(j) Contact with an infectious disease.

(k) Homoeopathy: the Council of the Faculty of Homoeopathy strongly supports the vaccination programme and has stated that vaccinations should be carried out in the normal way using the conventionally tested and approved vaccines, in the absence of medical contraindications.

Contraindications to vaccination

(a) Immunosuppressed children should not be given oral poliomyelitis vaccine.
(b) Hypersensitivity to egg contraindicates influenza vaccine.
(c) HIV-positive individuals should not receive BCG.

Anaphylaxis

Although not a common occurrence, anaphylactic reaction can occur as a result of vaccination and can be fatal. In the period 1978–79, in the UK, 118 cases were reported.

Acquired immune deficiency syndrome (AIDS) 📖 *Pages 712–3*

If you have grasped the basic structure and function of the immune system, you should understand the problems associated with one of the worst viral infections of mankind, this century. What follows in this study, is not a detailed description of **AIDS**, but some interesting facts which should enhance your knowledge of the immune system. You should achieve this, through working on Question 35.

Q35. Complete the following exercise on AIDS.

AIDS refers to (a) _____ _____ _____ syndrome. The condition was first recognised in the United States by Centres for Disease Control in the year (b) _____ following an increase of **two** relatively rare conditions which were found in AIDS patients. These conditions are (c) _____ _____ _____ (a specific type of respiratory infection) and (d) _____ _____ (a type of skin cancer).

The causative agent for AIDS is known as the (e) _____ _____ _____ virus. It has an incubation period (from HIV infection to full-blown AIDS) of about 7–10 (f) _____.

The virus is a type of virus known as a (g) _____, since it carries its genetic material in (h) _____ and copies this genetic coding into (i) _____ by using an enzyme called (j) _____ _____.

HIV primarily affects (k) _____ lymphocytes, since these cells display the receptor or (l) _____ proteins, and the number of lymphocytes are therefore reduced, resulting in progressive collapse of the immune system (both specific and nonspecific defence mechanisms are affected). The infected individual becomes susceptible to infection caused by organisms that are usually harmless, and this is referred to as (m) _____ infections.

Formation of antibodies in the infected person usually occurs within (n) _____ weeks after viral exposure. The presence of HIV (o) _____ is commonly used to diagnose AIDS. If a person was infected with HIV 18 days ago, the person is likely to test (p) _____ for HIV but (q) _____ (can? cannot?) transmit the virus.

It is now recognised that four main types of body fluids can transmit the virus and they are : (r) _____, _____, _____, and _____.

ALLERGIC RESPONSES, TRANSPLANTATION AND SOME MEDICAL TERMINOLOGIES 📖 *Pages 715–7*

By now you should have discovered that the immune system plays a significant role in the maintenance of an individual's health. However, there are times when instead of being beneficial to the host, the immune system may make things worse for an individual, for example those people who suffer from **hay fever** or **asthma** or those who experience the problems of rejection following transplantation.

In the last part of this study, you will meet **four** types of **allergic responses**. You will also be introduced very briefly to tissue transplantation and some medical conditions.

Q36. **Match the four types of allergic responses in the box with the correct descriptions below.**

> **1. Type I 2. Type II 3. Type III 4. Type IV**

☐ a. Known as cell-mediated reactions, or delayed-type hypersensitivity reactions, these lead to responses such as those that occur after exposure to poison ivy or after tuberculin testing.

☐ b. Antigen–antibody immune complexes trapped in tissues activate complement and lead to inflammation, as in systemic lupus erythematosus or rheumatoid arthritis.

☐ c. Caused by IgG or IgM antibodies against red blood cells or other cells, as in, for example, a response to an incompatible transfusion; called a cytotoxic reaction.

☐ d. Involves IgE produced by mast cells and basophils; effects may be localised (such as swelling of the lips) or systemic (such as acute anaphylaxis).

Questions 37 and 38 refer to transplantation.

Q37. **Complete this exercise about tissue rejection.**

Transplantation is likely to lead to tissue rejection, because the transplanted organ or tissue serves as an (a) _____ . The body tries to reject this foreign tissue by producing (b) _____ .

Q38. **Match the types of transplants in the box with descriptions below.**

> **1. Allograft 2. Isograft 3. Xenograft**

☐ a. Between animals of different species.
☐ b. The most successful type of transplant.
☐ c. Between two people with different genetic backgrounds.

Q39.   Match the condition in the box with the description below.

> **1. Autoimmune disease 2. Severe combined immune deficiency 3. Hodgkin's disease**
>
> **4. Systemic lupus erythematosus 5. Lymphangioma 6. Splenomegaly**

☐   a. A curable malignancy usually arising in lymph nodes.

☐   b. Multiple sclerosis, rheumatoid arthritis and systemic lupus erythematosus.

☐   c. Benign tumour of lymph vessels.

☐   d. Characterised by lack of both B and T cells.

☐   e. Autoimmune, inflammatory disease with skin and joint changes, and possibly serious effects on organs such as kidneys; skin lesions may resemble wolf bites, and part of the name is Latin for 'wolf'.

☐   f. Enlarged spleen.

Now that you have completed your study on the immune system, you should be able to check you progress by completing the Checkpoints Exercise.

CHECKPOINTS EXERCISE

Q40.   Arrange the following statements, which refer to activities in humoural immunity, in the correct chronological sequence.

a.   B cells develop in bone marrow or other parts of the body.

b.   B cells differentiate and divide (clone), forming plasma cells.

c.   B cells migrate to lymphoid tissue.

d.   B cells are activated by specific antigen that is presented.

e.   Antibodies are released and are specific against the antigen that activated the B cell.

_____   _____   _____   _____   _____

Q41.   Which one of the following is the correct answer?

Both the thoracic duct and the right lymphatic duct empty directly into:

a.   Axillary lymph nodes.

b.   Superior vena cava.

c.   Cisterna chyli.

d.   Subclavian arteries.

e.   Junction of internal jugular and subclavian veins.

Q42.   Which one of the following are the most numerous phagocytic cells?

a.   Monocytes.

b.   Basophils.

c.   Lymphocytes.

d.   Neutrophils.

e.   Eosinophils.

Q43. **Which one of the following is not an example of nonspecific defences?**

  a. Antigens and antibodies.

  b. Saliva.

  c. Complement.

  d. Interferon.

  e. Skin.

  f. Phagocytes.

Q44. **Which one of the following is not true of lymphocyte functions?**

  a. Helper T cells: stimulate B cells to divide and differentiate.

  b. Cytotoxic (killer) T cells: produce lymphokines that attract and activate macrophages and lymphotoxins that directly destroy antigens.

  c. Natural killer cells: suppress action of cytotoxic T cells and B cells.

  d. B cells: become plasma cells that secrete antibodies.

Q45. **Which one of the following is not a correct description of a type of allergic reaction?**

  a. Type I: anaphylactic shock, for example from exposure to iodine or bee venom.

  b. Type II: transfusion reaction in which recipient's IgG or IgM antibodies attack donor's red blood cells.

  c. Type III: involves Ag–Ab–complement complexes that cause inflammation, as in SLE or rheumatoid arthritis.

  d. Type IV: cell-mediated reactions that involve immediate responses by B cells, as in the tuberculin skin test.

Q46. **Which one of the following is a false statement about T cells?**

  a. T_c cells are best activated by antigens associated with **both MHC-I and MHC-II** molecules.

  b. T_H cells are activated by antigens associated with **MHC-II** molecules.

  c. For T_c cells to become cytolytic, they need **co-stimulation by IL-2**.

  d. Perforin is a chemical released by T_H cells.

Q47. **Which one of the following is the false statement about lymphatic vessels?**

  a. Lymph capillaries are more permeable than blood capillaries.

  b. Lymphatics have thinner walls than veins.

  c. Like arteries, lymphatics contain no valves.

  d. Lymph vessels are blind-ended.

Q48. **Which one of the following is a false statement about T cells?**

  a. Some are called memory cells.

  b. They are called T cells because they are processed in the thymus.

  c. They are involved primarily in antibody-mediated immunity.

  d. Like B cells, they originate from stem cells in the bone marrow.

Q49. **Which one of the following is a false statement?**

  a. Skeletal muscle contraction aids lymph flow.

  b. Skin is normally more effective than mucous membranes in preventing entrance of micro-organisms into the body.

  c. Interferon is produced by viruses.

  d. An allergen is an antigen, not an antibody.

Q50.   Circle 'T' (true) or 'F' (false) for the statements below.

T   F   a. Antibodies are usually composed of one light and one heavy polypeptide chain.

T   F   b. T_c cells are specially active against slowly growing bacterial diseases, some viruses, cancer cells associated with viral infections and transplanted cells.

T   F   c. Immunogenicity means the ability of an antigen to react with a specific antibody or T cell.

T   F   d. A person with autoimmune disease produces fewer than normal antibodies.

This concludes the main study on the immune system. Well done. If you now wish to test your progress in relation to many areas on the immune system, you could attempt the questions on the patient scenario.

PATIENT SCENARIO

David aged 32, is married to Jane aged 25, who has just given birth to baby Sarah via a caesarean section. A few days following the caesarean operation, Jane developed a slight bacterial wound infection, which did eventually heal satisfactorily within a couple of days. Sarah is to be breastfed.

David has been suffering from hay fever since he was eight years of age. He is allergic to grass pollen. When his hay fever flares up, he takes Triludan (an antihistamine). David has recently been diagnosed as suffering from chronic renal failure and is awaiting a kidney transplant. He is also known to be allergic to penicillin.

Q51.   Which type of resistance is Jane's bacterial infection likely to be? Give reasons for your answer.

_____

_____

_____

Q52.   Following surgery, Jane's abdominal wound is likely to show signs of inflammation. Referring to four symptoms of inflammation, explain how these are manifested.

_____

_____

_____

_____

_____

Q53.   Is hay fever a beneficial immune response by the host? Give the rationale for your answer.

_____

_____

_____

Q54.   In immunological terms, briefly explain how grass pollen is responsible for David's hay fever.

_____

_____

_____

_____

Q55.   Giving the rationale for your answer, at what time of the year is David likely to develop hay fever?

_____

_____

Q56.   Which type of immune response can be assigned to hay fever?

_____

Q57.   What is the name given to an antigen that induces an allergic response?

_____

Q58.   Discuss the physiological changes that occur in David's body during an acute episode of hay fever, and suggest how these may affect him.

_____

_____

_____

Q59.   Give a single explanation as to why Triludan relieves some of the symptoms of hay fever.

_____

_____

_____

Q60.   Name the two types of immunoglobulins that Sarah would have acquired in the first three
       months of life and suggest their likely sources. What is this type of immunity referred to as?

_____

_____

_____

Q61.   Sarah is to commence on her immunisation programme. She receives her first dose of D/T/P
       (diptheria, tetanus, pertussis) and polio at two months of age. With reference to B and T
       lymphocytes and macrophages, describe how antibodies are produced in Sarah's body
       following her first immunisation. What is this type of immunity referred to as?

_____

Q62.   Tetanus vaccine is a toxoid. Briefly explain the meaning of toxoid and suggest why it causes
       an immune response.

_____

_____

_____

Q63.   Sarah receives her second dose of D/T/P and polio at three months of age. Is this booster
       likely to give rise to a primary or a secondary response? Briefly discuss.

_____

_____

_____

To answer the following questions, see 📖 *Pages 702–15.*

Q64. From question 61, you know that antibodies are produced in response to vaccination.

a. Antibodies are known by what other names?

_____

b. Which types of antibodies first appear during a primary response?

_____

c. Assuming that Sarah's antibodies are of the same types, following the immunisation with D/T/P, briefly explain in what way these antibodies would differ in relation to the binding sites. Hint: Think of the structure of the antibody.

_____

_____

_____

d. For antibodies belonging to the same class, would you expect the constant regions to differ?

_____

Q65. David is very interested in obtaining as much information as possible with regard to his anticipated kidney transplant. For example, he wishes to know if his kidney transplant is going to be 100% successful. What sensible explanation should you give to David with reference to his transplant, bearing in mind some of the immunological responses that occur in transplantation.

_____

_____

_____

_____

Q66. One of the potential problems of transplantation is that of rejection. Discuss the immune responses associated with tissue rejection. You must describe the various T cells that are involved in this process.

_____

_____

_____

_____

_____

Q67. To reduce the risk of tissue rejection, David will receive immunosuppressant drugs and steroids. Briefly explain the possible actions of such drugs on the immune system.

_____

_____

_____

_____

_____

Q68. How would you explain to a nurse colleague the mechanism of anaphylactic shock, that might occur if David is given an injection of penicillin?

_____

_____

_____

_____

_____

Answers to questions

Q1. Lymphatic capillaries unite to form larger tubes called lymphatic vessels. They also contain valves to prevent back flow of lymph fluid. Two main vessels (thoracic and right lymphatic ducts) are involved in the drainage of lymph fluid from all parts of the body. The **thoracic duct** receives lymph from the left side of the head, neck, chest and the left upper extremity and the entire body below the ribs. The thoracic duct begins as a dilatation sac called the **cysterna chyli**, which in fact receives lymph fluid from the gastrointestinal tract and other organs. *Page 687, Figure 22.4.*

    The right lymphatic duct drains lymph from the upper right side of the body. The thoracic duct empties into the **left subclavian vein**, whilst the right lymphatic duct empties into the **right subclavian vein**.

Q2. Transporting dietary fats and protection of the body from invading micro-organisms.

Q3. a, Proteins; b, lipids; c, T; d, antibodies.

Q4. Lymph nodules are oval-shaped and consist primarily of lymphatic tissue, but are not covered by a capsule; whereas lymph nodes are also oval-shaped, but are covered with a capsule. Lymph nodules are usually solitary, whilst lymph nodes are usually in groups.

Q5. A, Afferent vessels; B, Germinal centres; C, Efferent vessels; D, Sinuses; E, Medullary cords.

Q6. A lymph node is covered by a capsule of dense connective tissue. The extensions of the connective tissue within the node are called **trabeculae**. Within the capsule is a large network of reticular fibres and fibroblasts. The parenchyma consists of **two** main areas, the **cortex** and **medulla**. In the outer cortex are lymphocytes arranged in masses called **follicles**. Each follicle contains **T cells**, **macrophages,** and **follicular dendritic cells** on the outside. During an immune response, the centre of the follicles contain **B cells** which produce **plasma cells.** In the medulla there are strands called **medullary cords** which contain lymphocytes. Each lymph node contains one or more **afferent** lymphatic vessels (these have valves that open toward the node), and one or two **efferent** vessels (these have valves that open away from the node). Lymph nodes act as filters and are assisted by macrophages; they produce lymphocytes, plasma cells and antibodies.

Q7. B cells and T cells develop from stem cells in the red bone marrow. They are also produced in lymph nodes. B cells complete their development in the marrow. Immature T cells, on the other hand, migrate to the thymus gland to develop **immunocompetence** (*Page 698).* T cells acquire several distinctive surface proteins. Some T cells also carry either CD4 or CD8.

Q8. a, upper left; b, diaphragm; c, lymphatic; d, white pulp; e, red pulp.

Q9. B lymphocyte and antibody production. Acts as a reservoir for blood, red blood cells and platelets. Plays a role in phagocytosis of micro-organisms.

Q10. a, Mediastinum; b, sternum; c, lungs; d, large; e, cortex; f, lymphocytes; g, T cells.

Q11. Nonspecific resistance comprises defence mechanisms that provide a general response against invasion by a wide range of pathogens as follows:

Skin – epidermis provides a barrier against entry of micro-organisms. This is partly due to the protein **keratin**. **Lysozyme** in perspiration can break down the bacterial cell wall, because of its antimicrobial activity. **Sebum**, an oily secretion contains unsaturated fatty acids which can inhibit growth of pathogenic bacteria and fungi.

Mucous membrane in many body systems – contains glands that secrete mucus. Mucus is slightly viscous and therefore traps foreign particles and micro-organisms.

Respiratory system – contains cilia that can propel inhaled dust and organisms to the outside environment.

Digestive tract – saliva contains lysozyme, which can destroy micro-organisms. Gastric juice contains **hydrochloric acid** which can also destroy bacteria.

Vagina – contains an acidic secretion on account of **lactic acid** produced by bacteria called Doderlein's bacilli.

The body can also produce antimicrobial substances such as transferrins, interferons, complement and properdin that can inhibit growth of bacteria or viruses as appropriate.

Phagocytosis – also provides a nonspecific defence to the host.

Q12. 5a, 8b, 1c, 2d, 4e, 3f, 6g, 7h.

Q13. a, Virus; b, I; c, Kaposi's sarcoma; d, natural killer; e, lymphocyte; f, cytolytic; g, AIDS; h, cancer.

Q14. a, Neutrophils; b, eosinophils; c, monocytes; d, macrophages; e, mononuclear phagocytic.

Q15. Role of complement – C3 is a key member of the complement system and is activated by both the classical and the alternative pathway. Once activated, it activates other complement proteins that play an important role in destroying micro-organisms. C3a contributes to the development of inflammation by causing dilatation of arterioles, increasing blood flow to the area; and the release of histamine, which increases the permeability of blood capillaries, enabling white blood cells to move in. C3b is important for opsonisation, that is the binding to the surface of micro-organisms and the interacting with the receptor on phagocytes to promote phagocytosis. Several complement proteins (*Page 693*) form the membrane attack complex and punch holes in the plasma membrane of micro-organisms, thereby causing them to rupture, a process called cytolysis.

Q16. 1a, 1b, 1c, 1d, 2e, 3f.

Q17. 5a, 2 and 7b, 6c, 4d, 1 and 4e, 8f, 1g, 3h.

Q18. Antibody-mediated immunity (also known as humoural immunity) and cell-mediated immunity.

Q19. a, lymphocytes; b, stem; c, bone marrow; d, lymph; e, T; f, perform immune functions against specific antigens, if properly stimulated; g, CD8$^+$; h, antigen receptor protein; i, bone marrow.

Q20. CMIa, AMIb, AMIc, CMId, both AMI and CMI for e.

Q21. a, Foreign; b, proteins; c, lipoproteins; d, glycoproteins; e, immunogenicity; f, reactivity; g, complete antigen or immunogen; h, hapten; i, immunogenicity; j, protein; k, allergic; l, epitopes.

Q22. There are two types of MHC antigens and they are referred to as class I and class II. Class I MHC (MHC-I) are built into the plasma membrane of all body cells, except red blood cells.

Class II (MHC-II) molecules appear on the surface of antigen presenting cells. MHC-I are associated with self antigens, the so-called endogenous antigens. MHC-II are associated with exogenous proteins and are responsible for tissue rejection.

Q23. Antigen from intruders outside body cells, such as bacteria, pollen, foods, cat hair, etc.

Q24. Macrophages, B cells and dendritic cells (including Langerhans cells in the skin).

Q25. e, d, c, a, b, f.

Q26. Those that are released by lymphocytes are known as lymphokines and those that are released by monocytes are referred to as monokines.

Q27. 3a, 5b, 2c, 1d, 4e.

Q28. A, antigen binding site; B. variable light chain; C, constant light chain; D, hinge region; E, carbohydrates; F, fragment crystallisable; G, disulphide bonds; H, constant heavy chain; I, variable heavy chain.

Q29. a, Immunoglobulins; b, four; c, 450; d, 200; e, variable; f, constant; g, bivalent; h, five; i, IgM.

Q30. IgM a, IgG b, IgA c, IgE d, IgD e.

Q31. 3a, 2b, 4c, 5d, 1e.

Q32. During activation of B cells, antigens bind to antigen receptors on their cell surface. However, their response is much more intense when antigens are first processed in follicular dendritic cells nearby and presented to them.

Antigens taken into the B cells are broken down into peptide fragments and combined with MHC-II self-antigen, and moved to the B cell surface. Helper T cells recognise the antigens MHC-II complex and respond through costimulation (e.g. producing interleukin II and other cytokines) which is needed for B cell proliferation and differentiation.

B cells proliferation and differentiation give rise to plasma cells and this is also influenced by interleukin II from the macrophages. The plasma cells produce antibodies for four to five days until they die.

The antibodies secreted are identical in their specificity to the antigen receptor displayed by the progenitor B cell that responded to the antigen in the first place. Antibodies that are produced enter the circulation and form antigen-antibody complexes. The latter can activate complement enzymes components.

The B cells that do not differentiate into plasma cells remain as memory B cells.

Q33. a, Memory cells; b, slowly; c, titre; d, IgM; e, IgG; f, booster; g, secondary; h, higher; i, primary.

Q34. 2a, 4b, 1c, 3d.

Q35. a, Acquired immune deficiency; b, 1981; c, Pneumocystis carinii pneumonia; d, Kaposi's sarcoma; e, human immunodeficiency virus; f, years; g, retrovirus; h, RNA; i, DNA; j, reverse transcriptase; k, T-helper; l, docking CD4; M, opportunistic; n, 3-20 weeks; o, antibodies; p, negative; q, can; r, blood, semen, vaginal fluid, breast milk.

Q36. 4a, 3b, 2c, 1d.

Q37. a, Antigen, b, antibodies or T lymphocytes against the tissues.

Q38.   3a, 2b, 1c.

Q39.   3a, 1b, 5c, 2d, 4e, 6f.

Q40.   a, c, d, b, e.

Q41.   e.

Q42.   d.

Q43.   a.

Q44.   c.

Q45.   d.

Q46.   d.

Q47.   c.

Q48.   c.

Q49.   c.

Q50.   Fa, Tb, Fc, Fd.

Q51.   It is nonspecific resistance. This is because it comprises defence mechanisms that provide a general response against a wide range of pathogens. No antibodies are produced and therefore no immunity is acquired. Consequently Jane is likely to become infected again with the same type of organisms at any time in the future.

Q52.   Four symptoms are: redness, swelling, pain and heat.

Redness – this is due to vasodilatation of blood vessels in the area of the incision. Therefore more blood flows through to the damaged area and brings with it important defensive mediators such as antibodies, phagocytes and clotting factors. There is also increased permeability of blood vessels which allows proteins to move into the area. Amongst the chemicals that contribute to vasodilatation and increased permeability are histamine, kinins, prostaglandins, leukotrienes and complement.

Swelling – this is obviously due to the increase in blood flow and the increased permeability that allows more blood to move from blood vessels into the tissue spaces. This swelling can also be called **oedema**.

Pain – this can result from injury of nerve fibres or from irritation by toxic chemicals from micro-organisms. Many of the chemical mediators such as kinins or prostaglandins can affect nerve endings directly and induce pain. Pain can also occur as a result of pressure from oedema.

One reason why **aspirin** is an effective analgesic is because it interferes with the synthesis of **prostaglandins**.

Heat – this is also due to the dilatation of arterioles and increased permeability of capillaries, which bring to the area a large amount of warm blood. The increase in local temperature causes an increase in reactions, that produce additional heat.

Q53.   It is not beneficial to the host, as there is indeed no special benefit to be gained by such an abnormal immune response. The severity of the symptoms varies from individual to individual, but the common symptoms are runny nose, itchy eyes, cough, irritation in the throat, wheeziness and itchiness of mucous membranes of the respiratory tract, causing increased production of mucus.

Q54. Grass pollen, which in this case can also be called an allergen, acts as the antigen and triggers an immune response. The antibodies that are producd are IgE. IgE causes mast cells to rupture, thus releasing **histamine**. It is the histamine that gives rise to the various signs and symptoms of hay fever. Histamine increases the permeability of the capillaries, thus allowing proteins to leak into the local tissues, in this case, the mucosa of the respiratory tract. This can cause swelling of the mucosa and increases the secretion of mucus by the goblet cells. Histamine can also cause bronchoconstriction, which can lead to wheeziness.

You can now appreciate the reason why **antihistamine** is used in the management of allergic reations.

Q55. Most likely to get hay fever in late spring and early summer, because this is the time when grass is likely to flower and therefore produce pollen.

Q56. Hay fever occurs as a result of humoural immunity.

Q57. An allergen.

Q58. This has been explained in question 54.

Q59. Triludan is an antihistamine and it therefore neutralises the histamine that has been released. It is reported to be non-sedating. An adult is usually prescribed 60mg twice daily.

Q60. Sarah would have received IgG which was passed from the mother via the placenta. Since Sarah is also breast-fed, she would receive IgA from the colostrum. Both of these antibodies are in this case acquired as a result of **natural passive immunity**.

Q61. Active artificial immunity.

Q62. A toxoid is a chemically treated toxin of micro-organisms, which when administered in the body can stimulate the body to produce its own antibodies (promotes active artificial immunity). The toxins are usually inactivated by formaldehyde.

Q63. This gives rise to a secondary response. By now Sarah's body should have both B and T memory cells to D/T/P and following the booster dose, the memory cells can proliferate rapidly and give rise to specific antibodies. Antibodies produced during a secondary response have a higher affinity for the antigen than those secreted during a primary response.

Q64. a. Immunoglobulins.
b. IgM.
c. These antibodies would differ at their variable regions which contain the antigen binding site. The variable region is different for each kind of antibody. How they differ would be in their primary structure, that is the sequence of amino acid in the chain. A change in the primary structure will obviously change the three-dimensional structure and therefore will alter the configuration of the antigen binding site.
d. No.

Q65. This is a very difficult question to tackle, even for the most experienced nurse, but patients who are awaiting a transplant do ask various questions relating to transplantation, and obviously the 'one million dollar question' 'is: 'Is the transplant likely to be successful ?'

David might not have specific knowledge related to human tissue transplant and its medical and surgical management. He might appreciate that the most successful transplants are autografts and isografts. As he is waiting for a kidney, it is most likely to be an allograft (📖 *pages 716–7)* and consequently there will be the problem of rejection. The tissue rejection response depends on how closely matched the MHC (HLA) antigens are between donor and recipient.

David's immune system will recognise the proteins in the transplanted kidney as foreign and therefore trigger both CMI and AMI against them. Cytotoxic T cells recognise the foreign antigens combined with MHC-I molecules on the surface of cells of a tissue transplant. They can activate phagocytic cells and this causes inflammation that destroys the transplant.

To reduce the risk of tissue rejection, David should be given explanations as to the medication that is used to suppress the immune response. These drugs are known as **immunosuppressants.**

Information should be clearly presented to David, in a manner that will promote understanding, but should not increase the level of stress and anxiety. The facts should be presented as they are, as it is not in the best interest of the individual for the nurse to be economical with the truth. The patient has a right to know the facts about his illness. A good rapport is essential between the nurse and David. Most kidney units operate within a multidisciplinary team approach.

Q66. This is a cell-mediated immune response. The foreign tissue, the antigen, is first recognised by T cell receptors of a small number of T cells. This is the first signal in the activation of the T cell. A second signal, the co-stimulator, is also needed and the T cell becomes activated. It can now start to proliferate and differentiate, producing **clones** of cells that can now recognise the same antigens. In this process, different types of T cells are produced. They are helper T cells, cytotoxic T cells, suppressor T cells and memory T cells. Helper T cells secrete interleukin-2, an important co-stimulator for cytotoxic T cells, the T cells which are mostly involved in tissue rejection. Cytotoxic T cells are also known as killer T cells, and they recognise foreign antigen combined with MHC-I molecules on the surfaces of body cells of the transplant. Maximal activation of cytotoxic T cells requires presentation of antigen associated with both MHC-I and MHC-II molecules.

Cytotoxic cells employ **two** killing mechanisms. The first is the release of granules containing **perforin** which forms holes in the plasma membrane of the target cells, therefore destroying them by **cytolysis.**

The second mechanism is the secretion of **lymphotoxin** that activates damaging enzymes within the target cells. This interferes with DNA, causing fragmentation, and therefore the target cells die.

Cytotoxic T cells promote the inflammatory processes within the area by secretion of gamma-interferon which activates neutrophils and macrophages, enhancing phagocytic activity.

Q67. Many of the immunosuppressants work by depressing the bone marrow and thereby reducing the number of T and B lymphocytes. In so doing, the immune responses (both AMI and CMI are affected) are diminished. The medications are not specific and they can therefore destroy or interfere with the production of other important cells, such as erythrocytes and platelets.

One immunosuppressant used widely is **azathioprine** (Imuran®) and although its precise mechanism of action is not determined, it is believed that it antagonises purine metabolism and appears to inhibit DNA, RNA and normal protein synthesis in rapidly growing cells and suppresses T cell effects before transplantation (i.e during the induction phase of the antibody response). It is usually given 1 to 5 days before kidney transplantation and restarted within 24 hours post-transplantation. Side effects are many, and may include: nausea, vomiting, anorexia, diarrhoea, leukopenia, various types of anaemia, thrombocytopenia and alopecia.

Steroids may also be used as immunosuppressants and the one commonly used is **prednisolone.** As it may be administered in large doses, side effects may appear very quickly. For example, the classical 'moon face' shape may occur, and there is also increased breakdown of tissue proteins, especially in muscles of the lower limbs. This can cause severe weakness and affect mobility. One immunosuppressant called **cyclosporine** is also favoured, as it inhibits secretion of IL-2 by helper T cells, and has only a minimal effect on B cells. It therefore still maintains resistance against some infections.

Due to the immunosuppressive effects, the patient becomes very susceptible to opportunistic infections.

Q68. Anaphylactic shock is a **Type I** hypersensitivity reaction and is a life-threatening emergency. It can occur within a few minutes after the person has been administered the allergen.

Penicillin by itself does not trigger an immune response, but in a person such as David who is allergic, the penicillin combines with proteins in his body and forms a complex which is **immunogenic.** In this case, penicillin is acting as a **hapten**. As David is allergic to penicillin, his body contains IgE antibodies that bind to the surface of mast cells and basophils. If he is administered penicillin, this interacts with IgE antibodies, which in turn cause mast cells to degranulate and release **histamine**, a mediator of anaphylaxis. Other mediators are prostaglandins, leukotrienes and kinins.

The mediators are powerful vasodilators, and they therefore cause vasodilatation of blood vessels. They increase blood capillary permeability, increase smooth muscle contraction of the bronchioles and increase mucus secretion. Constriction of the bronchioles may cause wheeziness and difficulty with breathing.

Severe anaphylactic shock can cause swelling of the lips, tongue and glottis, and this can give rise to **asphyxia**. Circulatory collapse (low blood pressure, reduced cardiac output) can also occur.

The management of anaphylactic shock includes administration of adrenaline by injection. This relaxes the smooth muscles of the bronchioles and assists with breathing. For severe swelling of the glottis, an airway should be provided, e.g by an emergency tracheostomy. Hydrocortisone (a steroid) may also be administered by injection. Antihistamines may also be given. To combat hypovolaemic shock, intravenous fluids are also administered. Oxygen therapy may also assist with breathing.

As caring professionals, nurses must always ask patients when planning their care, if they are allergic to any medications, foods or any other substance. They should ensure that everyone in the multidisciplinary team is aware of this. Nurses should also perhaps be very cautious when administering an antibiotic to a new patient, especially if it is by the intravenous route. It is also imperative that they are aware of the symptoms of anaphylactic shock and are able to provide cardiopulmonary resuscitation should this be required.

Overview and key terms

The respiratory system

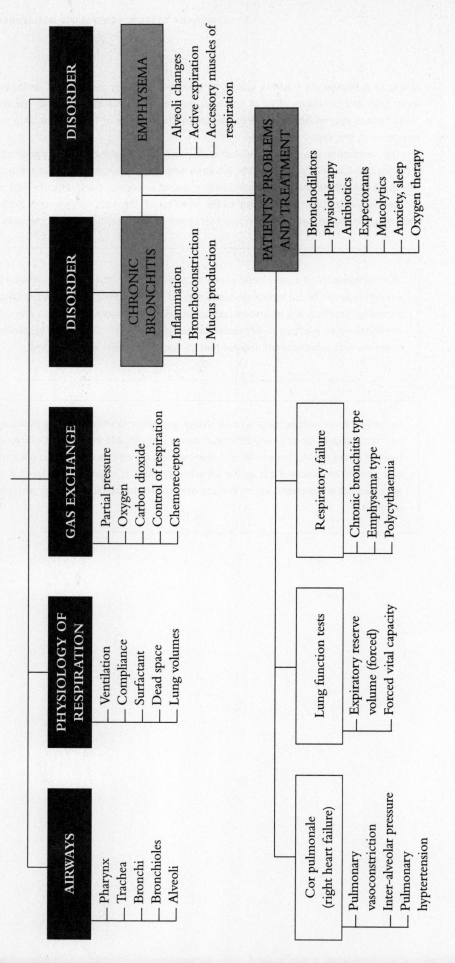

15. The Respiratory System

Learning outcomes

1. To understand basic lung structure and function.

2. To describe the respiratory and other changes that occur as a result of chronic bronchitis and emphysema.

3. To relate these changes to the problems that a sufferer of these diseases may exhibit.

4. To explain the rationale for the care and treatment in chronic bronchitis and emphysema.

5. To explain the long-term consequences of these conditions.

Chapter 23

INTRODUCTION

Respiratory disorders are very common in the UK. They range from the simple cold to serious conditions, such as pneumonia and bronchitis. The latter provides the focus for the patient scenario in this chapter. It was the association with our climate that led to bronchitis being called the 'English disease'.

The chapter begins with questions on several topics that will help you to explore the relevant anatomy and physiology of the respiratory system. These begin with the upper airways and then the lungs. The mechanics of lung movements are dealt with next, and then there are some questions on gas exchange and the transport of gases in the blood. The intake of gases like oxygen, and the excretion of carbon dioxide, are the prime purpose of the lungs. Finally, there are some questions that deal with the neurological control of breathing.

This knowledge is then used to link to, and describe, the nature of bronchitis; and examine why it produces the sorts of patient problems that it does. Following this, some aspects of the care and treatment of patients with chronic bronchitis are discussed. The chapter ends by briefly dealing with two complications of chronic bronchitis – respiratory failure and heart disease (cor pulmonale), a topic that was also dealt with in the cardiovascular chapter.

THE UPPER AND LOWER AIRWAYS 📖 *Pages 721–36*

Q1.   Write 'L' (laryngopharynx), 'N' (nasopharynx), or 'O' (oropharynx) to indicate the locations of each of the following structures.

☐   a. Adenoids.

☐   b. Palatine tonsils.

☐   c. Lingual tonsils.

☐   d. Opening (fauces) from oral cavity.

☐   e. Opening into larynx and oesophagus.

Q2.   On Figure 15.1, cover the key and identify all structures associated with the nose, palate, pharynx, and larynx.

Q3.   Explain how the larynx prevents food from entering the trachea. (Hint: notice the arrow on Figure 15.1).

_____

_____

_____

Figure 15.1.
Sagittal section of
the right side of the
head with the nasal
septum removed.

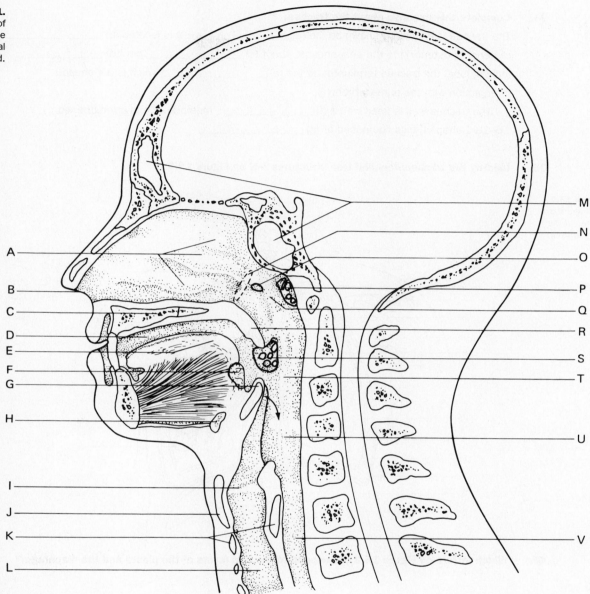

Figure 15.1.
Sagittal section of the right side of the head with the nasal septum removed.

KEY

A. Conchae

B. External naris

C. Hard palate

D. Oral cavity

E. Tongue

F. Lingual tonsil

G. Epiglottis

H. Hyoid bone

I. Vocal folds (true vocal cords)

J. Thyroid cartilage

K. Cricoid cartilage

L. Trachea

M. Paranasal sinuses

N. Internal naris

O. Orifice of auditory tube

P. Pharyngeal tonsil (adenoid)

Q Nasopharynx

R. Soft palate

S. Palatine tonsil

T. Oropharynx

U. Laryngopharynx

V. Oesophagus

Q4. **Complete this exercise about the trachea.**

The trachea is commonly known as the (a) _____ . It is located (b) _____ (anterior? posterior?) to the oesophagus. About (c) _____ cm ((d) _____ inches) long, the trachea terminates at the (e) _____ , which is a Y-shaped intersection with the primary bronchi.

The trachea wall is lined with a (f) _____ membrane, and strengthened by 16–18 C-shaped rings composed of (g) _____ .

Q5. **Identify the tracheobronchial tree structures J–N on Figure 15.2.**

Figure 15.2.
Diagram of structures of the respiratory system.

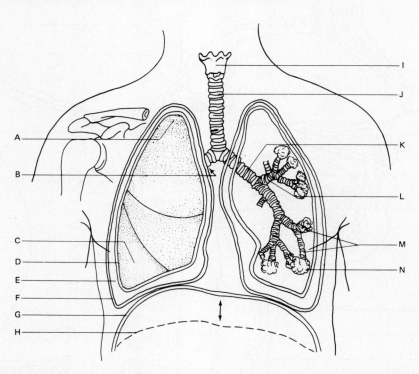

Q6. **Which letters on Figure 15.2 correspond to the two layers of the pleura and the diaphragm?**

_____

Q7. **Answer these questions about the lungs. (As you do the exercise, locate the parts of the lung on Figure 15.2.)**

The broad inferior portion of the lung that sits on the diaphragm is called the (a) _____ . The upper narrow apex of each lung extends just superior to the (b) _____ . The costal surfaces lie against the (c) _____ .

Along the mediastinal surface is the (d) _____ , where the root of the lung is located. This root consists of (e) _____ .

Answer these questions with **right** or **left.** In which lung is the cardiac notch located? (f) _____ . Which lung has two lobes and so only two lobar bronchi? (g) _____ . Which lung has a horizontal fissure? (h) _____ .

Write 'S' (superior), 'M' (middle) and 'I' (inferior) on the three lobes of the right lung, on Figure 15.2.

Figure 15.3.
Diagram of alveoli
and pulmonary
apillary. The insert
enlarges the
alveolar–capillary
membrane.

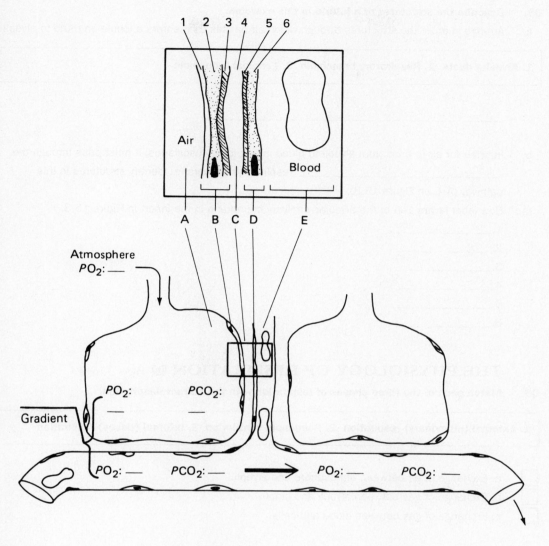

KEY

A. Alveolus

B. Alveolar wall

C. Interstitial space

D. Capillary wall

E. Blood plasma and blood cells

Q8. **Describe the structures of a lobule in this exercise.**

a. Arrange in order the structures through which air passes as it enters a lobule en route to alveoli.

| **1. Alveolar ducts 2. Respiratory bronchiole 3. Terminal bronchiole** |

_____ _____ _____

b. In order for air to pass from alveoli to blood in pulmonary capillaries, it must pass through the
_____ – _____ (respiratory) membrane. Identify structures in this
pathway (A–E on Figure 15.3).

c. Now label layers 1–6 of the alveolar–capillary membrane in the insert in Figure 15.3.

1._____ .

2._____ .

3._____ .

4._____ .

5._____ .

6._____ .

THE PHYSIOLOGY OF RESPIRATION 📖 *Pages 736–43*

Q9. **Match each of the three phases of respiration with the correct description.**

| **1. External (pulmonary) respiration 2. Pulmonary ventilation 3. Internal (tissue) respiration** |

☐ a. Exchange of air between atmosphere and alveoli.

☐ b. Exchange of gas between alveoli and blood.

☐ c. Exchange of gas between blood and cells.

Q10. **Refer to** 📖 *Page 739, Figure 23.14,* **and describe the process of ventilation in this exercise.**
In diagram (**a**), just before the start of inspiration, pressure within the lungs (called
(a) _____) is (b) _____ mmHg. This is (c) _____ (more
than? less than? the same as?) atmospheric pressure.

At the same time, pressure within the pleural cavity (called (d) _____ pressure)
is (e) _____ mmHg. This is (f) _____ (more than? less than? the same
as?) alveolar and atmospheric pressure.

The first step in inspiration occurs as the muscles in the floor and walls of the thorax
contract. These are the (g) _____ and (h) _____ muscles. Note in
diagram (**b**) that the size of the thorax (i) _____ (increases? decreases?). Since the
two layers of pleura tend to adhere to one another, the lungs will (j) _____
(increase? decrease?) in size also.

Increase in volume of a closed space such as the pleural cavity causes the pressure there
to (k) _____ (increase? decrease?) to (l) _____ mmHg. Since the lungs
also increase in size (due to pleural cohesion), alveolar pressure also (m) _____

(increases? decreases?) to (n) _____ mmHg. This inverse relationship between volume and pressure is a statement of (o) _____ 's Law.

A pressure gradient is now established. Air flows from a high pressure area (p) _____ (alveoli? atmosphere?) to a low pressure area (q) _____ (alveoli? atmosphere?). So air flows (r) _____ (into? out of?) the lungs. Thus (s) _____ (inspiration? expiration?) occurs. By the end of inspiration, sufficient air will have moved into the lungs to make pressure there equal to atmospheric pressure, that is (t) _____ mmHg

The process of inspiration is (u) _____ (active? passive?), whereas expiration is normally (v) _____ (active? passive?). In certain respiratory disorders, such as chronic bronchitis, accessory muscles help to force air out. Name two of these: (w) _____ and (x) _____ .

Q11. Answer these questions about compliance.

Imagine trying to blow up a new balloon. Initially, the balloon resists your efforts. Compliance is the ability of a substance to yield elastically to a force; in this case, it is the ease with which a balloon can be inflated. So a new balloon has a (a) _____ (high? low?) level of compliance, whereas a balloon that has been inflated many times has (b) _____ (high? low?) compliance.

Similarly, alveoli that inflate easily have (c) _____ (high? low?) compliance. The presence of a coating called (d) _____ lining the inside of alveoli prevents alveolar walls from sticking together during ventilation, and so (e) _____ (increases? decreases?) compliance.

Surfactant production is especially developed during the final weeks before birth. A premature infant may lack adequate surfactant; this disorder is known as (f) _____ .

Collapse of all or part of a lung may occur as a result of lack of surfactant or other factors. This lung collapse is known as (g) _____ .

Q12. Of the total amount of air that enters the lungs with each breath, about (a) _____ (99%? 70%? 30%? 5%?) actually enters the alveoli. The remaining amount of air is much like the last portion of a crowd trying to rush into a store. It does not succeed in entering the alveoli during an inspiration, but just reaches the airways and then is quickly ushered out during the next expiration. Such air is known as anatomic (b) _____ and constitutes about (c) _____ ml of a typical breath.

Q13. Match the lung volumes and capacities with the descriptions given. You may find it helpful to refer to 📖 *Page 742, Figure 23.16.*

> **1. Expiratory reserve volume 2. Total lung capacity 3. Functional residual capacity 4. Tidal volume 5. Inspiratory reserve volume 6. Vital capacity 7. Residual volume**

☐ a. This is the amount of air taken in with each inspiration during normal breathing.

☐ b. At the end of a normal expiration, this is the volume of air left in the lungs. Emphysemics who have lost elastic recoil of their lungs cannot exhale adequately, so this volume will be large.

☐ c. Forced exhalation can remove some of the air in the functional residual capacity. This is the maximum volume of air that can be expired beyond normal expiration. This volume will be small in emphysema patients.

☐ d. Even after the most strenuous expiratory effort, some air still remains in the lungs; this amount cannot be removed voluntarily.

☐ e. This is the volume of air that represents a person's maximum breathing ability. It is the sum of 1, 4, and 5.

☐ f. Adding 7 to 6 gives this.

☐ g. This is the excess air a person can take in after a normal inhalation.

GAS EXCHANGE AND TRANSPORT 📖 *Pages 743–51*

Q14. **Answer these questions about external and internal respiration.**

A primary factor in the diffusion of gas across a membrane is the difference in concentration of the gas (reflected by (a) _____ pressure) on the two sides of the membrane.

On the left side of Figure 15.3, write values for pO_2 (in mmHg) in each of the following areas (*see* 📖 *Page 745, Figure 23.17* for help):

Atmospheric air

Alveolar air (note that this value is lower than for atmospheric pO_2 since some alveolar O_2 enters blood).

Blood entering lungs.

Calculate the pO_2 difference (gradient) between alveolar air and blood entering lungs (b):

_____ mmHg – _____ mmHg = _____ mmHg

Three other factors that increase exchange of gases between alveoli and blood are:

(c) _____ (large? small?) surface area of lungs; (d) _____ (thick? thin?) respiratory membrane; and (e) _____ (increased? decreased?) blood flow through lungs (as in exercise).

By the time blood leaves the lungs to return to the heart and systemic arteries, its pO_2 is normally (f) _____ (greater than? the same as? less than?) pO_2 of alveoli. Write the correct value on Figure 15.3.

Now fill in all three pcO_2 values on Figure 15.3.

Q15. **Answer these questions about oxygen transport.** 📖 *Page 746 Figure 23.18.*

One hundred millilitres of blood contains about (a) _____ ml of oxygen. Of this, about 19.7 ml is carried as (b) _____ . Only a small amount of oxygen is carried in the dissolved state, since oxygen has a (c) _____ (high? low?) solubility in blood or water.

Oxygen is attached to the (d) _____ atoms in haemoglobin. The symbol for oxyhaemoglobin is (e) _____ . When haemoglobin carries all of the oxygen it can hold, it is said to be fully (f) _____ . High pO_2 in alveoli will tend to (g) _____ (increase? decrease?) oxygen saturation of haemoglobin.

Q16. **Complete this exercise about transport of carbon dioxide.**

Write the percentage of CO_2 normally carried in each of these forms: (a) _____ % is present in bicarbonate ion (HCO_3^-), (b) _____ % is bound to the globin portion of haemoglobin, and (c) _____ % is dissolved in plasma.

Carbon dioxide (CO_2) produced by cells of your body diffuses into red cells (RBCs) and combines with water to form (d) _____ . Carbonic acid tends to dissociate into two products. One is H^+, which binds to (e) _____ . The other product is (f) _____ , which is carried in (g) _____ (RBCs? plasma?) in exchange for a (h) _____ (K^+? Cl^-?) ion that shifts into the RBC.

THE CONTROL OF RESPIRATION 📖 *Pages 750–5*

Q17. **Complete the table about respiratory control areas. Indicate whether the area is located in the medulla (M) or pons (P).**

Name	M/P	Function
a.	M	Controls rhythm; consists of inspiratory and expiratory areas
Pneumotaxic	b.	c.
d.	e.	Prolongs inspiration and inhibits expiration

Q18. **Answer these questions about respiratory control.**

The main chemical change that stimulates respiration is an increase in blood level of (a) _____ , which is directly related to a (b) _____ (decrease in pO_2? increase in pCO_2?) of blood. Cells most sensitive to changes in blood CO_2 are located in the (c) _____ (medulla? pons? aorta and carotid arteries?).

An increase in arterial blood pCO_2 is called (d) _____ . Write an arterial pCO_2 value that is hypercapnic: (e) _____ . (f) _____ mmHg (even slight? only severe?) hypercapnia will stimulate the respiratory system, leading to (g) _____ (hyper? hypo?)-ventilation.

State two locations of chemoreceptors sensitive to changes in pO_2: (h) _____ and (i) _____ . (j) _____ (even slight? only large?) decreases in the pO_2 level of blood will stimulate these chemoreceptors and lead to hyperventilation. Give an example of a pO_2 level low enough to evoke such a response. (k) _____ mmHg.

Increase in body temperature (as in fever), as well as stretching of the anal sphincter, will cause (l) _____ -crease in the respiratory rate.

Take a deep breath. Imagine the (m) _____ receptors in your airways being stimulated. These will cause (n) _____ (excitation? inhibition?) of the inspiratory and apneustic areas, resulting in expiration. This reflex, known as the (o) _____ reflex, prevents overinflation of the lungs.

CHECKPOINTS EXERCISE

Q19. Which passageway is common to both the respiratory and digestive systems?

_____

Q20. Name the air passages between the larynx and the alveoli.

_____

Q21. What are the two muscles of respiration called?

_____

Q22. What is the driving force for the uptake of oxygen from the alveoli into the lungs?

_____

Q23. What is the tidal volume?

_____

Q24. What is the name for the maximum amount of air that can be inspired?

_____

Q25. What substance in red blood cells carries oxygen?

_____

Q26. Where is the control (respiratory) centre located?

_____

Q27. A rise in which gas provides the main stimulus to respiration?

_____

PATIENT SCENARIO

Mr Broster is a 55-year-old train driver, who suffers from chronic bronchitis. He has been a heavy cigarette smoker for over 30 years, and for the last ten years has tended to suffer from a 'winter cough'.

This cough has not always disappeared during the summer,in the past 2–3 years, and now he has a year-round cough. This is especially bad in the morning – when he suffers from tightness in the chest and **dyspnoea** (dys = difficulty, i.e. with breathing).

This tends to improve as the day wears on, as Mr Broster expectorates a large amount of sputum. At the present time, his sputum shows all the signs of an added infection – something that occasionally adds to chronic bronchitis.

Mr Broster lives at home with his wife. They have no children, but have a number of relatives living close by.

CHRONIC BRONCHITIS

Through many years of breathing in cigarette smoke and/or industrial pollution, Mr Broster has inflamed and damaged his air passages, and the ciliated columnar epithelial lining.

Q28.   What are the characteristic features when tissue becomes inflamed? 📖 *Page 695*

_____

_____

These changes are due to an increased blood flow **(vasodilatation).** The blood vessels that supply the lining of the bronchi have increased in diameter. Additionally, the capillaries have an increased permeability.

Q29.   What substances normally escape through the wall of the capillary? 📖 *Pages 632–3*

_____

This means that blood cells and proteins are normally contained within the circulatory system. With increased permeability, these can now escape into the tissues, allowing white blood cells to pursue foreign invaders.

Q30.   What action do white blood cells have on foreign substances? 📖 *Page 697*

_____

_____

The increased blood flow also helps to remove the white cells, and foreign invaders such as bacteria.

The chemicals that mediate these changes include histamine, prostaglandins and kinins. These last two are involved in the transmission of pain impulses. Histamine can be directly counteracted by substances called **anti-histamines** (creams, tablets or injections), and these are used to dispel the inflammatory changes resulting from allergic reactions such as skin rashes. But inflammation (and swelling) in a hollow tube tends to lead to narrowing, and in this case the trapping of air (emphysema).

Bronchial narrowing

Swelling is probably one of the most important consequences of these inflammatory changes. The internal diameter of the bronchi is now narrowed.

Q31. **What effect is this going to have on external respiration?** 📖 *Page 744–5*

_____

_____

Q32. **What changes will occur in the blood gases, as a result of reduced air flow?** 📖 *Page 746–7*

_____

_____

Q33. **What effect will these gas changes have on respiration?** 📖 *Page 752–3*

_____

_____

_____

This is another example of feedback control, in the attempt to regulate homeostasis 📖 *Page 10*. The second reason for a decrease in the diameter of the air passages is an accumulation of mucus, which clogs the bronchioles.

Q34. **What structures produce mucus in the bronchi and bronchioles? And what is the function of mucus?** 📖 *Pages 724 & 729*

_____

_____

_____

It is the accumulation of mucus that provides the basis for Mr Broster's cough, and the expectoration of sputum. Mucus is normally colourless and clear in appearance, but when it becomes infected by bacteria – as is now the case with Mr Broster – it turns a characteristic yellow/green colour. It is an important nursing role to observe and report on these colour changes. An infected sputum requires treatment with antibiotics.

At the same time as there is an increase in mucus production, there is usually a loss of cilia. These microscopic hair-like processes are another part of the lung's defence against foreign invaders. They trap, and propel upwards, any such material. Their loss means that lung irritants – in smoke, etc. – will become trapped in the lungs.

Emphysema

This word literally means 'inflation', and the condition occurs as a result of a collection of air in the tissues. It refers to the destruction of lung tissue (the alveoli), and thus the formation of large pockets of air in the lung tissue (see Figure 15.4).

Figure 15.4.
Normal and emphysematous alveoli. Note that the normal architecture of the alveoli has now been lost.

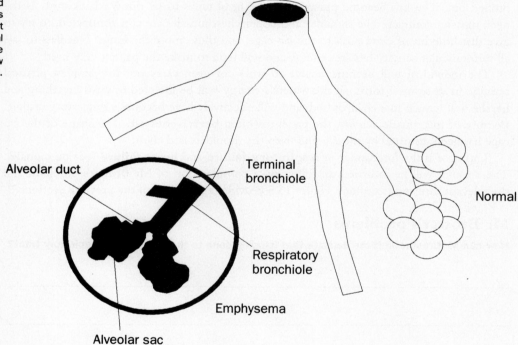

Alveolar duct

Terminal bronchiole

Normal

Respiratory bronchiole

Emphysema

Alveolar sac

Q35. **What is the effect of this change on gas exchange?**

_____

_____

_____

Emphysema represents a worsening of the chronic bronchitic's condition. Why has emphysema occurred? Because of the narrowing in the bronchi and bronchioles (from inflammatory changes and mucus accumulation), air flow out of the alveoli is reduced, and because air is still coming in – with each inspiration – the volume of air in the alveoli is increased. Thus – like an over-inflated balloon – the alveoli walls are stretched, and begin to break down, giving rise to the appearance in Figure 15.4.

Q36.   What takes place during the normal process of expiration? 📖 *Page 738–9*

_____

_____

_____

In emphysema, expiration becomes an **active** process, so that air which is trapped can be pushed out. The lips become pursed, and the head tends to be thrown backwards as the neck muscles contract. The shoulder and upper chest muscles are also contracted, to try to give that little bit of extra push to the rib cage, and thus empty the lungs. Needless to say, all this muscular activity requires energy and will tend to make the patient very tired.

The individual will become unable to work, or even carry out the simplest physical activity. In its severest form, all the patient's energy will be directed towards breathing and he/she will remain in a chair or bed; and will effectively have become a respiratory cripple. Because of this muscle activity, the patient is often **barrel-chested.** The shape of the rib cage has been distorted by muscle pull from the shoulders and chest.

This state is the forerunner of **respiratory failure** and **heart failure** (cor pulmonale). These topics will be returned to, following a consideration of Mr Broster's problems and the relevant care and treatment. Figure 15.5 provides a summary of the previous sections.

Mr Broster's problems

Q37.   How can Mr Broster limit the damage that is being done to the lining of his respiratory tract?

_____

_____

_____

_____

Q38.   Bronchodilator drugs work by stimulating the sympathetic nervous system. What other effects are they likely to have on Mr Broster? 📖 *Page 512, Exhibit 17.3.*

_____

_____

_____

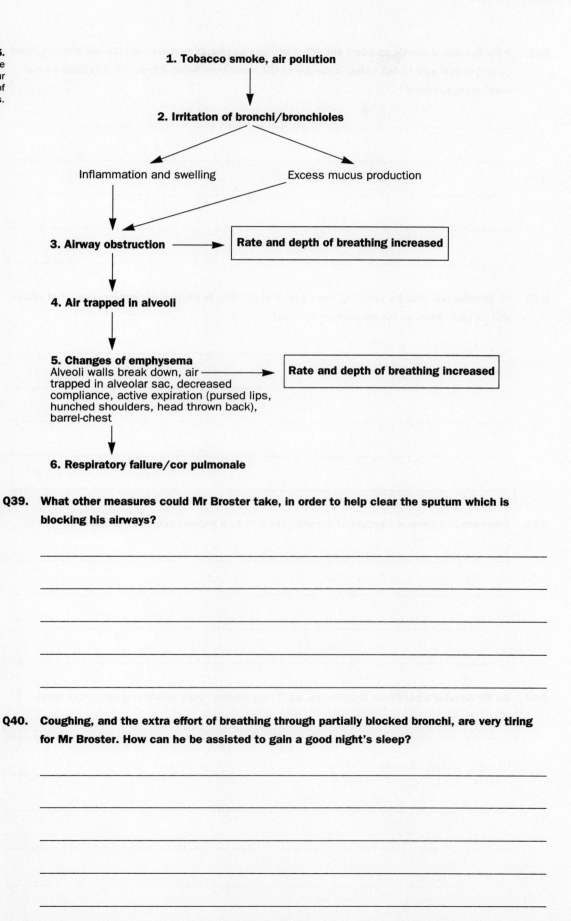

Figure 15.5.
A summary of the changes that occur the progression of chronic bronchitis.

1. Tobacco smoke, air pollution

2. Irritation of bronchi/bronchioles

Inflammation and swelling

Excess mucus production

3. Airway obstruction → **Rate and depth of breathing increased**

4. Air trapped in alveoli

5. Changes of emphysema
Alveoli walls break down, air trapped in alveolar sac, decreased compliance, active expiration (pursed lips, hunched shoulders, head thrown back), barrel-chest

Rate and depth of breathing increased

6. Respiratory failure/cor pulmonale

Q39. What other measures could Mr Broster take, in order to help clear the sputum which is blocking his airways?

_____

_____

_____

_____

_____

Q40. Coughing, and the extra effort of breathing through partially blocked bronchi, are very tiring for Mr Broster. How can he be assisted to gain a good night's sleep?

_____

_____

_____

_____

_____

Q41. If Mr Broster is unable to carry out adequate gas exchange because of blocked airways, then he will turn a pale bluish colour because of CO_2 retention. What effect will this have on his respiratory system?

_____

_____

_____

_____

Q42. Mr Broster will also be suffering from a lack of O_2. Why is oxygen necessary, and what effect will its lack have on his respiratory system?

_____

_____

_____

_____

_____

Q43. What are the general dangers of administering O_2 to a patient such as Mr Broster?

_____

_____

_____

_____

Q44. As Mr Broster's condition progresses, so it may worsen. How would you recognise this?

_____

_____

_____

_____

_____

Q45. One way of testing the functional capacity of Mr Broster's lungs is to measure the amount that he is able to exhale forcibly. What is this known as? 📖 *Page 742*

_____

_____

_____

_____

Q46. Cor pulmonale (right heart failure) is a complication of chronic bronchitis and emphysema. Can you say how lung disease gives rise to cor pulmonale, and what are the problems that Mr Broster will exhibit if he develops this condition.

_____

_____

_____

_____

_____

QUESTIONS FOR DISCUSSION

1. Using a nursing model, such as the Roper ADL format, devise a plan of care for Mr Broster, on his admission to hospital.

2. Find out what lung function tests are commonly performed in your hospital – and why.

3. Various types of inhalers are in use for chest diseases, e.g. Ventihaler, Spinhaler, and Rotahaler. Find out exactly what each of these uses, and what it is designed to do. Contrast their actions with those of humidifiers.

4. Acidosis of the blood may occur for reasons other than chest diseases. Explain what they are.

5. Compare and contrast chronic bronchitis and emphysema, with pulmonary tuberculosis and with pneumonia.

Answers to questions

Q1. Na, Ob, Oc, Od, Le.

Q2. See 📖 *Page 723, Figure 23.2.*

Q3. When food is swallowed and enters the pharynx, the swallowing reflex ensures that the flap of tissue called the epiglottis (labelled G on Figure 15.1) descends and closes the entry to the larynx (and respiratory system). Thus food can only go one way – down the oesophagus.

Q4. a, windpipe; b, anterior; c, 12; d, 4.5; e, carina; f, mucous; g, cartilage.

Q5. J. Trachea; K. Primary bronchus; L. Secondary (lobar) bronchus; M. Tertiary (segmental) bronchi and bronchioles; N. Alveoli.

Q6. D, F, G, H.

Q7. a, base; b, clavicle; c, ribs; d, hilus; e, bronchi, pulmonary vessels and nerves; f, left; g, left; h, right. 📖 *Page 733, Figure 23.9.*

Q8. a. 3, 2, 1.
b. Alveolar–capillary.
c. 1. Surfactant; 2. Alveolar epithelium; 3. Epithelial basement membrane; 4. Interstitial space; 5. Capillary basement membrane; 6. Capillary endothelium.

Q9. 2a, 1b, 3c.

Q10. a, alveolar or intrapulmonary; b, 760; c, the same as; d, intrapleural; e, 756; f, less than; g, diaphragm; h, external intercostal; i, increases; j, increase; k, decrease; j, 754; m, decreases; n, 758; o, Boyle, p, amosphere; q, alveoli; r, into; s, inspiration; t, 760; u, active; v, passive; w, abdominal; x, internal intercostals.

Q11. a, low; b, high; c, high; d, surfactant; e, increases; f, respiratory distress syndrome (RDS) or hyaline membrane disease (HMD); g, atelectasis.

Q12. a, 70% (350ml/500ml); b, dead space; c, 150.   **Q13.** 4a, 3b, 1c, 7d, 6e, 2f, 5g.

Q14. a, partial; b, 105 – 40 = 65 mmHg; c, large; d, thin; e, increased; f, the same as.
Alveolar air = 40.
Deoxygenated blood = 45.
Oxygenated blood = 40.

Q15.   a, 20; b, oxyhaemoglobin; c, low; d, iron; e, HbO_2; f, saturated; g, increase.

Q16.   a, 70; b, 23; c, 7; d, H_2CO_3 (carbonic acid); e, haemoglobin (as H·Hb); f, $H_2CO_3^-$; g, plasma; h, Cl^-.

Q17.   a, medullary rhythmicity; b, P; c, Limits inspiration and facilitates expiration; d, Apneustic; e, P.

Q18.   a, H^+; increase in pCO_2; c, medulla; d, hypercapnia; e, any value higher than 40; f, even slight; g, hyper; h, aortic bodies; i, carotid bodies; j, only large; k, usually below 60; l, in; m, stretch; n, inhibition; o, inflation (Hering–Breuer).

Q19.   The pharynx.   **Q20.** Trachea, bronchi and bronchioles.

Q21.   The intercostal muscles and the diaphragm.   **Q22.** Partial pressure of the gas (oxygen).

Q23.   The amount of air inspired (or expired) during normal breathing.   **Q24.** Inspiratory reserve volume.

Q25.   Haemoglobin.   **Q26.** The medulla oblongata.

Q27.   Carbon dioxide.   **Q28.** Redness, pain, heat, swelling and loss of function.

Q29.   Water, electrolytes and gases.

Q30.   Phagocytosis – which means to 'eat' (ingest) the foreign substance and destroy it.

Q31.   Airflow into and out of the lungs (increased airway resistance 📖 *Page 741*) is reduced by this internal swelling, and this will lead to an increase in the rate of respiration.

Q32.   Blood oxygen level will fall and blood carbon dioxide level will rise.

Q33.   The rise in blood CO_2 level (and to a lesser extent the fall in O_2 level) will stimulate the medulla and the chemoreceptors. These will, in turn, send messages to the respiratory centre. This will then increase the rate and depth of breathing, in an effort to remove CO_2 from the blood and take in O_2.

Q34.   The goblet cells. Mucus is there to moisten the air and trap dust particles. It is therefore a part of the body's defence system.

Q35.   Emphysema represents a loss of the surface area (alveoli walls), that is available for gas exchange. This will lead to a worsening of the blood gas changes as noted above, and the rate and depth of breathing will further increase. **Compliance** (📖 *Page 740)* also decreases, because of the destruction of elastic fibres in lung tissue. So the lungs become more difficult to inflate.

Q36.   Air is expelled from the lungs, because the diaphragm and intercostal muscles relax. This allows the elastic recoil of the thoracic cavity, and thus the lungs are squeezed and emptied. This is a passive process, i.e. the muscles of respiration relax and allow it to happen.

Q37.   He could stop smoking, and he could also consider moving to an environment where there is less pollution – perhaps the seaside.

    If his sputum is infected, then he can be prescribed antibiotics. He can also be prescribed **bronchodilator** drugs. These will widen (dilate) the bronchi, and thus allow more air to pass in and out of the lungs.

    These drugs work by relaxing the smooth muscle lining of the bronchi 📖 *Page 731*. The smooth muscle is controlled by the autonomic nervous system 📖 *Page 512, Exhibit 17.3*. Drugs which stimulate the sympathetic branch (e.g. **aminophylline**), will lead to bronchodilation. Thus more O_2 can then be taken in, and more CO_2 expired.

Q38. Sympathetic stimulation may result in: palpitations (a rapid heart rate), hand tremor and nervousness. When given by aerosol, these side effects appear to be lessened, but patients are still warned against excessive use of these inhaler devices, because of the possibility of abnormal heart rhythms, known as **arrhythmias**. These symptoms are, of course, a part of the normal 'fight or flight' reaction, which is the result of sympathetic stimulation.

Q39. Encouraging Mr Broster to cough and expectorate the sputum, will do much to clear his air passages. Physiotherapists are skilled in techniques such as **postural drainage**, which is aimed at helping the patient drain sputum from the lungs. The patient is positioned in various ways, depending on the portion of the lung to be drained. In addition, the physiotherapist can show Mr Broster how to breathe more effectively.

Many traditional 'cough' remedies are claimed to be expectorants, and thus to aid this process, but most pharmacology textbooks are somewhat dismissive of the scientific basis of such remedies. Their effect, if any, may be more psychological, than physical.

On the other hand, there are drugs called **mucolytics,** which will reduce sputum viscosity (thin it out). The traditional remedy is one of breathing in steam, either from a bowl or through the mouthpiece of an inhaler. This is also useful for blocked nasal sinuses. Substances such as menthol crystals can be added to the steam, to try to enhance the effect. However, the pharmacological action of these substances is somewhat doubted.

Q40. Reassurance, and thus building his confidence, can do much to help put Mr Broster's mind at rest, and thus allow him to sleep. This can be assured by giving him information about his care and treatment, and generally answering his questions. If he is 'on edge', or unsure about some of these aspects, then he is likely to be somewhat anxious and frightened. This will have the effect of promoting the release of hormones, such as **adrenaline** (epinephrine 📖 *Page 549*), which will induce general arousal (fight or flight response). This will certainly help to prevent him from resting.

Other factors, such as an annoying cough – which is valuable during the day, for getting rid of sputum – can keep Mr Broster awake at night. To suppress a cough, a linctus can be taken at night. This is usually a sweet liquid such as codeine linctus. Codeine is related to morphine, but is not as powerful. However, the action of this group of drugs, is primarily one of relieving pain (**analgesic**). Because they work by depressing the workings of the brain and central nervous system, they also suppress other events controlled from there, such as the cough.

The only danger of this is that it may be more important, even at night, to try to keep his airways clear of sputum, and thus ensure adequate gas exchange. Therefore, there is a delicate balance to try to maintain, between sedating Mr Broster (perhaps, also, using sleeping tablets) and ensuring his ability to keep his air passages clear. If these become severely blocked, respiratory failure could ensue.

Q41. The first effect of retaining CO_2 in the bloodstream is that it will increase the acidity of the blood (📖 *Page 749*); 70% of the CO_2 in the blood is carried as carbonic acid (H_2CO_3), which dissociates to H^+ and HCO_3^-. Therefore, any increase in CO_2 will lead to an increase in hydrogen ions (H^+) and thus to an increase in acidity (📖 *Page 39*).

The effect of a falling blood pH will be to stimulate the medulla and peripheral chemoreceptors in the carotid bodies (📖 *Page 654, Figure 21.22(b)*), and also the chemoreceptors in the aortic arch (📖 *Figure 21.10 Page 650*). This will lead to central stimulation of the respiratory centre in the medulla oblongata (📖 *Page 751, Figure 23.24*). Both the rate and depth of Mr Broster's breathing will increase (he will be starting to **hyperventilate**).

You can experience this effect for yourself, by simply holding your breath (as you would in swimming under water). As a result, the blood CO_2 level rises, the pH falls, and the respiratory centre is stimulated and breathing occurs!

The point at which breathing occurs can be delayed by starting with a very low blood CO_2 level. This can be achieved by forced hyperventilation, which will 'wash out' the CO_2 from the blood. It will then take that much longer for the blood CO_2 level to reach the point at which it triggers breathing. This can be a useful technique, if one is concerned to swim distances under water.

However, prolonged hyperventilation can cause blood chemistry changes, which may lead to unconsciousness and fits. This is usually associated with a hysterical attack (**hysterical overbreathing**). This progression to fits can be prevented, by getting the person to breathe in and out of a paper bag. The bag will form a CO_2 reservoir, and therefore breathing in CO_2-enriched air will prevent a fall in blood pH and the consequent risk of fits.

Q42. Oxygen is necessary for the full liberation of energy from glucose metabolism (📖 *Page 826*) – so-called cellular respiration. Without this, the cells will die.

A low blood O_2 level will stimulate the chemoreceptors, and have the same effect as a raised CO_2 level. As blood O_2 level rises, this stimulus is lost.

The O_2 can be administered to Mr Broster via a face mask. The mask will allow a certain amount of atmospheric air (with 21% O_2) to be drawn in. This will dilute the effect of the mask O_2, (as will breathing via the mouth) and so masks are usually calibrated as delivering a known percentage of O_2 (at a specified flow rate, in litres per minute). Masks can deliver between 24% and 60% O_2. The relevant percentage should be prescribed by a doctor.

Generally speaking, the more O_2, the better it is for the person – like Mr Broster – who has breathing difficulties. The one exception to this, is that patients like Mr Broster (with chronic bronchitis) have become adjusted to higher than normal blood CO_2 levels. After a while, the chemoreceptors and the medulla fail to respond to this situation. The respiratory centre then appears to respond only to a low blood O_2 level.

If the blood O_2 level is raised, by receiving O_2 to breathe, then the raised blood O_2 level will no longer stimulate breathing. And so, because of a reduced rate and depth of breathing, CO_2 will be retained in the blood, and the pH will start to fall. The respiratory centre is no longer responding to this. So much of the body's chemistry is dependent on correct pH levels (📖 *Page 39–40*), and only a small fall in blood pH levels, say from 7.4 to 7.1, can be incompatible with cellular functions – and thus lead to death.

To prevent this from happening, Mr Broster would be given a little extra O_2, but not enough to abolish his chemoreceptor 'drive'. He would probably be given a mask that is calibrated to deliver 28% O_2, at a known flow rate (e.g. of 5 litres/minute). Hence the importance of using the correct mask for patients (like Mr Broster), and acting upon the physician's prescription.

Q43. Oxygen in pure form (100%) is both irritant and toxic. It has been known, at these levels, to cause blindness in babies and to irritate the lungs of patients who are artificially ventilated. Thus, O_2 is never given in concentration greater than 60–70%.

Also, O_2 supports combustion and a spark, glowing cigarette or match end can burst into flames in the presence of O_2. Needless to say, patients and visitors need warning of these dangers. Written hazard signs are used in many hospitals. Special care is taken not to generate sparks in operating theatres – where many gases of an explosive nature are in use – and to this end, the staff are required to wear antistatic footwear. Trolley wheels and mattresses are also composed of antistatic materials.

Q44. He may require continuous O_2, whilst at rest in bed or chair. Whilst at rest, he may continually have difficulty in breathing (**dyspnoea**). This can make what are relatively simple activities, such as talking or eating, very difficult. Recall the **accessory muscles of respiration** (📖 *Page 740*), which lead to tightening of the neck and shoulders, as well as the abdominal muscles, which aid expiration.

The brain will very quickly suffer from a lack of O_2 – its cells are extremely sensitive to both O_2 and nutrient supply, e.g. glucose. An early sign of this is a slight clouding of consciousness, followed by confusion. In response to questions, Mr Broster may find it difficult to respond or not know where he is, or what day it is. As this worsens, so he may become semiconscious.

This picture now points to Mr Broster as being in **respiratory failure**. Measurement of his blood gas levels (raised CO_2, low O_2), will confirm this. The decision may then be taken to ventilate him artificially.

Patients with **chronic obstructive airways disease** (COAD) fall into two categories:

The chronic bronchitis type

Here, the patient is cyanosed (blue from O_2 lack and CO_2 build up). Emphysema is usually slight, and there is a development of right ventricular failure (which will be dealt with shortly).

These patients are often thick set, and are sometimes referred to as 'blue bloaters'.

The emphysema type

The patient has severe emphysema, but no cyanosis. They are hyperventilating, and are sometimes referred to as 'pink puffers'.

In the chronic bronchitis type, the low blood O_2 level triggers the release of erythropoietin (📖 *Page 570*) by the kidneys. This stimulates red cell production by the bone marrow. This means that the red cell count rises, and more oxygen can then be carried by a given volume of blood. This will compensate, to a certain extent, for the reduced O_2 uptake by the lungs (by increasing the O_2-carrying capacity of the blood). Therefore, this is another example of a **homeostatic** response (📖 *Page 11, Figure 1.3*), in which the body is trying to return to a normal blood O_2 level.

Erythropoietin is normally released when we suffer low oxygen levels – as when ascending a mountain – in an attempt to increase our O_2-carrying capacity. People who live at high altitudes have a greater number of red cells in their circulation, in contrast to those of us living at lower altitudes.

Athletes have taken (illegally) erythropoietin for the same reasons, in an attempt to boost performance. Unfortunately, once the red cell numbers rise (known as **polycythaemia**), so the blood becomes more viscous and prone to clotting. Unexpected deaths, in otherwise healthy professional cyclists, have been attributed to strokes/heart attacks caused by blood clots from taking erythropoietin.

In patients like Mr Broster, the increase in blood viscosity (stickiness) will increase the workload of the heart (flow along a tube is more difficult if the liquid is viscous. See 'resistance' 📖 *Page 631*. This, in turn, will add to the right ventricular failure (cor pulmonale).

Also, there is an increased risk of deep vein thrombosis (discussed in Chapter 13), as a consequence of increased blood viscosity.

Q45. This is the **expiratory reserve volume** (📖 *Page 742, Figure 23.16*). A 'forced' expiratory volume (in other words, what Mr Broster is capable of) is known as **FEV.** It is measured by blowing into a machine for one second. (FEV_1), and a graph is produced (Figure 15.6).

The other volume that is measured is the **forced vital capacity** (FVC). In essence, this is the sum of the total volume that can possibly be inhaled, **plus** what can be exhaled with force. Hence, it is the overall lung volume. However, at the end of the forced expiration there is still air in the lungs, because the lungs are not fully collapsible. It is not possible to flatten the rib cage.

Figure 15.6. Forced vital capacity and forced expiratory volume.

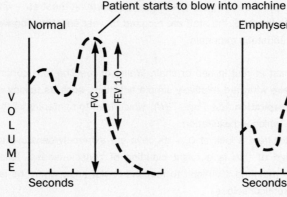
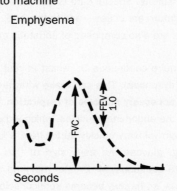

Figure 15.6 shows a normal and an emphysema-type FVC and FEV_1. Notice the steeper fall in the 'normal' curve, representing a greater fall in volume (of air expired) in one second. Also, the normal has a larger lung volume (FVC). The ratio of FEV_1/FVC can be expressed as a percentage. Normal people can expel between 65% and 80% of the FVC in one second. Mr Broster's percentage may be reduced, by up to 40%. In other words, he can only expel, in one second, about half of the volume of air that he used to be able to expel. Hence, the term **chronic obstructive airways disease** (COAD).

The FEV_1 may be improved by drugs, such as bronchodilators. Measuring the FEV before and after taking the drug would provide an objective measure of its efficacy.

Blood samples from his femoral artery (📖 *Page 656, Figure 21.23*) would also reveal any improvement in O_2 and CO_2 levels. Note that venous blood would be of no use for this type of testing. It is only arterial blood that reflects the efficiency of the lungs, in the uptake of the O_2, and CO_2 excretion.

Q46. With these lung disorders, Mr Broster will be subject to CO_2 retention and a low blood O_2 level, because of airways obstruction. In addition, emphysema leads to a loss of alveoli and the formation of large air sacs in the lungs. The loss of alveoli means that the surface area in the lungs, available for gas exchange, is now reduced. This makes the CO_2 retention, (and O_2 lack) worse.

These changes have three complications:

(a) Pulmonary vasoconstriction will increase the pressure in the pulmonary circulation, and is primarily a result of the blood gas changes.

(b) The above-mentioned diseases lead to an overall reduction in the volume of the pulmonary circulation. This is due to loss of alveoli and their surrounding capillaries.

(c) Airways obstruction raises the pressure inside the remaining alveoli. This increases the pressure on the remaining capillaries within them.

The net effect of these three changes is **pulmonary hypertension.** The right ventricle (📖 *Page 647, Figure 21.19*) is now having to work harder (against this pressure), to pump the same volume of blood through the lungs. Its muscle enlarges, because of this extra effort, and eventually – when it can no longer enlarge – it fails. This is **cor pulmonale,** or right-sided heart failure.

The features will be those of cyanosis – due to blood gas changes. As cardiac output falls, so the extremities will become cold and the pulse weak. Also, peripheral oedema may develop. This is a collection of fluid in the tissues, caused by back pressure in the venous system (see Chapter 13, the scenario on Mr Brown). The sacrum and ankles will swell, and if gently pressed upon with the thumb, then a small hollow will remain.

In addition to the treatment already mentioned, Mr Broster may now be prescribed **digoxin,** to strengthen and steady his failing heart. **Diuretics** will be prescribed. These are drugs that increase the volume of urine output, and thus lead to a decrease in oedema.

Figure 15.7 provides a summary of Mr Broster's problems and treatment.

Figure 15.7.
Mr Broster's problems and treatment.

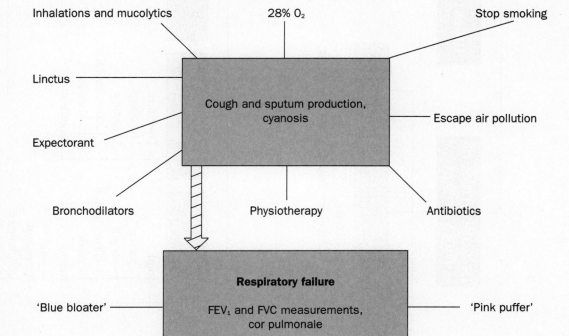

Overview and key terms

Digestive system

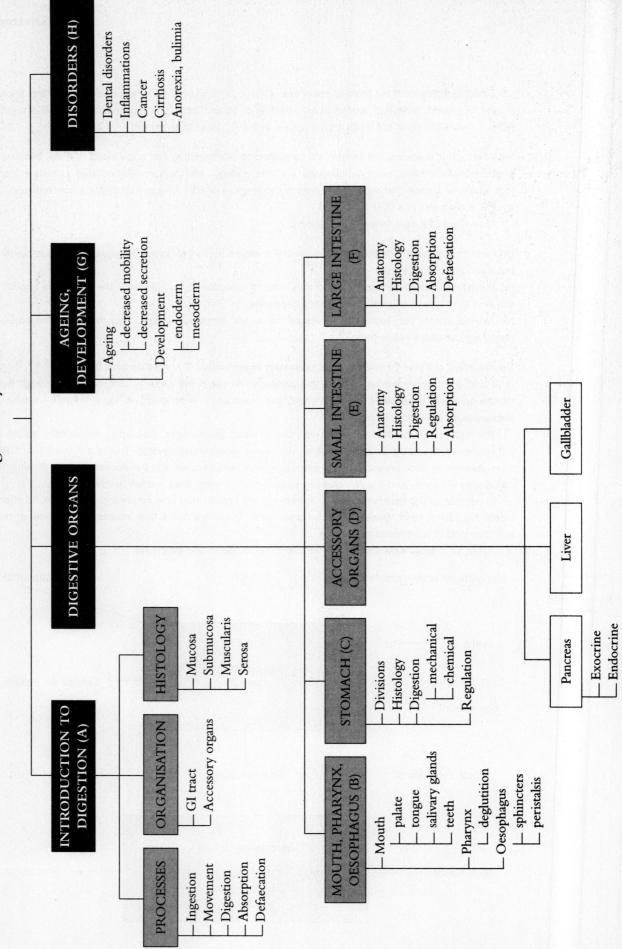

INTRODUCTION TO DIGESTION (A)

PROCESSES
- Ingestion
- Movement
- Digestion
- Absorption
- Defaecation

ORGANISATION
- GI tract
- Accessory organs

HISTOLOGY
- Mucosa
- Submucosa
- Muscularis
- Serosa

DIGESTIVE ORGANS

MOUTH, PHARYNX, OESOPHAGUS (B)
- Mouth
  - palate
  - tongue
  - salivary glands
  - teeth
- Pharynx
  - deglutition
- Oesophagus
  - sphincters
  - peristalsis

STOMACH (C)
- Divisions
- Histology
- Digestion
  - mechanical
  - chemical
- Regulation

ACCESSORY ORGANS (D)
- Pancreas
  - Exocrine
  - Endocrine
- Liver
- Gallbladder

SMALL INTESTINE (E)
- Anatomy
- Histology
- Digestion
- Regulation
- Absorption

LARGE INTESTINE (F)
- Anatomy
- Histology
- Digestion
- Absorption
- Defaecation

AGEING, DEVELOPMENT (G)
- Ageing
  - decreased mobility
  - decreased secretion
- Development
  - endoderm
  - mesoderm

DISORDERS (H)
- Dental disorders
- Inflammations
- Cancer
- Cirrhosis
- Anorexia, bulimia

16. The Digestive System

Learning outcomes

1. To describe the structures and functions of the organs (including accessory organs) forming the digestive tract.

2. To outline the mechanical movements of the gastrointestinal tract.

3. To explain how salivary secretion, gastric secretion, gastric emptying, pancreatic secretion, bile secretion and small intestinal secretion are regulated.

4. To define absorption and explain how the end products of digestion are absorbed.

5. To outline the processes involved in the formation of faeces and defaecation.

6. To outline the role of hormones in digestion.

7. To describe the effects of ageing on the digestive system.

8. To outline some of the clinical symptoms in the following disorders: dental caries, periodontal disease, peptic ulcer, appendicitis, diverticulitis, cirrhosis, hepatitis, gallstones, anorexia nervosa and bulimia.

Chapter 24

INTRODUCTION

Important nursing skills, such as feeding the patient, assessing their nutritional needs, giving the appropriate amount and types of foods, observing the product of elimination, and giving the appropriate advice with regard to diet and health, form part of good principles of caring. It is therefore essential that a nurse fully understands the structure and normal functions of the digestive system, if he or she is to be able to formulate care plans when caring for patients with various digestive tract disorders. The guided study which follows will enable you to gain the desired knowledge on the digestive system.

STRUCTURE AND FUNCTIONS OF THE DIGESTIVE SYSTEM

Q1.   List the five basic activities of the digestive system.

_____

_____

Q2.   **Figure 16.1 shows organs of the digestive system.**

a.   Label the structures A to T from the list given below:

parotid gland, sublingual and submandibular glands, oesophagus, liver, gallbladder, duodenum, colon (ascending), caecum, vermiform appendix, mouth, pharynx, stomach, pancreas, colon (transverse), jejunum, ileum, colon (sigmoid), rectum, anus.

b.   Name the structures which are referred to as accessory organs of the digestive system.

_____

For questions 2–9, see 📖 *Pages 770–5*

Q3.   **Figure 16.2 shows the oral cavity. Label the following structures:**

hard palate, palatoglossal arch, uvula, palatine tonsils, lingual frenulum, vestibule, incisor tooth, canine tooth and molar tooth.

Q4.   **Outline some of the important functions of the tongue.**

_____

_____

_____

Figure 16.1.
Organs of the
digestive system.

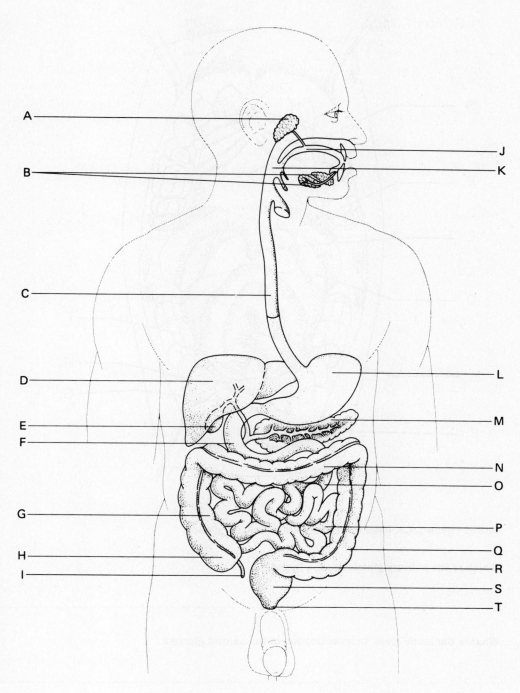

A

B

C

D

E

F

G

H

I

J

K

L

M

N

O

P

Q

R

S

T

Figure 16.2.
Diagram of the oral
cavity.

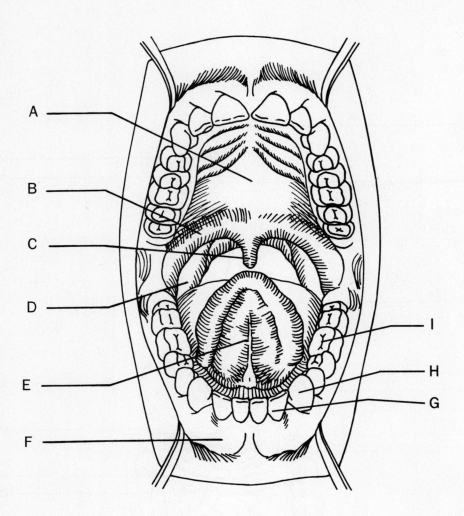

A

B

C

D

E

F

I

H

G

Q5.   On the Figure 16.3, label the three pairs of salivary glands.

Q6.   Which of the salivary glands are the largest?

_____

Q7.   What is the name given to inflammation of the parotid glands?

_____

Q8.   Briefly describe the constituents and functions of saliva.

_____

_____

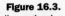

Figure 16.3.
ne salivary glands.

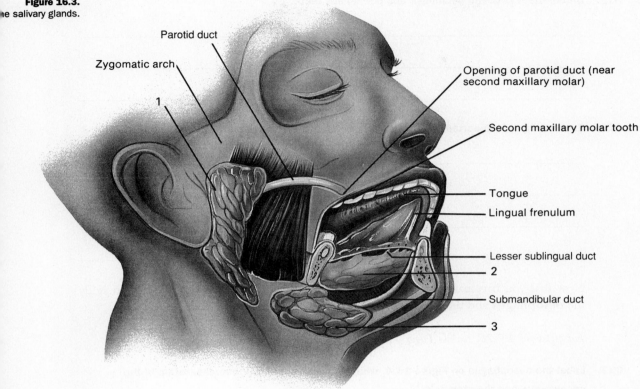

Parotid duct

Zygomatic arch

1

Opening of parotid duct (near
second maxillary molar)

Second maxillary molar tooth

Tongue

Lingual frenulum

Lesser sublingual duct

2

Submandibular duct

3

Q9.   Outline the three principal portions of a tooth.

_____

Q10. Arrange each of the following structures in the correct sequence.

a.   From the most superficial to the deepest.

1. Root 2. Neck 3. Crown

_____   _____   _____

b.   From the most superficial to the deepest within a tooth.

1. Enamel 2. Dentine 3. Pulp cavity

_____   _____   _____

c.   From the hardest to the softest.

1. Enamel 2. Dentine 3. Pulp cavity

_____   _____   _____

Q11. **Differentiate between deciduous and permanent teeth.**

_____

_____

_____

Q12. **Explain why it is important for a nurse to give mouth care to patients who require it.**

_____

_____

_____

_____

Now that you have gained some knowledge on the oral cavity, you can proceed to study the **oesophagus** and the **stomach**.

For questions 13–26, see 📖 Pages 776–87

Q13. **Label the oesophagus on Figure 16.4, which shows a schematic representation of the oesophagus and the stomach.**

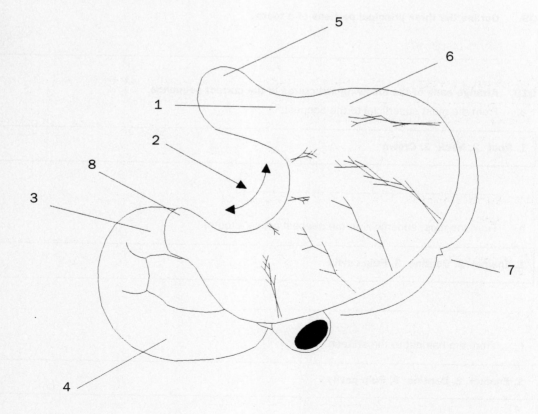

Figure 16.4.
A schematic representation of the oesophagus and stomach.

Q14. Outline the structure of the oesophagus, indicating its anatomical position in relation to structures that are very close to it.

_____

_____

_____

Q15. Complete the exercise below, which describes the act of deglutition.

The term **deglutition** means (a) _____ . It can be divided into three stages. The first stage, the (b) _____ stage, occurs when the bolus is forced to the back of the oral cavity and into the oropharynx by the movement of the tongue against the palate. The second stage, the (c) _____ stage, occurs when the soft palate and epiglottis close off the respiratory passageways and (d) _____ temporarily ceases. During the second stage, receptors in the oropharynx are stimulated and they send impulses to the deglutition centre in the (e) _____ and lower pons of the brainstem. The third stage, the (f) _____ stage, involves peristaltic contractions which push the bolus from the pharynx to the (g) _____ .

Q16. Summarise digestion in the mouth, pharynx and oesophagus by completing parts a and b of Table 16.1, next page. (The other sections will be completed later.)

Q17. Label the following on Figure 16.4: fundus, duodenum, cardia, lesser curvature, greater curvature, pylorus and pyloric sphincter. _Page 781, Figure 24.11._

Q18. Arrange the regions of the stomach according to the pathway of food from first to last :

1. Body 2. Fundus 3. Pylorus 4. Cardia

_____   _____   _____   _____

Q19. Complete the table below, which refers to types of cells and their functions in gastric secretions.

Name of cell	Type of secretion	Function of secretion
Chief (zymogenic)	a. b.	c.
Mucous	d.	e.
f.	HCl g.	h.
i.	Gastrin	j.

Table 16.1 Summary of Digestion

Digestive Organs	Carbohydrate	Protein
a. Mouth, salivary glands	Salivary amylase: digests starch to maltose	
b. Pharynx, oesophagus		
c. Stomach		
d. Pancreas		
e. Intestinal juices		
f. Liver	No enzymes for digestion of carbohydrates	
g. Large intestine	No enzymes for digestion of carbohydrates	No enzymes for digestion of protein

Lipid	Mechanical	Other functions
	Deglutition, peristalsis	
		1. Secretes intrinsic factor 2. Produces hormone stomach gastrin
Pancreatic lipease: digests about 80% of fats		
No enzymes for digestion of lipids		

Q20. **Complete the exercise below, which relates to chemical digestion in the stomach.**

Pepsin is most active at very (a) _____ pH. Two important factors that enable the stomach to digest protein without digesting its own cells are firstly, that pepsin is released in the inactive form known as (b) _____ , and secondly, that mucus is present, secreted by the (c) _____ glands. If mucus fails to protect the gastric lining, the condition known as (d) _____ may result.

Another enzyme produced by the stomach is (e) _____ , which digests (f) _____ . In adults it is quite ineffective because it works best at an optimum pH of (g) _____ or (h) _____ .

Q21. **Complete the exercise below, which is about the control of gastric secretion.**

The **three** phases of gastric secretion are (a) _____ , (b) _____ and (c) _____ . The first phase causes release of gastric secretion even before the food enters the stomach, and this is due to the (d) _____ , (e) _____ , (f) _____ or thought of food.

Gastric glands are stimulated mainly by the (g) _____ nerves, which consist of (h) _____ fibres and therefore form part of the (i) _____ nervous system.

Three emotions that inhibit production of gastric secretions are (j) _____ , (k) _____ and (l) _____ . Distension of the stomach triggers the (m) _____ phase. Two effects of this stimulus are the (n) _____ (increase? decrease?) in parasympathetic impulses and release of the hormone (o) _____ . This hormone, together with the effects of the vagus, causes the production of (p) _____ , which is essential to activate pepsinogen.

When **chyme** reaches the intestine, nerves initiate the (q) _____ reflex, which (r) _____ (stimulates? inhibits?) further gastric secretion.

Three hormones released by the intestine also inhibit gastric secretion as well as gastric motility, so their effect is to (s) _____ (stimulate? delay?) gastric secretion. The **three** hormones are : (t) _____ , (u) _____ and (v) _____ .

Q22. **Complete the following exercise, which relates to gastric function.**

Food stays in the stomach for about (a) _____ to (b) _____ hours. Food rich in (c) _____ spends less time in the stomach than food that contains a large amount of (d) _____ .

Q23. **Discuss the functions of the enzymes secreted by the gastric glands.**

_____

_____

_____

Q24. Outline the function of the intrinsic factor, identifying the cells that are responsible for its secretion.

_____

_____

_____

Q25. Discuss the effects of prolonged vomiting with reference to homeostasis.

_____

_____

_____

_____

Q26. What is the name given to the group of drugs that can reduce or prevent vomiting?

_____

For what reason would a premedication drug such as 'papaveretum and scopolamine' be administered to a patient before he goes for surgery? The term 'premedication' is fully explained in the answer section.

_____

_____

Having studied the oral cavity, oesophagus and stomach, you should now proceed to the small intestine (duodenum, jejenum, and ileum) and also the accessory structures (pancreas, liver and gallbladder).

Q27. Anatomically the duodenum, jejunum and ileum have a similar cross-section, consisting of an inner layer, the mucosa, a middle layer, the submucosa, and an outermost layer, the serosa. Between the serosa and the submucosa lies the muscularis ▱▱ *Pages 799–800.*

a.   Figure 16.5 shows a cross section of the small intestine. Label the circular layer, longitudinal layer, mucosa, submucosa and serosa.

Figure 16.5.
Diagram of cross section of the small intestine.

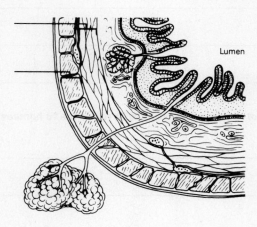

Lumen

b.   Briefly describe each of the three layers mentioned above, indicating their specific functions.

_____

_____

_____

_____

PERITONEUM

Having studied the cross section of the intestine, it is well to consider the **peritoneum** 📖 *Pages 768–9*. The peritoneum is a double serous membrane forming a closed sac within the abdomen. In fact, it is one of the largest membranes in the body. The part of the membrane that lines the abdominal cavity is called the **parietal** peritoneum and the part that covers the organs in the abdominal cavity is referred to as the **visceral** peritoneum. There is a potential space between the visceral and parietal peritoneum.

Q28.   What is the name of this potential space?

_____

The peritoneum has some useful functions, which are as follows:

(1) It protects all the organs in the abdominal cavity, for example in the limitation of the spread of infection.

(2) It acts as a fat store.

(3) It keeps the organs in the abdominal cavity in position.

Use of the peritoneum as an aid to medical intervention/therapy

Due to its large surface area, the peritoneum can actually play a significant role as a membrane that can allow the process of diffusion to take place and thus can be used in some cases to allow exchanges of various ions. For example, in renal diseases where patients are accumulating large amount of urea, creatinine, potassium, sodium and water in their blood, the procedure known as **peritoneal dialysis** may be used in order to reduce the level of these ions. In this process, water is also lost. For more information on peritoneal dialysis, please refer to Chapter 18.

Peritonitis

It is very important to realise that the peritoneum can become inflamed (**peritonitis**) and if this is not treated promptly, it can be life-threatening. Peritonitis may occur as a result of bacterial or chemical irritation. It can occur following a burst appendix, perforation of an ulcer or rupture of the bowel or gallbladder.

The management of peritonitis involves pain control, drugs for the control of infection (antimicrobial agents), and replacement of fluids and electrolytes, usually by intravenous infusions. A patient may also require emptying of the stomach, which is usually done via a nasogastric tube.

Q29.   Match the names of these peritoneal extensions with the correct descriptions.

---

1. Falciform ligament 2. Greater omentum 3. Lesser omentum 4. Mesentery 5. Mesocolon

---

☐   a. Attaches liver to anterior abdominal wall.

☐   b. Binds intestine to posterior abdominal wall; provides route for blood and lymph vessels and nerves to reach small intestine.

☐   c. Binds part of large intestine to posterior abdominal wall.

☐   d. 'Fatty apron'; covers and helps prevent infection in small intestine.

☐   e. Suspends stomach and duodenum from liver.

Q30.   You will have discovered that the mucosa consists of a large number of structures called villi. They have an important function in the absorption of digested foods. Briefly outline the structure of a villus 📖 *Pages 797–9.*

PANCREAS

It is appropriate at this stage to look at the structure and functions of the **pancreas.**

Q31. **On Figure 16.6 below, label the following: body of pancreas, main pancreatic duct, duodenum, right and left lobe of the liver, gallbladder, cystic duct, common bile duct, ampulla of Vater, right and left hepatic duct.**

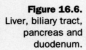

Figure 16.6.
Liver, biliary tract,
pancreas and
duodenum.

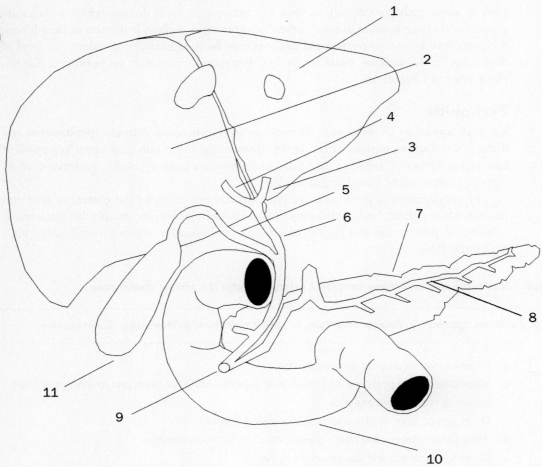

Q32. **Complete the exercise below, which relates to the structure and function of the pancreas.**

The pancreas lies in the (a) _____ and is posterior to the (b) _____ .
Anatomically, it may be divided into three main parts namely, the (c) _____ which is
in close proximity to the first part of the small intestine, the (d) _____ , the body
and the (e) _____ , which lies very close to the (f) _____ .

The pancreas contains two types of glands, 1% of which has cells that are organised into
clusters called (g) _____ _____ and 99% of which has the cells
arranged in clusters called (h) _____ . These cells secrete a mixture of fluid and
enzymes called (i) _____ . One type of these secretions is (j) _____
fluid to neutralise the chyme entering from the stomach.

One enzyme in the pancreatic secretions is trypsin; it digests (k) _____ . Trypsin
is formed initially in the inactive form, which is called (l) _____ and it becomes
activated by the action of (m) _____ . Trypsin itself activates (n) _____
to (o) _____ , which behaves as a protease. The pancreas also secretes
(p) _____ , which digests carbohydrates, and (q) _____ , which digests fats.

All (r) _____ secretions (produced by glands with ducts) of the pancreas empty into a very large duct known as the duct of (s) _____ or the (t) _____ and these ultimately reach the first part of the small intestine, the (u) _____ .

Q33. **Discuss the exocrine and endocrine functions of the pancreas.** 📖 *Pages 549–51*

_____

_____

_____

_____

Q34. **Which two hormones influence the exocrine secretions of the pancreas?** 📖 *Pages 790*

_____

Q35. **Outline the digestion and absorption of carbohydrates, lipids and proteins in the small intestine.** 📖 *Pages 801–6*

_____

_____

_____

_____

Q36. **Summarise digestion in the stomach and pancreas, to include functions of the intestinal juices, by completing sections c, d and e of Table 16.1.**

LIVER AND BILARY TREE

Now that you understand the physiological processes that take place in the upper part of the digestive tract and the pancreas, it is appropriate to study the liver and biliary tree, which are also accessory organs of digestion. Refer to Figure 16.6.

For questions 37–40, see 📖 *Pages 790–6*

Q37. **Answer this question, which relates to the anatomical position and structure of the liver.**
The liver weighs about (a) _____ kg and is situated in the right (b) _____ just beneath the (c) _____ . The right (d) _____ lies beneath the liver. It consists of (e) _____ lobes, the (f) _____ is the largest. The liver is almost covered by a membrane called the (g) _____ . The (h) _____

ligament separates the right and left lobes. At the edge of this ligament is the ligamentum teres (round ligament of the liver), which is the obliterated (i) _____ vein.

The liver receives its main oxygenated blood supply from the (j) _____ artery, which is a branch of the abdominal (k) _____ . It also receives a large blood supply from the (l) _____ _____ vein, which connects it to the small (m) _____ .

Q38. Complete the exercise below, which should enhance your knowledge of the microscopic structure of the liver and some of its functions. 📖 *Pages 791–5.*

The functional unit of the liver is known as a (a) _____ . Each (b) _____ consists of hepatic cells called (c) _____ . These have a central (d) _____ and blood reaches them via the (e) _____ .

The hepatic cells also secrete bile, which is poured into small vessels called (f) _____ . The bile secreted from the liver is composed largely of the pigment named (g) _____ , which is a breakdown product of (h) _____ . Excessive amounts of this pigment give skin a yellowish colour, a condition known as (i) _____ .

The hormone (j) _____ is responsible for the release of bile from the (k) _____ . Two functions of bile are (l) _____ of fats and (m) _____ of fat-soluble vitamins.

Liver cells also produce several plasma proteins, two of which are essential for blood clotting. They are (n) _____ and (o) _____ . The most abundant of the plasma proteins is (p) _____ .

The liver also plays an important function in the metabolism of proteins. It removes the amino group (NH_2) from the amino acids, a process known as (q) _____ . The product formed in this process is later converted into (r) _____ and this is excreted in the (s) _____ .

Q39. Outline some of the other functions of the liver, which are not mentioned in question 38. Also complete part f of Table 16.1.

_____

_____

_____

Q40. Outline the constituents and functions of bile.

_____

_____

_____

_____

LARGE INTESTINE

Now that you have studied the pancreas, liver and biliary tree, you can move on to the **large intestine**, the last part of the digestive tract.

For questions 41–44, see 📖 *Pages 806–11*

Q41. **On Figure 16.7, which shows an anterior view of the large intestine, label the following: transverse colon, ascending colon, caecum, vermiform appendix, rectum, descending colon, taenia coli, sigmoid colon, anus, hepatic flexure and splenic flexure.**

Figure 16.7.
Anterior view of large intestine.

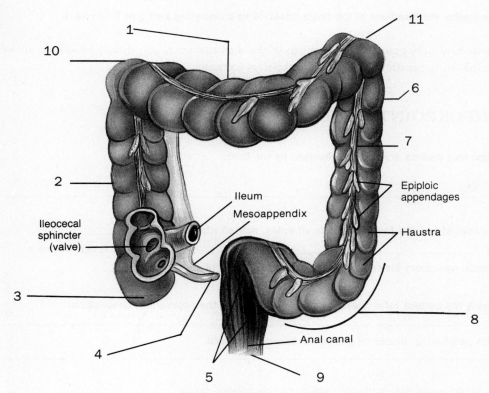

Q42. **With reference to anatomical structures, differentiate between the large intestine and the ileum.**

_____

_____

_____

_____

Q43. **Describe the physiology of defaecation.**

_____

_____

_____

Q44. **Summarise the functions of the large intestine by completing part g of Table 16.1.**

If you have fully grasped the functions of the digestive tract, you should be able to answer the following questions from the Checkpoints Exercise.

CHECKPOINTS EXERCISE

Q45. **Name four plasma proteins synthesised by the liver.**

_____

Q46. **The liver stores the four fat-soluble vitamins, named vitamins (a) _____ ,
(b) _____ , (c) _____ and (d) _____ . It also stores a
vitamin necessary for erythropoiesis, namely vitamin (e) _____ .**

Q47. **Match the correct term related to the intestine with the appropriate description.**

1. Peyer's patches 2. Duodenal glands 3. Microvilli 4. Villi

☐ a. Submucosal glands that secrete protective alkaline fluids.
☐ b. Fingerlike projections up to 1mm high that give the intestinal lining a velvety appearance and increase absorptive surface.
☐ c. Aggregated lymphatic follicles located primarily in the wall of the ileum.
☐ d. Fingerlike projections of plasma membrane.

Q48. **For extra review of secretions involved with digestion, give the appropriate name of the secretions that match the descriptions below.**

a. _____ Stimulates production of alkaline pancreatic fluids and bile.
b. _____ Increases gastric activity (secretion, motility).
c. _____ Activates pepsinogen.
d. _____ The active form of this enzyme starts protein digestion.
e. _____ Activates the inactive precursor to form trypsin.

f. _____ A storage form of carbohydrates.

g. _____ Most effective enzyme in the digestion of fats.

h. _____ Emulsifies fats before they can be digested effectively.

i. _____ Starch-digesting enzymes secreted by salivary glands and pancreas.

Q49. **All of the following chemicals are produced by the walls of the small intestine except:**

a. Lactase.

b. Secretin.

c. CCK.

d. Trypsin.

e. Brush border enzymes.

Q50. **Choose the false statement about layers of the wall of the GI tract.**

a. Most large blood and lymph vessels are located in the submucosa.

b. The myenteric plexus is part of the muscularis layer.

c. Most glandular tissue is located in the layer known as the mucosa.

d. The mucosa layer forms the peritoneum.

Q51. **Match each structure in the large intestine with the description.**

---

1. Anal canal 2. Ileocaecal valve 3. Hepatic flexure 4. Appendix

---

☐ a. Valve between small and large intestine.

☐ b. Blind-ended tube attached to caecum.

☐ c. Portion of colon located between ascending and transverse colon; also called right colic flexure.

☐ d. Terminal 3cm of rectum.

Q52. **Contrast different portions of the GI tract by identifying structures or functions associated with each.**

---

1. Large intestine 2. Small intestine 3. Stomach

☐ a. Has thickened bands of longitudinal muscle known as taeniae coli.

☐ b. Pouches give this structure its puckered appearance.

☐ c. Its fat-filled peritoneal attachments are known as epiploic appendages.

☐ d. Bacteria here decompose bilirubin to urobilinogen, which gives faeces its brown colour.

☐ e. Involved in gastrocolic reflex (two answers).

☐ f. Has rugae.

☐ g. Has villi and microvilli.

Q53.   Arrange the following answers in the correct sequence.

a.   Pathway of bile:

1.   Bile canaliculi.

2.   Common bile duct.

3.   Common hepatic duct.

4.   Right and left hepatic ducts.

5.   Hepatopancreatic ampulla and duodenum.

_____   _____   _____   _____   _____

b.   Pathway of chyme:

1.   Ileum.

2.   Jejunum.

3.   Caecum.

4.   Duodenum.

5.   Pylorus.

_____   _____   _____   _____   _____

c.   Pathway of wastes:

1.   Ascending colon.

2.   Transverse colon.

3.   Sigmoid colon.

4.   Descending colon.

5.   Rectum.

_____   _____   _____   _____   _____

d.   GI tract wall, from deepest to most superficial layer:

1.   Mucosa.

2.   Muscularis.

3.   Serosa.

4.   Submucosa.

_____   _____   _____   _____

Q54.   Match the terms with the descriptions.

1. Anorexia nervosa 2. Bulimia 3. Cholecystitis 4. Colitis 5. Colostomy 6. Constipation 7. Diarrhoea 8. Dysphagia 9. Flatus 10. Haemorrhoids 11. Hepatitis 12. Heartburn (dyspepsia) 13. Peptic ulcer

☐   a.   Incision of the colon, creating artificial anus.

☐   b.   Inflammation of the liver.

☐ c. Inflammation of the colon.

☐ d. Burning sensation in region of oesophagus and stomach; probably due to gastric contents in lower oesophagus.

☐ e. Frequent defaecation of liquid faeces.

☐ f. Inflammation of the gallbladder.

☐ g. Infrequent or difficult defaecation.

☐ h. Craterlike lesion in the GI tract due to acidic gastric juices.

☐ i. Excess air (gas) in stomach or intestine, usually expelled through anus.

☐ j. Binge–purge syndrome.

☐ k. Loss of appetite and self-imposed starvation.

☐ l. Difficulty in swallowing.

If you have had an opportunity to gain some practical experience within the clinical areas, you should attempt to answer the questions in the two patient scenarios which follow.

PATIENT SCENARIO 1

Simon is a ten-year-old boy who is very keen on participating in various sporting activities. Two years ago he was diagnosed as suffering from diabetes mellitus and was put on insulin, which he administers to himself three times daily before meals. With some restrictions of carbohydrates and fats, Simon is able to eat a normal diet.

Simon at times is very frustrated as he constantly has to adjust his insulin and diet in order to be able to maintain his sporting activities. He is very conscientious about his health and is always keen to follow appropriate advice, especially in relation to his diabetes.

Q55. Based on your knowledge of carbohydrate, fat and protein metabolism, discuss some of the physiological changes (you may refer to signs and symptoms) that could have taken place within Simon's body before the diagnosis was made. Give the rationale for your answer.

_____

_____

_____

_____

_____

Q56. Simon enjoys a baked potato now and then with his meals. Briefly outline the digestion of the carbohydrate component in baked potato, until its final constituents.

_____

_____

_____

Q57. If Simon had omitted his insulin, suggest the possible consequence on the homeostatic control of his carbohydrate metabolism, following the consumption of two very large baked potatoes.

_____

_____

_____

Q58. Write notes on insulin and indicate if it is secreted via a negative or positive feedback mechanism.

_____

_____

_____

Q59. Which other hormone from the pancreas plays a role in the control of carbohydrate metabolism?

_____

Q60. Suggest how Simon may be affected if he omits his breakfast following his insulin injection.

_____

_____

Q61. What appropriate advice should you give to Simon with regard to his insulin management?

_____

_____

_____

_____

_____

Q62. Briefly explain why Simon needs to adjust his insulin and diet prior to rigorous physical activities.

_____

_____

_____

_____

Q63. List some of the complications that Simon may face later in life as a result of his diabetes.

_____

_____

_____

_____

_____

_____

Overview: diabetes mellitus

Diabetes mellitus is a chronic metabolic disorder that occurs as a result of dysfunction, mainly of the endocrine part of the pancreas. The **beta cells of the Islets of Langerhans** in the pancreas fail to secrete enough insulin, or secrete no insulin at all. Thus, carbohydrate metabolism is affected.

The symptoms of diabetes may also be produced by a number of factors, such as increased activity of **glucocorticoids, catecholamines, growth hormone,** and **glucagon.** The symptoms of diabetes mellitus vary with the severity of the disease, but the manifestations are those of hyperglycaemia, glycosuria, increased protein breakdown, ketosis and acidosis.

Diabetes may be classified into three types. **Type I** is the juvenile onset diabetes and is insulin-dependent; **Type II** is the adult or maturity onset (onset after 40 years and 70% of affected individuals are obese) and **Type III** is the maturity onset diabetes of youth.

The causes of diabetes are not known, although such factors as inheritance, viral infections, autoimmunity and nutrition have been implicated.

Inheritance

There is some evidence that among the relatives of affected individuals, diabetes mellitus was found to be four- to tenfold greater than in relatives of unaffected controls. Evidence for genetic inheritance has also been shown in twin studies. It is interesting to note that diabetes is nonexistent in Eskimos.

Infection

Various studies have indicated that infections may be responsible for the development of diabetes in children. For example an association has been found between juvenile diabetes and previous infections with **coxsackie B₄ virus**, and also between congenital rubella syndrome and diabetes. The prevalence in these children could exceed 20%.

Autoimmune disorders

There is some indication that there may be a statistical association between insulin-dependent diabetes and autoimmune organ-specific disease, such as Hashimoto's thyroiditis or pernicious anaemia.

Nutrition

It is believed that diabetes mellitus could occur as a result of over-nutrition, since in individuals who suffer from diabetes in their 40s, 80% are obese.

Management

The management is primarily the relief of symptoms through controlling the diet and thereby maintaining a reasonable weight acceptable for the individual, and the administration of insulin or the sulphonylureas or biguanides, where this is indicated. The essential advice to be given to patients is that of minimising the risk of infection, especially of the foot, to monitor both the blood and urine for the presence of glucose and urine also for the presence of ketones.

Patients should also take great care of their health, since there are diabetic changes that occur in the capillaries and other small blood vessels, the so-called diabetic microangiopathy. These may lead to vascular diseases affecting the eyes (diabetic retinopathy), kidneys (diabetic nephropathy), blood vessels of the legs (can lead to intermittent claudication, and later gangrene). Patients should also be very vigilant, and report any ill health to their general practitioner, since infection may exacerbate the symptoms of diabetes.

QUESTIONS FOR DISCUSSION

1.   Discuss how other hormones (excluding insulin and glucagon) may assist in the control of blood sugar level.

2.   Identify all the relevant factors that you would take into consideration when planning an education programme for Simon and his parents.

PATIENT SCENARIO 2

Mrs Ethel Daniels, aged 55, has been admitted to a surgical ward with severe intermittent colicky pain, radiating to the right shoulder. She had been vomiting copiously for several hours before hospital admission.

Following several tests and a full medical history, it has been confirmed that Mrs Daniels is suffering from obstructive jaundice which in her case is due to a gallstone completely blocking the common bile duct. She is prescribed medication which will help to ease her pain.

She is to be under close observation and her condition is to be monitored for any sign of deterioration. She is to receive no food or fluid orally, as she may require an emergency operation. She is commenced on an intravenous infusion of normal saline (500ml four-hourly).

Q64. Explain why Mrs Daniels is being administered intravenous fluids.

_____

_____

_____

Q65. Giving the rationale for your answer, explain why Mrs Daniels looks jaundiced.

_____

_____

_____

Q66. With specific reference to gallstones, describe three other symptoms that are likely to be present in Mrs Daniels. Give the rationale for your answer.

_____

_____

_____

_____

Q67. What specific nursing observations would Mrs Daniels require and why?

_____

_____

_____

_____

Q68. Prior to hospital admission, Mrs Daniels had been complaining of nausea and vomiting, whenever she consumed foods containing fats. With reference to her illness, briefly explain the possible cause of the nausea and vomiting.

_____

_____

_____

Q69. List the general nursing care (other than those mentioned in question 67) that Mrs Daniels may require prior to surgery.

_____

_____

_____

_____

_____

Q70. Prior to surgery, Mrs Daniels is prescribed intramuscular injection of vitamin K. Explain the reason for the administration of vitamin K.

_____

_____

_____

_____

Q71. Mrs Daniels is to receive a total of 2000ml of fluids intravenously. Calculate at what time she would have received the 2000ml, if the infusion is 500ml in four hours and commenced at 8 a.m on a Monday morning.

_____

_____

_____

QUESTIONS FOR DISCUSSION

1. Discuss the possible complications that could occur with Mrs Daniels following surgery. As a nurse, what measures could you take to minimise the risk of the complications that you have mentioned?

2. If Mrs Daniels had undergone a cholecystectomy with exploration of the common bile duct, she would have a T tube _in situ_. Giving the rationale for your answer, explain the reason for the T and discuss all the specific nursing management that Mrs Daniels would require.

Some facts about gallstones (cholelithiasis)

Gallstones in the biliary tract can occur at any age, and in either sex, but they are more common in women. It is not known why stones form, but the following factors may contribute to the formation of gallstones: inflammation, stasis and metabolic factors.

Metabolic factors

These are many, but in the main it is the precipitation of bile salts, bile pigments and cholesterol that cause the formation of the stones. Most gallstones in Western society are cholesterol stones (75%).

Biliary stasis

This leads to stagnation of bile in the gallbladder and to excessive absorption of water and therefore gives rise to stone formation.

Inflammation

When the gallbladder is inflamed, the mucosa can absorb more of the bile acids and this may act as a focus for formation of gallstones.

One important symptom associated with gallstones is **biliary colic.** Biliary colic is caused by spasm of the ducts as they attempt to move the stone. The pain is felt under the scapula and the right shoulder. During an attack, the patient may sweat profusely.

Cholecystitis

This is inflammation of the gallbladder and is often associated with cholelithiasis. There is often a history of intolerance of fatty foods, abdominal distension, flatus and diarrhoea. The patient may present with an acute phase (acute cholecystitis), but can progress on to chronic cholecystitis.

During an acute attack, the individual experiences severe abdominal pain, mainly in the right hypochondrium, and this radiates to the back. There may be nausea and vomiting and also an elevation of temperature. The medical management usually consists of intramuscular injection of analgesia, such as pethidine, an antiemetic such as metoclopramide and an antimicrobial agent to treat the infection. The patient will be on bedrest and will require intravenous fluid management. It is essential for the nurse to monitor pain, fluid balance, oral hygiene and the vital signs.

Removal of gallstones

Although there are various ways by which gallstones are removed (ERCP and lithotripsy, as explained below), the commonest procedure is surgery and this involves the removal of the gallbladder (**cholecystectomy**). In this operation there may be exploration of the common bile duct via an incision (**choledochotomy**) and a tube called a T tube is then inserted to maintain the patency of the common bile duct and to ensure the drainage of bile. To ensure that the tube is in position, a **cholangiogram** is performed (radio-opaque dye is inserted through the T tube) and X-rays are taken.

Endoscopic Retrograde Cholangiopancreatography

ERCP is the procedure used for the removal of a stone located within the bile ducts. A fibrescope is passed through the oral pharynx to the duodenum and into the biliary and pancreatic tracts. Contrast media may also be injected through the endoscope.

Lithotripsy

This is an advanced technique for the removal of gallstones. It involves a machine (lithotripter) which produces shock waves to dislodge and disintegrate the stones. It is a noninvasive procedure and is advantageous for the elderly and for those persons who may have respiratory problems. There is less risk of complications.

Specific care with regard to biliary drainage

If a patient has a T tube *in situ* following surgery, specific nursing management is required.

(1) Measure and record drainage of bile as directed by the surgeon.
(2) Monitor the amount and colour of the drainage frequently.
(3) Explain to the patient the importance of avoiding kinks or pulling the tube.
(4) Monitor the colour of urine and stools. Stools should be a light colour if bile is flowing out of the drainage tube.
(5) Report any signs or symptoms which may indicate **peritonitis** (abdominal pain or rigidity, nausea or vomiting, elevated temperature).

Possible investigations to detect the presence of gallstones

These may include the following: ultrasonography, computerised axial tomography (CAT scan), radionuclide scan, percutaneous transhepatic cholangiography and cholecystography. In percutaneous transhepatic cholangiography a dye is injected through the skin and abdominal wall into a blood vessel or bile duct.

Answers to questions

Q1. Ingestion, movement of food, digestion, absorption and defaecation. For more explanation see 📖 *Page 766.*

Q2. a. A, parotid gland; B, sublingual and submandibular glands; C, oesophagus; D, liver; E, gall bladder; F, duode-num; G, ascending colon; H, caecum; I, vermiform appendix; J, mouth; K, pharynx; L, stomach; M, pancreas; N, transverse colon; O, jejunum; P, ileum; Q, descending colon; R, sigmoid colon; S, rectum; T, anus.

b. The accessory structures include the teeth, the tongue, the salivary glands, the liver, the gallbladder and the pancreas.

Q3. A, hard palate; B, palatoglossal arch; C, uvula; D, palatine tonsils; E, lingual frenulum; F, vestibule; G, incisor tooth; H, canine tooth; I, molar tooth.

Q4. The tongue contains powerful muscles which are responsible for chewing (mastication) and the transformation of the food into a **bolus**. It also contains the taste buds (fungiform papillae and the circumvallate papillae), and therefore plays an essential part in taste sensations. The tongue is also important for swallowing and speech.

Q5. 1, Parotid; 2, Sublingual; 3, Submandibular.

Q6. The parotid glands.

Q7. Infective parotitis, which is also commonly known as mumps.

Q8. Saliva contains about 99% water, in which there are sodium, potassium, chloride, bicarbonate and phosphate ions. It also contains an enzyme known as salivary amylase and a bacteriolytic enzyme, which is called **lysozyme.** Bacteriolytic means capable of destroying bacteria. Amongst the other substances present in saliva are: urea, uric acid, mucin and globulin. Also present in saliva are the **glycoproteins** that are responsible for the type of blood group to which we belong. Glycoprotein means a substance that contains both protein and carbohydrate.

Q9. The crown, the neck and the root.

Q10. a. 3, 2, 1.
b. 1, 2, 3.
c. 1, 2, 3.

Q11. Deciduous or milk teeth appear at about six months of age. There are 20 in number. Permanent teeth are those that appear following the loss of the deciduous teeth. This usually takes place between age 6 and adulthood. *For more information,* 📖 *Pages 774–5.*

Q12. Oral hygiene is very important and is an essential nursing intervention, especially in those patients who are unable to care for themselves, e.g. if they are unconscious. Oral hygiene might improve salivation and therefore improves the function of the taste buds. Many ill patients cannot taste their foods and this can also occur in patients who have fevers.

Oral hygiene may prevent the development of thrush (**candidiasis**) which is a fungal infection. This infection can affect very ill patients, especially those who are taking antibiotics or immunosuppressants (medications used in the management of cancer patients and also to reduce the risk of rejection of transplanted organs). Another common infection that can occur in patients whose resistance is reduced is the viral infection commonly known as 'cold sores' (**Herpes simplex**). These are extremely painful and can prevent the patients from eating.

Oral hygiene will also reduce the problem of bad breath (**halitosis**). Some patients may have offensive breath as a result of their illness. For example, patients with kidney failure may have a 'fishy' smell on their breath (due to the excess of urea in their blood), whilst diabetic patients may have 'pear smell' on their breath (due to the presence of ketone).

Oral hygiene will also keep the mouth moist and this will assist with speech. A dry mouth (for example when you have been severely stressed or anxious) makes speech difficult.

On the whole, oral hygiene, apart from removing food particles and other debris, will promote hydration, moisten the oral mucosa and prevent dental caries and other problems of the gums and the tongue. Inflammation of the gums is known as **gingivitis** and inflammation of the tongue is known as **glossitis**.

Q13. 1, cardia; 2, lesser curvature; 3, pylorus; 4, duodenum; 5, oesophagus; 6, muscularis; 7, greater curvature; 8, pyloric sphincter.

Q14. The oesophagus is a muscular structure situated in the thoracic cavity, behind the trachea. It is about 25cm in length in the adult. It is connected to the pharynx above, and the superior portion of the stomach below. It passes through the diaphragm to reach the stomach. It is lined by stratified squamous epithelium.

Q15. a, swallowing; b, voluntary; c, pharyngeal; d, respiration; e, medulla; f, oesophageal; g, stomach.

Q16. a. Mouth, salivary glands: *protein* – no enzymes for digestion of proteins; *lipid* – lingual lipase breaks down triglycerides and other lipids to fatty acids and monoglycerides; *mechanical* – deglutition; *other functions* – secretes saliva; important for mastication, speech, tasting; softens, moistens and dissolves food, cleanses mouth and teeth.

b. Pharynx, oesophagus: *carbohydrate* – no enzymes for digestion of carbohydrates; *protein* – no enzymes for digestion of proteins; *lipid* – no enzymes for digestion of lipids; *other functions* – closes air passageways and therefore prevents foods from entering into respiratory tract; relaxation of the lower oesophageal sphincter allows bolus to pass into the stomach.

Q17. 1, Cardia; 2, lesser curvature; 3, pylorus; 4, duodenum; 5, oesophagus; 6, fundus; 7, greater curvature; 8, pyloric sphincter.

Q18. 4, 2, 1, 3.

Q19.

Name of cell	Type of secretion	Function of secretion
Chief (zymogenic)	Pepsinogen Gastric lipase	Precursor of pepsin
Mucous	Mucus	Protects gastric lining from acid and pepsin
Parietal (oxyntic)	HCl intrinsic factor	Activates pepsinogen to pepsin. Facilitates absorption of vitamin B_{12}
G cells	Gastrin	Stimulates secretion of HCl and pepsinogen; contracts lower oesophageal sphincter, increases gastric motility and relaxes pyloric sphincter

Q20. a, acid; b, pepsinogen; c, mucous; d, ulcer; e, gastric lipase; f, fats; g, 5; h, 6.

Q21. a, cephalic; b, gastric; c, intestinal; d, sight; e, smell; f, presence; g, vagus; h, parasympathetic; i, autonomic; j, anger; k, fear; l, anxiety; m, gastric; n, increase; o, gastrin; p, HCl; q, enterogastric; r, inhibits; s, delay; t, gastric inhibitory peptide; u, secretin; v, cholecystokinin.

Q22. a, 2; b, 6; c, carbohydrates; d, fats.

Q23. The enzymes are pepsinogen and gastric lipase. Pepsinogen is inactive and becomes activated under the influence of HCl. It digests protein into peptides (which consist of chains of amino acids). The chemical reaction in this digestion is the breakdown of peptide bonds between amino acids (📖 *Page 46*).

Gastric lipase splits the short chain triglycerides in butterfat molecules found in milk. This is perhaps more important in babies, since the pH of gastric juice is much higher than in the adult stomach. Gastric lipase works best at pH 5–6.

Q24. Intrinsic factor is a glycoprotein secreted by the parietal cells of the stomach and it is important for the absorption of vitamin B_{12}. Vitamin B_{12} promotes erythropoiesis, the formation of red blood cells in the bone marrow. Lack of vitamin B_{12} causes **pernicious** or **megaloblastic** (this term means the presence of large red cells, which are immature) anaemia.

Someone who suffers from pernicious anaemia would need to receive vitamin replacement and this is given as an injection. One of these preparations is **Cytamen®**.

Q25. Prolonged vomiting obviously causes excessive loss of fluids and electrolytes such as potassium, sodium and chlorides. HCl is also lost. Loss of excessive fluids causes dehydration. In dehydration, the fluid compartment of the body is affected. For example, fluids will leave the cell (intracellular fluid), with serious consequences on homeostasis of water balance. The individual may go into shock (recognised by a rapid pulse rate, a decrease in blood pressure, profuse sweating, also possibly being cold and clammy to the touch) as a result of a decreased cardiac output.

As more fluid is lost, the patient may become lethargic and disorientated. Urine output will be diminished. This is referred to as **oliguria.** Excessive loss of HCl may give rise to metabolic alkalosis. This is due to the large amount of hydrogen ions that are lost.

Vomiting is a common symptom in many gastrointestinal disorders, but can also occur in food poisoning, in motion sickness, following ingestion of a large amount of alcohol and also when patients are given cytotoxic drugs. These are drugs that are administered in many types of cancer.

Q26. Antiemetics. Examples of antiemetics are: Stemetil® (prochlorperazine), scopolamine (hyoscine), chlorpromazine hydrochloride (Largactil®).

A premedication is usually given to individuals prior to surgery (at least 2–3 hours before surgery). The action of the medication is to inhibit the vagus (also called parasympathetic) nerve activity, and thereby reduce salivary and gastric secretion. It also delays gastric emptying.

The reason a premedication is given is to prevent or reduce the risk of vomiting during or immediately following surgery. This therefore prevents inhalation of vomitus which could lead to asphyxia and death. The medication papaveretum (Omnopon®) also provides sedation and will contribute to postoperative pain relief. It is an opiate drug.

Q27. a.

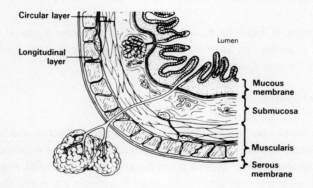

b. Outer layer is the **serosa,** an outer protective layer which may be a serous membrane or fibrous tissue. In the abdominal cavity the serosa is in fact the **visceral peritoneum.** The serosa prevents friction during gut motility. Middle layer is the **submucosa,** consisting of areolar connective tissue which contains many blood vessels, lymphatic vessels and nerves.

Inner layer is the **mucosa,** containing many cavities lined with glandular epithelium. They also form the intestinal glands that secrete intestinal juice. The types of gland may vary in the different parts of the intestine. For example, the duodenum contains the Brunner's glands, which secrete an alkaline mucus that neutralises gastric acid. The mucosa also forms a series of villi, which are important for absorption of food nutrients.

Q28. Peritoneal cavity.

Q29. 1a, 4b, 5c, 2d, 3e.

Q30. A villus is a finger-like projection. Villi increase the surface area of the epithelium for absorption and digestion. Each villus has a core of lamina propria (📖 *Page 798, Figure 24.22(b)*), which contains the blood vessels and a central vessel known as the **lacteal** (it is in fact a lymphatic vessel), which drains fatty acids.

Q31. The labels for the diagram should be as follows: 1, left lobe; 2; right lobe; 3, left hepatic duct; 4, right hepatic duct; 5, cystic duct; 6, common bile duct; 7, body of pancreas; 8, main pancreatic duct (or duct of Wirsung); 9, ampulla of Vater; 10, duodenum; 11, gallbladder.

Q32. a. Abdominal cavity; b, stomach; c, head; d, duodenum; e, tail; f, spleen; g, Islets of Langerhans; h, acini; i, pancreatic juice; j, alkaline; k, proteins; l, trypsinogen; m, enterokinase; n, chymotrypsinogen; o, chymotrypsin; p, amylase; q, lipase; r, exocrine; s, Wirsung; t, main pancreatic duct; u, duodenum.

Q33. Endocrine functions – two main hormones, **insulin** and **glucagon,** are secreted. Insulin is secreted by the beta cells of the Islets of Langerhans. Its main function is the conversion of excess glucose into glycogen. It also promotes the entry of glucose and potassium into the cells. Glucagon is secreted by the alpha cells of the Islets of Langerhans. It increases the blood glucose level when it is low.

Exocrine functions – produce the enzymes trypsinogen, chymotrypsinogen, lipase, amylase, carboxypeptidases, ribonucleases and deoxyribonucleases. For functions of the first two enzymes mentioned here, see answer to question 32.

Lipase breaks down fats into fatty acids and glycerol. Amylase continues the digestion of cooked starch and converts it to maltose. Ribonucleases and deoxyribonucleases digest nucleic acids.

Q34.   Secretin and cholecystokinin.

Q35.   Carbohydrate – digested and absorbed as monosaccharides. Fructose and galactose are transported into epithelial cells of the villi by secondary active transport, coupled to the active transport of sodium ions.

Proteins – final digestion products are amino acids. These are absorbed by active transport into the duodenum and jejunum. Both monosaccharides and amino acids are absorbed by the villi and carried in the blood to the liver by the hepatic portal vein.

Lipids – all absorbed by simple diffusion, but the absorption of lipids is rather complex. For more information, refer to the terms **micelles** and **chylomicrons** (📖 *Pages 804–5*).

Q36.   c. Stomach: *carbohydrate* – no enzymes for digestion of carbohydrates; *protein* – secretes pepsinogen which when activated to pepsin, digests proteins into peptides; can also digest milk proteins; *lipid* – gastric lipase which splits the short-chain triglycerides in butterfat molecules found in milk; more important in babies; *mechanical* – peristaltic movements which mix foods with gastric juice to form chymes.

d. Pancreas: *carbohydrate* – pancreatic amylase which digests polysarchaide into maltose, maltriose and dextrins; *protein* – trypsinogen which activated to trypsin by enterokinase and breaks down proteins into peptides; chymotrypsinogen which is activated by trypsin and breaks down proteins to peptides; carboxypeptidase acts at carboxyl end of amino acid to yield peptides and amino acids; *mechanical* – none; *other functions* – endocrine functions; secreting insulin and glucagon.

e. Intestinal juices: *carbohydrate* – maltose which breaks down maltose into glucose; sucrase which breaks down sucrose into fructose and glucose; lactase which breaks down lactose into glucose and galactose; *protein* – peptidases continue digestion of proteins to yield amino acids; *lipid* – no enzymes for digestion of lipids (note: lipids are digested in the small intestine but by enzymes secreted elsewhere); *mechanical* – segmentation; peristalsis; *other functions* – absorption; nucleosases and phosphatases digest DNA to form pentoses, phosphates and nitrogenous bases.

Q37.   a, 1.4; b, hypochondrium; c, diaphragm; d, kidney; e, four; f, right. g, peritoneum; h, falciform; i, umbilical; j, hepatic; k, aorta; l, hepatic portal; m, intestine.

Q38.   a, lobule; b, lobule; c, hepatocytes; d, vein; e, sinusoids; f, bile canaliculi; g. bilirubin; h, red blood cells; i, jaundice; j, cholecystokinin; k, gallbladder; l, emulsification; m, absorption; n, fibrinogen; o, prothrombin; p, albumin; q, deamination; r, urea; s, urine.

Q39.   Converts glucose into glycogen. Converts amino acids into glucose (gluconeogenesis). Synthesises lipoproteins, which transport fatty acids. Removes drugs and hormones. Stores many fat-soluble vitamins (A, D, E and K). Also stores vitamin B_{12}. Plays a part in phagocytic action, on account of containing reticuloendothelial cells.

Q40.   Bile is an alkaline fluid, consisting of water, bile salts (sodium taurocholate and sodium glycocholate), cholesterol, lecithin, bile pigment (mainly bilirubin) and various ions. Bile plays an important role in the emulsification of fats and in the absorption of fat-soluble vitamins. It deodorises and colours the faeces.

Q41.   Labelling is as follows: 1, transverse; 2, ascending; 3, caecum; 4, vermiform appendix; 5, rectum; 6, descending; 7, taenia coli; 8, sigmoid; 9, anus; 10, hepatic flexure; 11, splenic flexure.

Q42.   The large intestine is about 1.5 metres whilst the ileum is about 3.6 metres. In cross section the colon has a much thicker wall than the ileum. The colon contains a series of pouches called haustrations, which are lacking in the ileum. The muscularis of both ileum and colon consists of an external layer of longitudinal muscles and internal circular muscles. However, the longitudinal muscles in the large intestine are arranged into three bands called taeniae coli. There are no villi in the colon as compared to the ileum. Both the ileum and colon contain simple columnar epithelium, amongst which there are numerous goblet cells. The submucosa is similar in both the ileum and the colon.

Q43. Defaecation occurs as a result of stimulation of stretch receptors in the wall of the rectum when this is distended. The receptors send nerve impulses to the sacral spinal cord. The motor impulses travel along the parasympathetic nerves back to the descending colon, rectum and anus. The motor activity causes contraction of the longitudinal muscles which therefore shorten and thus force the faeces through the anus. This is also assisted by contraction of the diaphragm and abdominal muscles. The act of defaecation itself is controlled by two sphincters; the internal and the external sphincters. The external sphincter is under voluntary control.

Q44. g. Large intestine: *mechanical* – peristalsis; haustral churning; mass peristalsis; defaecation; *other functions –* production of flatus; decomposition of bilirubin to urobilinogen by bacteria; absorption of vitamins B and K; absorption of water; production of faeces.

Q45. Albumin, fibrinogen, prothrombin and globulin.

Q46. a, A; b, D; c, E; d, K; e, B_{12}.

Q47. 2a, 4b, 1c, 3d.

Q48. a, Secretin; b, gastrin; c, HCl; d, pepsin; e, enterokinase; f, glycogen; g, lipase; h, bile; i, amylase.

Q49. d.

Q50. d.

Q51. 2a, 4b, 3c, 1d.

Q52. 1a, 1b, 1c, 1d, 1 and 3e, 3f, 2g.

Q53. a. 1, 4, 3, 2, 5.
b. 5, 4, 2, 1, 3.
c. 1, 2, 4, 3, 5.
d. 1, 4, 2, 3.

Q54. 5a, 11b, 4c, 12d, 7e, 3f, 6g, 13h, 9i, 2j, 1k, 8l.

Q55. Possible signs and symptoms: loss of weight, excessive thirst (polydipsia), excessive production of urine (polyuria), presence of glucose and ketone in the urine, sweet smell of ketone on the breath, episode of hypoglycaemia (low blood sugar level), weakness, tiredness and fatigue.

You know that diabetes is an endocrine disorder, due to the lack of or reduction in insulin secretion and it primarily affects carbohydrate metabolism. Since CHO is the main source of energy for the body, in its absence, fats will be metabolised instead. In the absence of glucose as prime source of energy, fat catabolism causes the formation of ketone bodies, which are then excreted in the urine. One simple reason why ketone is formed is because in the absence of glucose as the main source for **glycolysis, oxaloacetic acid** production is reduced. Oxaloacetic acid is the main substance that drives the **Kreb's cycle** through combining with **acetyl coenzyme A**. This is the last process in glycolysis, and when acetyl coenzyme A cannot combine with oxaloacetic acid, it then combines with other molecules of acetyl coenzyme A to form ketone bodies. You should understand this if you have studied glycolysis and the chapter on metabolism and nutrition.

The presence of glucose (glycosuria) and ketone in the urine is largely due to the failure of the body's cells to use glucose. When all the body's lipids have been used, proteins will be catabolised to provide energy. By this time, Simon would have lost large amount of body mass. This accounts for the weight loss.

Relating all the above to possible symptoms:

(1) Loss of weight is due to excessive catabolism of fats and proteins.

(2) Sweet 'pear' smell on the breath is the result of excess ketone in the blood.

(3) Polyuria is due to large amounts of glucose excreted in the urine. This causes a diuresis effect and more fluid is lost from the body. If the fluid is not replaced, it could lead to dehydration.

(4) Polydipsia – fluid loss causes disturbance of the homeostatic control of body fluid and therefore the thirst mechanism comes into play and patients drink large amounts of fluid.

(5) Passing of urine during the night is explained above for number (3).

(6) Periods of hypoglycaemia as a result of sympathetic activity – pallor, tachycardia, perspiration, hunger, palpitation, weakness; and a result of central nervous system activity – mental confusion, blurred vision, incoherent speech, fatigue, numbness of lips and tongue.

It is important to realise that if a diagnosis is not made promptly, it is possible that Simon could suffer from **ketoacidosis**. However, in most cases, with vigilant parents, they would have noticed that something was wrong with Simon.

Q56. Potato contains starch. Cooked starch is firstly broken down by the action of salivary amylase in the mouth and converted into dextrins and **maltose.** The digestion is continued in the small intestine, where maltose is broken down into two molecules of glucose by the enzyme **maltase.** Glucose is then absorbed by the villi of the intestine and is carried to the liver via the hepatic portal vein.

Q57. Following such a meal, the blood glucose level will rise. Under normal circumstances, i.e. in health, the body readjusts the glucose level through the secretion of insulin, which then converts excess glucose into glycogen in the liver. Since Simon is a diabetic, his pancreas is not secreting insulin and therefore his blood glucose will rise. This could lead to **hyperglycaemia** (high level of blood glucose), and **glycosuria.** The symptoms of hyperglycaemia are: dehydration, hypotension, anuria, elevated body temperature, circulatory collapse, coma etc.

Q58. Insulin is a hormone (it is a protein consisting of 51 amino acids). It is secreted by the beta cells of the Islets of Langerhans which are found in the pancreas. Its main function is to convert excess glucose into glycogen. It also facilitates the entry of glucose and potassium into the cell. It is secreted through a negative feedback mechanism. This is because when blood glucose level is low, insulin release is suppressed and when blood glucose level is high, this causes the release of insulin. It is in fact the blood level of glucose that controls the regulation of insulin secretion.

Q59. Glucagon.

Q60. This is perhaps the reverse of what has been discussed in question 57. Insulin reduces the blood level of glucose. So, if Simon has received his insulin injection, but has missed his breakfast, he may well develop **hypoglycaemia.**

Q61. It is important that Simon understands the role of insulin in relation to his diabetes. Is the type of insulin administered short- or long-acting? He should always ensure that he takes his meals regularly. It is also important for him to take his insulin even if he is not feeling too well, for example if he has a touch of flu. He must let his parents know if he is unwell.

He must also be given advice with regard to hygiene, so as to reduce the risk of infection at injection sites. He should always ensure that the insulin is the right strength. He must check that the insulin is not cloudy. He should ensure that the insulin injected is at room temperature. He must check for and remove any air bubbles after the insulin is drawn. He must rotate the sites of injection, because **lipodystrophy** may occur with repeated injections in the same sites. Two forms of lipodystrophy can occur: hypertrophy and atrophy. Hypertrophy is thickening of an injection site because of the development of fibrous scar tissue from the repeated injections in the same sites. Atrophy is the loss of cutaneous fats and again is as a result of repeated injection in the same sites.

Q62. Depending on the level of physical activities, the body's demands for glucose will increase as muscles need more glucose for their functions. Simon's body may not have this storage of glucose for this activity and he would need to increase his CHO intake. This will also need to be counterbalanced by an adjustment of his insulin. With careful management by the doctor and the dietitian, an approximate calculation (sometimes by trial and error) of CHO may be worked out. The insulin will be adjusted accordingly.

It is important that diabetic children are not deprived of exercise because they are diabetics. They must be encouraged to live a normal happy life.

Q63. Obviously, different individuals will have different complications. Diabetic persons develop **atherosclerotic** changes in large arteries. This could lead to hypertension, cerebrovascular disease, coronary artery disease or peripheral vascular disease. The last may give rise to gangrene. Blindness may occur as a result of diabetic retinopathy. Cataract may also occur and this may be caused by prolonged hyperglycaemia that results in swelling of the lens and formation of opacity. Nephropathy can also occur as a result of microvascular changes in the renal structure and function. This can lead to renal diseases. An earlier sign is the loss of protein (proteinuria) in the urine. Neuropathy may also occur and this can affect the peripheral nerves, the autonomic nervous system, the spinal cord, or the central nervous system. This can give rise to varied symptoms, such as pins and needles in the hands or the legs, and bilateral sensory loss in the distal lower extremities.

With early diagnosis and prompt treatment and regular medical examinations, many of these complications are less likely to occur.

Q64. As she has been vomiting, she would have lost a large amount of fluids and this could lead to dehydration. There would also be disturbance of electrolytes as potassium, sodium, chlorides and hydrogen ions are lost in the vomitus. Most of these ions can be replaced with the intravenous infusions.

Q65. Since the gallstone is blocking the common bile duct, bile cannot reach the duodenum. There is therefore reflux of bile on the biliary system and the liver, and the serum level of the bile pigment **bilirubin** will be increased. The normal serum level of bilirubin is 2–17μmol/l. In the situation here, the level may be as high as 35–50μmol/l. There is yellow discolouration of the skin, mucous membrane and sclera of the eyes.

Q66. All of the symptoms are as a result of the increase in bilirubin and its absence from the intestines.

Mrs Daniels may complain of **pruritus**, which is an intense skin irritation, as a result of the bilirubin in the blood. Her stools will be pale or clay coloured. This is due to the absence of **stercobilin**. Stercobilin is derived from **stercobilinogen**, which is present in bile when it can reach the duodenum in the normal pathway. Stercobilinogen is converted into stercobilin following bacterial activity in the gut and is responsible for the colouration of the faeces. The other substance responsible for colouration of the faeces is **urobilinogen**. It is only present when bile can enter the duodenum. Urobilinogen is reabsorbed from the gut and is usually excreted in the urine. Therefore it will be absent in Mrs Daniels' stools. Her urine will be very dark and on exposure will look a dark green colour. Urine contains bilirubin, but no urobilinogen. The explanation is the same as above.

Q67. Specific nursing observations:

(1) Monitor all vital signs.
(2) Monitor administration of intravenous fluids.
(3) Observe and record any vomitus.
(4) Measure and record fluid output.
(5) Observe colour of urine and stools.
(6) Assess and monitor any pain.

All observations should help in assessing Mrs Daniels' condition, to ensure that she is hydrated, that she is not going into hypovolaemic shock, and that early signs of peritonitis can be detected. These should help the surgeon in his decision as to whether she is fit for surgery.

Q68. Bile contains bile salts which play an important role in the emulsification of fats and therefore aid in its digestion. Since Mrs Daniels has obstructive jaundice, bile is not present in the duodenum and consequently the process of emulsification is missing. Fat digestion is impaired, and this can give rise to nausea and vomiting.

Q69. **(1)** Give as much explanation as possible, to reassure Mrs Daniels as to the reason for the surgery. This should reduce any fear or anxiety.

(2) Ensure that she understands what is involved before she consents to the operation.

(3) Prepare the skin site of the abdomen for surgery as per procedure.

(4) Ensure as far as is possible general hygiene, but without causing too much discomfort to the patient. Change into the operation gown.

(5) Give premedication as prescribed.

(6) Test the urine for any other abnormalities, such as the presence of blood or glucose.

(7) Remove any prosthesis and ensure that the identity bracelet is worn.

Q70. Vitamin K is a fat-soluble vitamin and is usually absorbed in the presence of bile. Once absorbed, vitamin K is stored in the liver, where its main function is the synthesis of **prothrombin**, which is an important clotting factor. Lack of prothrombin may cause bleeding following surgery.

Mrs Daniels may lack vitamin K on account of her obstructed bile duct. Since she cannot digest fats properly, there is therefore a reduction in the absorption of any fat-soluble vitamins.

Q71. If the infusion is 500ml in four hours, 2000ml should be delivered in 16 hours. If the infusion commenced at 8 a.m, it should be finished by midnight of the same day (Monday).

Overview and key terms

Metabolism

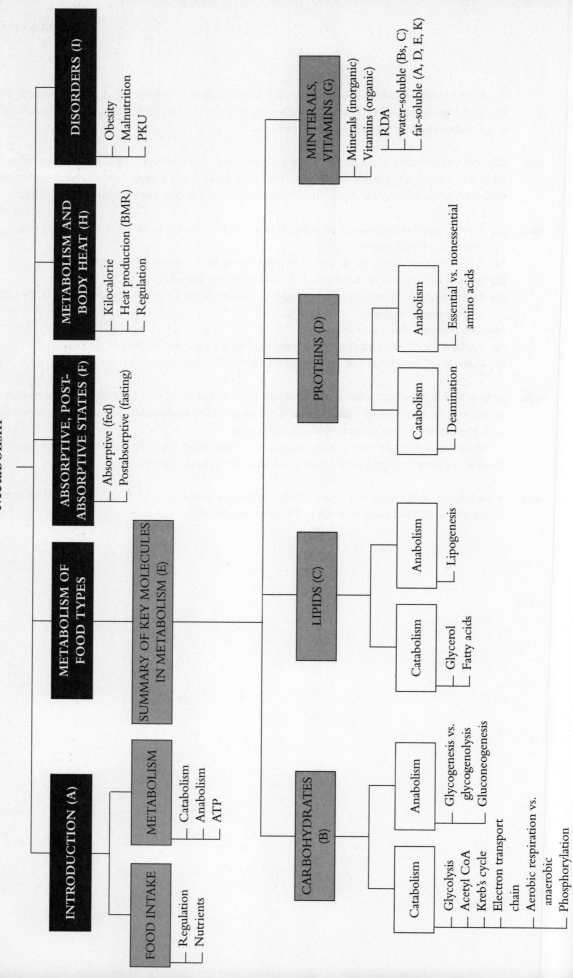

17. Nutrition and Metabolism

Learning outcomes

1. To explain how food intake is regulated.

2. To define a nutrient.

3. To list the functions of six principal classes of nutrients.

4. To define metabolism and explain the role of ATP in anabolism and catabolism.

5. To describe the metabolism of carbohydrates, lipids and proteins.

6. To differentiate between the absorptive (fed) and the postabsorptive (fasting) state.

7. To name the sources and outline the functions of minerals and vitamins in metabolism.

8. To outline the nutritional problems associated with phenylketonuria and coeliac disease.

9. To define the term malnutrition.

Chapters 2 & 25

INTRODUCTION

It is hoped that when you have completed this study, you will have a thorough knowledge of the constituents of food, and what happens to them when they have been ingested, digested, absorbed and utilised by the body's cells.

You will also understand the meaning of **metabolism**, which is defined as 'all the chemical reactions that take place in the body'.

To survive, all living organisms need foods from which they derive their energy. These foods are actually organic compounds and humans obtain them from plants and animals. Foods provide **nutrients**, of which there are six principal classes.

As you proceed through this study, you should uncover the complex nature of food utilisation and what this means for a living body.

METABOLISM

For questions 1–3 *Page 822*

Q1. List two primary functions of nutrients.

_____

_____

Q2. List the six principal classes of nutrients.

_____

Food will be utilised by the body after it has been ingested, but what mechanism governs food intake in the individual? This is still not well understood.

Read the section on regulation of food intake and then answer question 3.

Q3. The site within the brain that is the location of feeding and satiety centres is the (a) _____ . The satiety hormone is known as (b) _____ .

Q4. List five functions of water in the body.

_____

_____

Q5. Complete the table below, which compares catabolism with anabolism.

Process	Definition	Releases or uses of energy	Examples
a. Catabolism			
b. Anabolism			

In your answer to question 1, you would have included carbohydrates (CHO), proteins and fats. You will now explore in detail the compositions and functions of these three important nutrients and their significance to the body. The remaining three nutrients will be dealt with later.

CARBOHYDRATES

Carbohydrates are **organic** compounds, and amongst all the foods that we eat they are the most important in producing the energy which the body requires for its metabolic activities.

For questions 6–11 📖 *Page 41, Chapter 2.*

Q6.   **Explain what you understand by an organic compound.**

_____

_____

Q7.   **List four groups of chemicals that belong to CHO.**

_____

Q8.   **State the chemical composition of CHO.**

_____

Q9.   **List four common foods that contain CHO.**

_____

Q10.   **Carbohydrates are divided into three major groups depending on the number of carbon atoms in the molecule. Name the three major groups of CHO.**

_____

Q11.   **Complete the statements about CHO.**

The ratio of hydrogen to oxygen in all carbohydrates is (a) _____: (b) _____ . The general formula for carbohydrates is (c) _____. The chemical formula for a hexose is (d) _____. Two common hexoses are (e) _____ and (f) _____ One common pentose sugar found in DNA is (g) _____. Its name and its formula ($C_5H_{10}O_4$) indicate that it lacks one oxygen atom from the typical pentose formula, which is (h) _____.

When two glucose molecules ($C_6H_{12}O_6$) combine, a disaccharide is formed. Its formula is (i) _____, indicating that in a synthesis reaction such as this, a molecule of water is (j) _____.

Continued dehydration synthesis leads to enormous carbohydrates called (k) _____. One such carbohydrate is (l) _____. When a disaccharide such as sucrose is broken, water is introduced to split the bond linking the two monosaccharides. Such a decomposition reaction is termed (m) _____, which literally means 'splitting using water '.

By now you will have discovered that glucose, a hexose sugar, is the main energy-supplying molecule of the body. The other hexoses, such as fructose and galactose can also be used to provide energy, but only after they have been converted into glucose.

Q12.   In which organ are galactose and fructose converted into glucose? 📖 *Page 825.*

_____

Q13.   How do you explain the fact that glucose and galactose have the same chemical formula ? Hint: think in terms of the three-dimensional structure of a molecule.

_____

_____

_____

Disaccharides

Three disaccharides that are found in some foods are **lactose**, **sucrose** and **maltose**. They are broken down by enzymes in the digestive tract to yield mainly glucose and other hexoses.

Q14.   Give the name of the enzymes and the products of digestion of lactose, maltose and sucrose. (📖 *Page 801*)

Q15.   List one important polysaccharide that is stored in the liver and muscles. (📖 *Page 41*)

_____

Q16.   From your daily experience of eating, suggest two types of polysaccharides that you take in your diet (one a food source and the other providing roughage).

_____

Fate of CHO and glucose movement into cells

Now that you have grasped some essential facts about CHO, you can consider how the body utilises glucose for synthesising energy in the form of **adenosine triphosphate (ATP)**. Organisms use mainly two mechanisms of phosphorylation to generate ATP. Phosphorylation is the addition of a phosphate group to a chemical compound. This raises the energy level of the molecule .

For questions 17 and 18, 📖 *Page 825*

Q17. **List the two main mechanisms of phosphorylation that take place in the body to generate ATP.**

_____

_____

Q18. **List five possible outcomes of absorbed glucose in the body.**

_____

_____

_____

Q19. **Which hormone facilitates the entry of glucose into the cells?** 📖 *Page 826*

_____

Glycolysis

The section which follows is to assist you in understanding how the body utilises glucose to provide energy through the process of **catabolism**. As explained previously, and from question 17, you should know that this occurs in the cytosol and in the mitochondria. In the cytosol, the catabolism of glucose occurs mainly through **oxidation** in the process known as **glycolysis**, whilst in the mitochondria the process is referred to as the Kreb's cycle, citric acid cycle or tricarboxylic acid (TCA) Cycle.

The overall catabolic reaction of glucose may be represented by the following equation:

Glucose + oxygen ⟶ carbon dioxide + water + energy (stored in ATP).

Q20. **Write the chemical representation of the equation given above.**

_____

Both glycolysis and phosphorylation are very complex and involve many enzymes. In this study reference will only be made to the most important enzymes and the most important chemical reactions. In parts, simple explanations will be given so as to make your study easy and enjoyable.

Q21. **This question relates to glycolysis.** 📖 *Page 826.*

Glycolysis, which occurs in the cytosol of the cells of the body, is an (a) _____ process. It starts when (b) _____ enters the cytoplasm and combines with a phosphate group, a process known as (c) _____ to form (d) _____. The enzyme which is involved in this reaction is known as (e) _____. For each glucose molecule used (f) _____ (how many?) molecules of ATP are used and (g) _____ are produced. There is therefore a net gain of (h) _____ molecules of ATP. 📖 *Figure 25.2 Page 827.*

The process of glycolysis causes the six-carbon molecule of glucose to split into two, three-carbon molecules, known as (i) _____ acid. Many enzymes are involved in these chemical reactions. Steps 4 and 5 show that fructose 1, 6-biphosphate is converted into two three-carbon compounds known as dihydroxyacetone phosphate and (j) _____.

Several steps are involved before pyruvic acid is formed (end product of glycolysis). Once formed, pyruvic acid is ready to enter the mitochondria for the next stage in ATP production (the Kreb's cycle). If there is insufficient (k) _____, pyruvic acid is converted into another three-carbon compound which is known as (l) _____ acid. This is likely to occur during active exercise. The (m) _____ acid may be transported to the liver and is converted back to (n) _____. When oxygen is available, pyruvic acid through enzymatic reactions is converted into acetyl (o) _____.

Q22. **This question explains the fate of pyruvic acid.** 📖 *Page 829.*

The conversion of pyruvic acid to acetyl coenzyme A is a transitional stage that involves the loss of a molecule of (a) _____ to yield a two-carbon fragment, called an (b) _____ group. This fragment attaches to a carrier molecule called (c) _____ , to form (d) _____ . This compound attaches to a molecule known as (e) _____ acid and forms a new six-carbon molecule known as (f) _____ acid, which in fact is the first step in the so called Kreb's cycle.

Kreb's cycle

So far in this study concerning the catabolism of glucose, you have discovered that pyruvic acid is formed in the cytoplasm in the process of glycolysis. The pyruvic acid is then converted into acetyl coenzyme A and this enters the mitochondria. This is the beginning of the Kreb's cycle. The Kreb's cycle consists of a series of biochemical reactions that occur in the matrix of the mitochondria (📖 *Page 76, Figure 3.18*).

Q23. **Why is the Kreb's cycle referred to as a 'cycle'?** 📖 *Page 829*

_____

_____

The Kreb's cycle is very complex and consists of a series of **decarboxylation** and **oxidation–reduction reactions**, each controlled by a different enzyme.

Q24. What do you understand by the term decarboxylation?

_____

Q25. Explain the meaning of oxidation–reduction reaction.

_____

_____

_____

In the Kreb's cycle, a total of six molecules of **carbon dioxide** are formed from each glucose molecule that has entered the cytosol.

Q26. With reference to pyruvic acid, explain why a six-carbon glucose molecule gives rise to six molecules of carbon dioxide .

_____

_____

Q27. Explain what happens to the CO_2 that is formed in the Kreb's cycle. 📖 *Page 829.*

_____

_____

Q28. The Kreb's cycle is assisted by two important coenzymes. Name the two important coenzymes and briefly explain their significance in the Kreb's cycle. 📖 *Page 831.*

_____

_____

The reduced coenzymes from question 28 play a vital role in the production of ATP in the electron transport chain, since a series of reductions transfer the stored energy to ADP + P to form ATP.

Electron transport chain

The final stage in **ATP** production takes place on the **cristae** of the inner mitochondrial membrane and involves the **electron transport chain**. This is a very complex process involving various **electron carrier molecules**.

Q29.   List five of the electron carriers in the electron transport chain. 📖 *Page 832*

_____

_____

There are many steps in the electron transport chain, but you may find them very difficult to understand. However, when reading this section of the textbook (📖 *Page 832*) you should pay particular attention to the **cytochromes, iron–sulphur,** and **copper atoms, and ubiquinones.**

If you have understood the section on the electron transport chain, you can try question 30.

N.B. If you did not understand the section on the electron transport chain, you may need to seek assistance from your tutor or your colleagues. You may leave this question and move on.

Q30.   Complete the exercise below, which describes the electron transport chain.

The first step in the electron chain is transfer of high energy from NADH + H$^+$ to the coenzyme (a) _____. As a result, this carrier is (b) _____ to (c) _____. Vitamin (d) _____ is essential for the function of this particular carrier. As electrons are passed on down the chain, FMNH$_2$ is (e) _____ back to (f) _____.

The portion of cytochromes on which electrons are ferried contains the mineral (g) _____. Cytochromes are positioned toward the end of the transport chain. Two other minerals that are known to be involved in the electron transport chain and are hence necessary in the diet are (h) _____ and (i) _____. The last carrier in the chain is (j) _____. It passes H$^+$ and e$^-$ to (k) _____, the final oxidising molecule. This is a key step in the process of (l) _____ cellular respiration.

Electron carriers are located on the (m) _____ mitochondrial membrane (cristae). The carriers are grouped into (n) _____ complexes. Each complex acts to pump (o) _____ from the matrix into the (p) _____ mitochondrial membrane. As a result, a gradient of H$^+$ is set up across the (q) _____ mitochondrial membrane, resulting in potential energy known as the (r) _____ motive force. These protons travel across special (s) _____ in the inner (t) _____ membrane.

The channels through which H$^+$ diffuse contain the enzyme known as ATP (u) _____ . Since the formation of the resulting ATP is driven by an energy source that consists of a gradient and subsequent diffusion of H$^+$, this mechanism is known as (v) _____ generation of ATP.

After consideration of the catabolism of glucose, it is now appropriate to refer to glucose **anabolism.** This includes synthesis of **glycogen (glycogenesis)** and formation of glucose from fats and proteins (**gluconeogenesis**).

Consider glycogenesis first by working on question 31. 📖 *Page 835.*

Q31.   When glucose is not needed immediately for ATP production, it combines with many other
molecules of glucose to form (a) _____, which is stored in the liver and muscles. This process takes place in the (b) _____ and is assisted by a hormone from the

pancreas called (c) _____ . The body can store about (d) _____ g of glycogen, the majority of which is stored in the (e) _____ muscle fibres (what type of muscle fibres?)

Glycogenolysis

When the body needs energy, the substance in the liver (from question 31) is broken down to provide glucose.

For questions 32 and 33, 📖 *Page 835.*

Q32.   **Briefly outline how the process of glycogenolysis is achieved.**

_____

_____

_____

Q33.   **Briefly explain why muscle glycogen cannot yield glucose.**

_____

Gluconeogenesis

When the body is depleted of glucose, and liver glycogen is low, it can obtain energy by converting the catabolised products of triglycerides and proteins into glucose. This is known as **gluconeogenesis**.

Q34.   **Define gluconeogenesis and briefly discuss how it is related to other metabolic reactions.**

_____

_____

Q35.   **Name five hormones that stimulate gluconeogenesis.**

_____

Having completed the study on carbohydrates, you can now proceed to lipids. This is another group of important organic compounds. They can be used to provide energy when glucose level is low.

LIPIDS

For questions 36–38, 📖 *Pages 42–5.*

Q36. In terms of their chemical composition, how do lipids differ from carbohydrates? Hint: refer to the number of C, H and O atoms.

_____

_____

Q37. Lipids are hydrophobic. True or false?

_____

Q38. List the different types of lipids in the body.

_____

_____

You should now be familiar with the different types of lipids in the body. The most plentiful lipids in the body are the **triglycerides**.

Q39. What is the other name by which triglycerides are known?

_____

Q40. What is the link between saturated fat and ill health?

_____

_____

_____

Q41. Briefly explain what you understand by the terms saturated, monounsaturated and polyunsaturated fats.

_____

_____

_____

_____

Q42. **Where are lipids stored in the body?**

_____

Q43. **Figure 17.1, shows two different molecules which, when reacting with each other, form a lipid.**

Figure 17.1.
Structure of two
molecules.

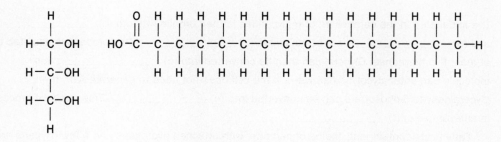

Molecule A   Molecule B

a.   Identify molecule A and B.

_____

b.   When A joins with B, a molecule of H_2O is formed. What is this reaction referred to as?

_____

c.   Is the compound that is formed a monoglyceride, a diglyceride or a triglyceride?

_____

Fate of lipids

Like CHO, lipids can be metabolised to produce ATP if the body has no immediate use for them. In this instance, they are stored in the **adipose tissue** throughout the body and in the liver.

Q44. **List three important substances that are derived from lipids.**

_____

Q45. **List some of the major functions of adipose tissue.** 📖 _Page 837._

_____

_____

Lipid catabolism

In the absence of glucose, the body can make use of triglycerides for the production of **ATP**.

Q46. **In terms of energy yield, how does lipid compare with CHO, gram for gram?**

_____

If the cell needs to produce more ATP, glyceraldehyde 3–phosphate can be broken down to pyruvic acid, in a very similar process to that which occurs during the catabolic pathway (glycolysis).

Complete question 47, which is an exercise that should enable you to understand how triglycerides can be metabolised as an energy source. You should note that it is a slightly complex process and occurs in two distinct phases. 📖 *Page 838.*

Q47. The initial step in the catabolism of triglycerides is their breakdown into (a) _____ and (b) _____ , a process called (c) _____. This process is assisted by at least five hormones. Glycerol can then be converted into (d) _____ ; this molecule can enter glycolytic pathways. If the cell does not need to generate ATP, then glyceraldehyde 3-phosphate can be converted into (e) _____. This anabolic process is an example of (f) _____.

Fatty acids contain long chains of carbons, with attached hydrogens and a few oxygens and they are catabolised differently from **glycerol**, yielding more ATP. This catabolic process occurs in the matrix of (g) _____ and is known as (h) _____ and results in formation of a two-carbon fragment. The two-carbon fragment (i) _____ acid, is attached to (j) _____ (an enzyme), forming (k) _____. The substance formed in (k) then enters the (l) _____ cycle and the electron transport chain.

However, if there are large numbers of (i), they tend to pair chemically to form a substance called (m) _____. Some of these substances formed in (m) can be converted into ß-hydroxybutyric acid and (n) _____. These three substances are collectively known as (o) _____ bodies and if present in excess, they can lead to what is known as (p) _____.

In this situation, the pH of the blood is lowered, giving rise to (q) _____.
(q) _____ can also occur in many clinical situations in which there is excessive beta oxidation, for example during fasting or starvation or in the disease **diabetes mellitus**.

Having completed the above exercise, you should now be aware of the importance of glucose as an energy source for the body. Question 48 should enable you to understand why a diabetic individual may be prone to develop ketosis. As a nurse you would be able to detect this by testing the individual's urine or by noticing the 'sweet smell' from the patient's breath.

Q48. **Briefly explain why a diabetic individual is very prone to develop ketosis, if his diabetes is not well controlled. Hint: think in terms of how the body obtains energy.**

_____

_____

_____

_____

You have now completed the exercises on lipid metabolism and you can proceed to **protein** metabolism, but before doing so, you need to be familiar with the chemical nature of proteins.

PROTEINS

For questions 49–55, 📖 Pages 45–6 & 840–1

Q49. List the four main atoms that are found in most proteins.

_____

Q50. List another atom that may be present in some proteins.

_____

Q51. Complete the exercise below, which relates to some important facts about proteins.

The building blocks of proteins are (a) _____ _____ , of which there are (b) _____ in nature. Each (a) _____ _____ has three important groups attached to a central carbon atom; an (c) _____ (NH$_2$) group, a (d) _____ (COOH) group and a side chain (R group).

   A protein may consist of several hundred of (a) _____ _____. It is synthesised through many steps, which initially include the combination of **one** (a) _____ _____ to a **second** (a) _____ _____, a **third** is then added to the first two, and so on. This chemical reaction between **two** (a) _____ _____ involves the formation of a covalent bond which is called a (e) _____ bond, and this occurs because a molecule of (f) _____ is removed by dehydration synthesis. The (f) _____ molecule is formed because the (g) _____ group of the carboxyl group of the first (a) _____ _____ joins the hydrogen of the (h) _____ group.

See 📖 *Page 47, Figure 2.13* for more information.

Q52. Consider Figure 17.2, which shows two amino acids, glycine and alanine. They are to join, thus forming a peptide bond. 📖 *Page 47, Figure 2.13.*

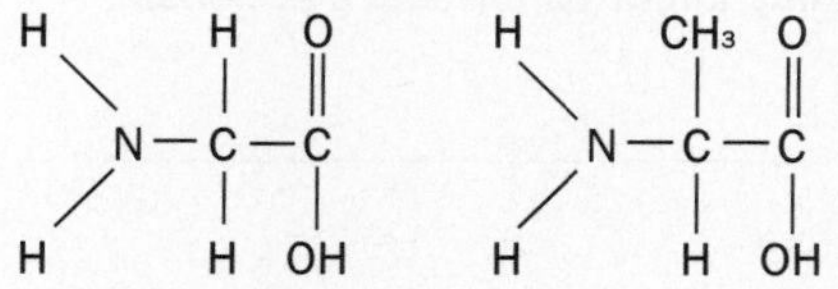

Figure 17.2. Structures of glycine and alanine.

a. Indicate on the diagram how a water molecule is formed during this process.

b. Draw a diagram to show the peptide bond which is formed between glycine and alanine.

Q53. Define the terms dipeptide, tripeptide and polypeptide.

More facts about amino acids ▭▭ *Page 840–1*

Of the **20** amino acids in the body, **10** are referred to as **essential amino acids**.

Q54. Why are the ten amino acids referred to as essential?

_____

_____

Q55. What are the remaining amino acids known as?

_____

Proteins are very important for the body. For example, there are many chemical processes that take place in the body in the presence of specific types of proteins called enzymes. *For questions 56 and 58,* ▭▭ *Page 49.*

Q56. Briefly define the term enzyme.

_____

Q57. Outline three factors that may affect an enzyme's actions.

_____

ABSORPTIVE AND POSTABSORPTIVE STATES

Having completed the study on carbohydrates, fats and proteins, you will now be introduced to absorptive and postabsorptive states, and minerals and vitamins.

For questions 58–59, 📖 *Pages 843–7*

Q58. Contrast these two metabolic states by writing 'A' if the description refers to the absorptive state and 'P' if it refers to the postabsorptive state.

☐ a. The period when the body is fasting and is challenged to maintain an adequate blood glucose level.

☐ b. The state during which glucose (stored in the liver and muscle) is released.

☐ c. The state during which most systems (excluding the nervous system) switch over to use fatty acids as energy sources.

☐ d. The time when the body is absorbing nutrients from the GI tract.

☐ e. The state during which the principal concern is formation of stores of glucose (as glycogen) and fat.

☐ f. The state when insulin is released under stimulation from gastric inhibitory peptide (GIP); insulin then facilitates the transport of glucose and amino acids into cells.

☐ g. The period dominated by anti-insulin hormones, such as glucagon.

Q59. List four sources of glucose that may be called upon during the postabsorptive state.

_____

_____

Q60. Can fatty acids serve as a source of glucose? Give the rationale for your answer.

_____

_____

_____

Q61. Complete the table which represents a summary of hormonal regulation of metabolism. Underline the hormones in the table that are hyperglycaemic.

Hormone	Source	Action
a.	g.	Stimulates glycogenesis in liver; stimulates glucose uptake in other cells
b.	Alpha cells of Islets of Langerhans in pancreas	j.
c. Human growth hormone	h.	k.
d. Glucocorticoids	i.	l.
e.	Thyroid gland	m.
f.	Adrenal medulla	n.

MINERALS 📖 *Pages 846–52*

Q62. Outline what you understand by the term mineral.

_____

_____

Q63. Match each of the minerals in the box below with the appropriate definition.

1. Calcium 2. Chlorine 3. Cobalt 4. Fluorine 5. Iron 6. Iodine 7. Potassium 8. Magnesium 9. Sodium 10. Phosphorous 11. Sulphur

☐ a. Main anion in extracellular fluid; part of HCl in stomach; component of table salt.

☐ b. Involved in the generation of nerve impulse; helps to regulate osmosis; acts in buffer systems.

☐ c. Most abundant cation in the body; found mostly in bones and teeth; necessary for normal muscle contraction and for blood clotting.

☐ d. Important component of haemoglobin and cytochromes.

☐ e. Main cation inside of cells; used in nerve transmission.

☐ f. Essential component of thyroxin.

☐ g. Constituent of vitamin B_{12}, so necessary for red blood cell formation.

☐ h. Important component of amino acids, vitamins and hormones.

☐ i. Improves tooth structure.

☐ j. Found mostly in bones and teeth; important in buffer system and in ATP processes; component of DNA and RNA.

VITAMINS 📖 *Pages 849–52*

Q64. In general, what are the functions of vitamins? This is a brief overview of functions and therefore you do not need to refer to all the vitamins.

_____

_____

Q65. Contrast the two principal groups of vitamins, and list the main vitamins in each group.

_____

_____

_____

Q66. From the list of vitamins in the box, select the one that fits each of the descriptions below.

1. A   2. B₁   3. B₂   4. B₁₂   5. C   6. D   7. E   8. K

☐ a. This serves as a coenzyme that is essential for blood clotting, so it is called 'antihaemorrhagic vitamin'; synthesised by intestinal bacteria.

☐ b. Its formation depends upon sunlight on skin, and also on activation of kidney and liver; necessary for calcium absorption.

☐ c. 'Riboflavin' is another name for it; a component of FAD; necessary for normal integrity of the skin, mucosa and eye.

☐ d. This vitamin acts as an important coenzyme in carbohydrate metabolism; deficiency leads to beriberi.

☐ e. Formed from carotene, it is necessary for normal bones and teeth; it prevents night blindness.

☐ f. This substance is also called 'ascorbic acid'; deficiency causes anaemia, poor wound healing and scurvy.

☐ g. This coenzyme, the only B vitamin not found in vegetables, is necessary for normal erythropoiesis; absorption from GI tract depends on intrinsic factor.

☐ h. Also known as 'tocopherol', it is necessary for normal red blood cell membranes; deficiency is associated with sterility in some animals.

This concludes your study on metabolism, and we hope that you have enjoyed it. Before moving on, perhaps you would like to test your progress by working on the Checkpoints Exercise.

CHECKPOINTS EXERCISE

Q67. **Contrast CHO with lipids in this exercise. Write 'C' next to any statement true of CHO, and write 'L' next to any statement true of lipids. Write 'C' and 'L' if both are true.**

☐ a. These compounds are insoluble in water (hydrophobic).

☐ b. These compounds are organic.

☐ c. These substances have a hydrogen : oxygen ratio of about 2 : 1.

☐ d. These substances have very few oxygen atoms (compared to the numbers of carbon and hydrogen atoms). (📖 *Page 44, Figure 2.9*)

Q68. **Match the types of lipids in the box with their functions given below.**

| 1. Bile salts 2. Carotene 3. Cholesterol 4. Oestrogen 5. Phospholipids 6. Prostaglandins |

☐ a. Present in egg yolk and carrots; leads to formation of vitamin A, a chemical necessary for good vision.

☐ b. The major lipid in cell membranes.

☐ c. Present in all cells, but can cause atherosclerosis.

☐ d. Substances that emulsify fats before their digestion.

☐ e. Steroid sex hormones produced in large quantities by females.

☐ f. Important regulatory compounds with many functions, including modifying responses to hormones.

Q69. **Complete this exercise about fat-soluble vitamins.**

The fat-soluble vitamin that helps with calcium absorption and is necessary for normal bone growth is vitamin (a) _____. Vitamin (b) _____ may be administered to a patient before surgery, in order to prevent excessive bleeding, since this vitamin helps in the formation of clotting factors.

Normal vision is associated with an adequate amount of vitamin (c) _____. Vitamin (d) _____ has a variety of possible functions, including the promotion of wound healing and the prevention of scarring.

Q70. **Match the types of proteins listed in the box with their functions given below. You have already met this question in Chapter 2, on the chemical level of organisation.**

| 1. Catalytic 2. Contractile 3. Immunological 4. Regulatory 5. Structural 6. Transport |

☐ a. Haemoglobin in red blood cells.

☐ b. Proteins, such as actin and myosin, in muscle tissue.

☐ c. Keratin in skin and hair; collagen in bone.

☐ d. Hormones, such as insulin.

☐ e. Defensive chemicals, such as antibodies and interleukins.

☐ f. Enzymes, such as lipase, which digests lipids.

Q71. **Contrast proteins with the other organic compounds you have studied so far, by completing this exercise.**

Carbohydrates, lipids and proteins all contain carbon, hydrogen and oxygen. A fourth element, (a) _____, makes up a substantial portion of proteins. Just as large carbohydrates are composed of building blocks called (b) _____, so proteins are composed of building blocks, called (c) _____ _____. As in the synthesis of carbohydrates or fats, when two amino acids bond together, a water molecule must be (d) _____. This is another example of (e) _____ synthesis. The product of such a reaction is known as a (f) _____.

When many amino acids are linked together in this way, a polypeptide results. One or more polypeptide chains form a (g) _____.

Q72. **Match the description below with the four levels of protein organisation in the box.**

> **1. Primary structure 2. Secondary structure 3. Tertiary structure 4. Quaternary structure**

☐ a. Specific sequence of amino acids.
☐ b. Twisted and folded arrangement (as in spirals or pleated sheets).
☐ c. Irregular three-dimensional shape.
☐ d. Two or more tertiary structures bonded together.

Q73. **Name two hormones that enhance the transport of amino acids into cells and also stimulate protein synthesis.**

_____

Q74. Amino acids derived, for example, from worn out muscle cells, may undergo a process known as (a) _____ to form new body proteins. If other energy sources are used up, amino acids may undergo catabolism. The first step is (b) _____, in which an amino group (NH_2) is removed and converted in the liver to (c) _____, a component of (d) _____, which exists in the urine. The remaining portion of the amino acid may enter (e) _____ pathways at a number of points. In this way, proteins can lead to the formation of (f) _____. (📖 *Page 841, Figure 25.12*).

Q75. **Which of these processes is anabolic?**
a. Pyruvic acid ⟶ $CO_2 + H_2O$ + ATP
b. Glucose ⟶ pyruvic acid + ATP
c. Protein synthesis.
d. Digestion of starch to maltose.
e. Glycogenolysis.

Q76. Which one of the following hormones is said to be hypoglycaemic, since it tends to lower blood sugar?

a.   Glucagon.

b.   Glucocorticoids.

c.   Growth hormone.

d.   Insulin.

e.   Adrenaline.

Q77. Which one of the following is not a product of the complete oxidation of glucose?

a.   ATP.

b.   Oxygen.

c.   Carbon dioxide.

d.   Water.

Q78. What is the name of the process that results in the formation of glucose from amino acids or glycerol?

a.   Gluconeogenesis.

b.   Glycogenesis.

c.   Ketogenesis.

d.   Deamination.

e.   Glycogenolysis.

Q79. Four of the processes mentioned above occur exclusively or primarily in the liver cells. Which one occurs in virtually all body cells?

_____

Q80. Which one of the following is not part of fat absorption or fat metabolism?

a.   Lipogenesis.

b.   Beta oxidation.

c.   Chylomicron formation.

d.   Ketogenesis.

e.   Glycogenesis.

Q81. Which one of the following involves a cytochrome chain?

a.   Glycolysis.

b.   Transition step between glycolysis and Kreb's cycle.

c.   Kreb's cycle.

d.   Electron transport system.

Q82. Arrange the following statements, which indicate steps in the complete oxidation of glucose, in the correct sequence.

a.   Glycolysis takes place.

b.   Pyruvic acid is converted to acetyl CoA.

c.   Hydrogens are picked up by NAD and FAD; hydrogens ionize.

d. Kreb's cycle releases CO_2 and hydrogens.

e. Oxygen combines with hydrogen ions and electrons to form water.

f. Electrons are transported along cytochromes, and energy from electrons is stored as ATP.

_____ _____ _____ _____ _____ _____

Q83. Circle 'T' (true) or 'F' (false) for each of the statements given below.

T   F   a. Coenzyme A is derived from pantothenic acid, also known as **vitamin C**.

T   F   b. Complexes of carrier molecules utilised in the electron transport system are located in the **mitochondrial matrix**.

T   F   c. Catabolism of carbohydrates involves **oxidation**, which is a process of **addition of hydrogens**.

T   F   d. Nonessential amino acids are those that **are not used in the synthesis of human protein**.

T   F   e. The complete oxidation of glucose to CO_2 and H_2O yields **four** molecules of ATP.

T   F   f. Anabolic reactions are **synthetic reactions that release energy**.

T   F   g. **Carbohydrates, proteins, and vitamins** provide energy and serve as building materials.

Q84. Briefly outline the altered physiology in the body of an individual who suffers from phenylketonuria.

_____

_____

_____

_____

Q85. The exercise below relates to coeliac disease.

Coeliac disease occurs when the body is unable to digest a water (a) _____ protein called (b) _____. Many types of (c) _____ contain the substance mentioned in (b).

In this condition there may be destruction of villi, leading to atrophy (reduction in size) of the intestinal mucosa, and this may give rise to (d) _____. The condition is easily managed by restriction in the types of food that contain the irritant substance. All cereal grains should be avoided, with the exception of (e) _____ and (f) _____.

During your nursing career, you are likely to meet patients with various types of metabolic disorders, especially those concerned with nutrition. Many of the disorders are genetically determined, and the cause is often the failure or lack of specific enzymes.

It is therefore important that as nurses you are aware of some of the basic principles with regard to these disorders, so that you are in a better position to care and advise the patients appropriately. Although this will often encompass the area of counselling for the individual and parents, this is not discussed here.

To assist you with the understanding of some nutritional problems, you will be presented with some short scenarios and questions, followed by an overview of the particular disorders. It is not intended here to give detailed analyses of diet management of the patients, but we hope that if you understand the basic principles, you will be motivated to undertake further reading (references are provided), so as to obtain a complete picture of the problem.

The main objective of the exercise is to enable you to work out from your knowledge of normal physiology, what particular problems may arise in the individual if functions are impaired specifically in relation to nutrition.

The scenarios to be discussed will include the following: phenylketonuria, cystic fibrosis, coeliac disease and nephrotic syndrome.

SCENARIO 1

Carl, who suffers from phenylketonuria, is five years of age and is soon to start at infant's school. He is well established on a low phenylalanine diet, but his mother fears that other school children might influence the pattern of his eating habits.

Carl is very active and enjoys all types of vigourous activities.

Q86.   What is the name given to the diagnostic test for the detection of phenylketonuria in babies?

_____

Q87.   Giving the rationale for your answer, discuss the importance of keeping Carl on a diet of low phenylalanine.

_____

_____

_____

Q88.   Suggest ways in which school children could influence Carl's dietary habits.

_____

_____

_____

Q89. **Suggest a day's menu for Carl, identifying the types and sources of the foods. Give the rationale for your answer.**

_____

_____

_____

_____

QUESTION FOR DISCUSSION

1. It is inevitable that Carl's parents are anxious about the likelihood of having another child with phenylketonuria. If you were to counsel Carl's parents with regard to the probability of having another child with phenylketonuria, what factors would you need to consider?

Overview of phenylketonuria

Phenylketonuria is inherited as an autosomal recessive disorder, and is one of the few causes of mental retardation. It is primarily due to failure of an enzyme in the liver known as **phenylalanine hydroxylase** to convert excess phenylalanine (an amino acid) to tyrosine (also an amino acid). Thus, the blood level of phenylalanine is increased and all the signs and symptoms in the affected individual are related to this. It is estimated that the normal blood level of phenylalanine is 180–480 μmol/l, but in individuals with phenylketonuria, the level may rise to 600μmol/l or more. A high level of phenylalanine also interferes with the metabolism of myelin and amines in the brain.

In a recent survey of a large number of patients, it was observed that children with phenylketonuria appeared to have normal I.Qs, but had educational problems and also an increased incidence of behavioural disorders, especially hyperactivity. There have also been suggestions that magnetic resonance imaging shows distinct abnormalities in the brain.

Phenylalanine is an essential amino acid and is contained in most proteins (1g of natural protein contains 50mg of phenylalanine). Phenylalanine is necessary for both physical and mental growth.

Some protocols in the management of individuals with phenylketonuria indicate that only one-third to one-tenth of the protein in the diet is required. Synthetic protein substances containing the amino acids leucine, isoleucine, valine, threonine, methionine, lysine and tryptophan are also administered. Additional supplements of calcium, magnesium, phosphate, potassium, sodium, zinc and iron may also be given. Women who are suffering from phenylketonuria and wish to have a child should strictly monitor their diet, some weeks before contraception is stopped. It is known that if mothers have phenylketonuria during pregnancy, there is an increase in the incidence of children born with congenital abnormalities such as microcephaly, heart defects and mental retardation.

As health promoters, nurses should also know that foods containing sweeteners such as **aspartame** (Canderel® and Nutrasweet®) contain phenylalanine.

SCENARIO 2

Debbie is eight years of age, and is admitted to the children's ward of the local hospital with a recurrent chest infection. She is very reluctant to eat, although she will tolerate various types of fluids.

Her management, which is not at all unfamiliar to Debbie, consists of postural drainage four times a day before meals, antibiotics and high-energy foods. Her parents are fully involved in her management and are allowed to participate in the various daily activities for Debbie.

Both parents are extremely anxious with regard to Debbie's progress and prognosis, as she has been hospitalised on several occasions, with severe chest infections. Despite Debbie's taking sufficient quantities of pancreatic enzymes, there is still the presence of steatorrhoea.

Q90. **Referring to the exocrine functions of the pancreas, describe the nutritional problems that may occur with Debbie. Giving the rationale for your answer, suggest how these may affect Debbie's health.**

_____

_____

_____

_____

_____

Q91. **To maintain nutritional balance, suggest the types of foods that would need to be included in Debbie's diet.**

_____

_____

_____

_____

_____

Q92. **Discuss the use of pancreatic enzymes (e.g Creon®, Cotazym®, Pancrease®, Nutrizym GR®) in the management of Debbie.**

_____

_____

_____

_____

Q93. What is the main cause of steatorrhoea in cystic fibrosis?

_____

_____

Q94. A junior nursing colleague is very keen to understand the condition, cystic fibrosis. She wishes to know how the mother would have recognised that there was something wrong with her child. Assuming that Debbie had some of the classical signs and symptoms of this condition, explain to the junior nurse what they would have been and why.

_____

_____

_____

Q95. Debbie's parents, who are very health orientated, find it very difficult to understand why Debbie needs foods that are 'high in energy'. They seek explanations from you, to establish whether this is the right management for their child. What reasonable explanations should you give them?

_____

_____

_____

_____

QUESTIONS FOR DISCUSSION

1. Explain why postural drainage is necessary in the management of Debbie.

2. Suggest factors that you would have needed to take into consideration when planning an educational programme for Debbie's parents when the diagnosis was first established.

3. Discuss some of the long-term complications that may occur with Debbie.

4. Relating to some of the diagnostic tests which are usually carried out to detect the presence of cystic fibrosis, discuss your role as a nurse in caring for both Debbie and her parents.

Overview of cystic fibrosis

Cystic fibrosis, one of the conditions associated with failure to thrive, is the most common autosomal recessive disease (incidence in Caucasians is 1 in 2500 live births). The incidence in the Black populations is 1 in 20000, and 1 in 100000 in Oriental populations.

It has been shown that the condition is caused by an abnormality of a single gene in the middle of chromosome 7.

It affects mainly the exocrine glands of the body. The two main organs affected are the pancreas and the lungs. The exocrine glands of these two organs secrete an abnormal composition of exocrine secretions (viscous and tenacious), which are responsible for the specific symptoms of the disease.

The sweat glands and salivary glands also excrete large amounts of sodium chloride. The exocrine functions of the pancreas are affected, and this gives rise to varying degrees of steatorrhoea. The respiratory tract is affected, and the child suffers from recurrent bouts of chest infections.

The medical and nursing management of these children is long-term, and this involves the dietary regime, which includes the use of pancreatic enzymes, vitamin supplements (especially vitamins A, D, and E), antibiotics for infections and postural drainage therapy. The aims of treatment are twofold: prevention of malnutrition, which occurs as a result of malabsorption, and the control of respiratory tract infections.

Cirrhosis may occur in some individuals, as a result of the blockage of bile ducts with tenacious mucus.

Symptoms of cystic fibrosis usually starts quite early in infancy. It is estimated that in Britain there is a 50% survival rate up to the age of 20 years. The survival rate is better in countries such as the USA, Canada and Australia.

SCENARIO 3

Tracy is a 12-year-old girl who has just been diagnosed as suffering from coeliac disease. She has been admitted to hospital on account of severe loss of weight and weakness. She has also been complaining of tiredness and has felt very breathless when engaging in physical activities at school. She has had frequent bouts of diarrhoea and abdominal fullness prior to hospital admission. At times, she had also noticed that her stools were rather bulky, offensive and greasy.

She is accompanied by her parents, who are extremely anxious about her condition. Tracy and her parents are seen by the dietitian and full explanations are given with regard to the dietary regime.

Q96. Tracy wants to know why she has lost a lot of weight, feels very tired and breathless, and is passing bulky, offensive, greasy stools. Giving the rationale for your answer, explain these symptoms to Tracy.

_____

_____

_____

_____

Q97. Discuss some of the problems that Tracy may face with regard to her new diet. In this question you need to refer to the psychological and biological factors that a teenager may face.

_____

_____

_____

_____

Q98. Explain why Tracy has been put on a gluten-free diet. Give examples of types of foods that she is able to eat.

_____

_____

_____

_____

Q99. In preparing an educational programme for Tracy and her parents with regard to her management, suggest all the relevant factors that you would include in such a programme.

_____

_____

_____

_____

QUESTIONS FOR DISCUSSION

1. Discuss some of the long-term complications that may occur with Tracy.

2. Tracy had a jejunal biopsy (use of 'Crosby capsule') performed before a diagnosis could be made. Discuss the essential nursing management of Tracy prior to and after the biopsy.

Overview of coeliac disease (gluten enteropathy)

Coeliac disease is a condition affecting the lining of the small intestine resulting in inflammation, destruction, atrophy and loss of villi. It can affect children, young adults and also the elderly.

The condition occurs in individuals who are sensitive to the **gliadin** (a protein) found in association with gluten, which is the main constituent of wheat flour, rye, barley and oats. Gluten is not present in rice or maize.

The prevalence of the condition is 1 : 2000 and it has been reported that there is a high incidence of coeliac disease (1 : 300) in the west of Ireland. The condition is very rare in Black and Oriental populations. There is some evidence based on twin studies that there may be a genetic factor. The disease also shows a familial tendency, although the mode of inheritance is not clear.

There are several theories to explain the pathological changes that occur in the small intestines of individuals with coeliac disease. These include an abnormal immunological response, and lack of specific enzymes.

The symptoms vary with the severity of the condition and usually arise within the first three years of life. Lesions develop in the small intestines which lead to diarrhoea and mal-absorption.

In children, the symptoms tend to occur between three and five months after consuming foods containing gluten. This is because most babies are weaned onto solid foods that contain gluten. Babies who have been growing well previously, on milk, start to become difficult, refuse to take their feeds and fail to gain weight. The symptoms include abdominal disten-sion, wasting and lethargy and the individual passes large bulky, sticky , offensive, pale stools. Steatorrhoea is also very common. Vomiting may occur and the baby could develop diar-rhoea and dehydration. Children who are affected fail to thrive and become wasted, especial-ly around the buttocks. This is partly due to the malabsorption of fats. Consequently, the absorption of fat-soluble vitamins (A, D and K) is also affected. There is also malabsorption of iron, folate and vitamin B_{12}. Iron deficiency anaemia may be present in some individuals.

In adults, the symptoms may present in different ways. In a large number of patients, there may be breathlessness, fatigue and general tiredness, especially at the end of the day. Some adults with coeliac disease may also complain of symptoms directly related to the effects of gluten on the small intestine, such as abdominal fullness, discomfort and vomiting.

Diagnosis is usually via jejunal biopsy using a 'Crosby capsule'. The biopsy usually reveals that the mucosa of the jejunum appears to be flat and the villi are blunted. The epithelial cells are flat instead of the columnar type. A large area of the jejunum may be devoid of villi. This is associated with lack of disaccharidases and peptidases. The manage-ment of patients with coeliac disease includes a gluten-free diet (many products arc avail-able on prescription) which should be continued for life. Vitamin supplements may be necessary for some patients.

Some patients with coeliac disease may also complain about constipation once they have been established on the gluten-free diet, and this may be due to lack of fibre in the diet.

A 'home test kit' is now available for patients with coeliac disease to monitor the effects of their diet.

SCENARIO 4

Jonathan is eight years of age and is admitted to the children's ward with a confirmed diagnosis of the nephrotic syndrome. He has gained 10kg in body weight due to oedema. His face and abdomen appear quite swollen. His normal weight is usually 25kg. He is very reluctant to eat, despite encouragement from both the nursing staff and his parents. He has been prescribed frusemide (a diuretic). His dietary regime will consist of protein (1g protein/kg body weight), high-energy fluids and a reduced fat intake. Both his parents are involved in his management and care.

Q100. Giving the rationale for your answer, outline a suitable diet for the day for Jonathan.

_____

_____

_____

_____

Q101. Discuss the nursing management to monitor Jonathan's fluid balance.

_____

_____

_____

_____

Q102. For what reason is frusemide prescribed for Jonathan?

_____

_____

Q103. How many litres of fluid would Jonathan need to lose in order to attain his usual weight?

_____

Q104. What is the approximate weight of protein that Jonathan should consume in his daily diet?

_____

QUESTIONS FOR DISCUSSION

1. Discuss the possible complications that Jonathan could be faced with, assuming that the nephrotic syndrome does not respond to treatment.

2. Jonathan may be prescribed steroids. Discuss the use of steroids in the nephrotic syndrome, identifying the possible side effects.

3. Jonathan's parents wish to know the reasons for his facial and abdominal oedema. What reasonable explanations should you give them, so that they are able to appreciate the nature of the oedema?

Overview of the nephrotic syndrome

The nephrotic syndrome is characterised by proteinuria (greater than 5g/l in adults), oedema, hypoalbuminaemia, hypercholesterolaemia and hyperlipidaemia. The hyperlipidaemia occurs because there is an increased hepatic secretion of lipoproteins. Nephrotic syndrome can occur in many diseases (e.g glomerulonephritis, diabetes mellitus, systemic lupus erythematosus, amyloidosis and sarcoidosis) in which there is loss of a large amount of albumin in the urine.

The oedema arises as a result of loss of albumin due to increased permeability of the glomerular basement membrane. The decrease in plasma albumin level causes a decrease in plasma colloid osmotic pressure. The hydrostatic pressures across the capillaries also change. These two factors promote the movement of water and solutes from the circulating blood plasma to the interstitial fluid. Plasma volume falls and this causes a decrease in cardiac output and blood pressure. Consequently, blood flow to the kidneys is reduced and this causes release of renin and aldosterone, which leads to salt and water retention.

Children affected by nephrotic syndrome usually have facial and abdominal oedema. In adults, the oedema is usually present in the legs.

The management of nephrotic syndrome involves the treatment of any underlying non-renal cause and the reduction of the oedema by using diuretics. Other drugs may be used, such as steroids or immunosuppressant agents such as cyclosphosphamide or cyclosporin A. The use of diuretics may lead to dehydration and also to the loss of potassium. Potassium supplement is often given when such drugs as frusemide are administered. Excess fluid loss may also lead to postural hypotension.

To replace the protein loss, a diet containing 1g of protein/kg of body weight is recommended. A low protein diet is indicated only when renal failure has developed. Patients are also advised to have a 'no added salt diet' especially those who need to limit their fluid intake. Patients who are malnourished should be encouraged to take high-energy drinks.

As a result of hyperlipidaemia, patients should monitor their fat intake by using polyunsaturated fats and reducing their intake of saturated fats.

Answers to questions

Q1. To supply energy for sustaining life processes (such as active transport, DNA replication, synthesis of proteins), and to synthesise structural or functional molecules.

Q2. Carbohydrates, lipids, proteins, minerals, vitamins and water.

Q3. a, Hypothalamus; b, cholecystokinin.

Q4. Acts as a solvent, participates in hydrolysis reactions, acts as a coolant, can lubricate, and helps to maintain a constant body temperature.

Q5. *Definition:* a. catabolism is the chemical reactions that break down complex organic compounds into simple ones; b. anabolism is the chemical reactions that combine simple substances into more complex molecules.
Releases or uses of energy: a. uses water to break chemical bonds (hydrolysis reactions); releases the available chemical energy in organic molecules; b. process often involve dehydration synthesis reactions (reactions that release water) and require energy to form new chemical bonds.
Examples: a. chemical digestion, cellular respiration; b, formation of peptide bonds between amino acids, fatty acids built into phospholipids, glucose formed into glycogen.

Q6. An organic compound is a substance that contains **carbon** and usually **hydrogen**. Many organic compounds also contain **oxygen** and sometimes **nitrogen**.

Q7. Cellulose, sugar, starch and glycogen.

Q8. Carbon, hydrogen and oxygen.

Q9. Sugars, most fruits, potatoes, bread, etc.

Q10. Monosaccharides, disaccharides and polysaccharides.

Q11. a, 2; b, 1; c, $(CH_2O)_n$; d, $C_6H_{12}O_6$; e, glucose; f, fructose (you may have included galactose and you would be correct); g, deoxyribose; h, $C_5H_{10}O_5$; i, $C_{12}H_{22}O_{11}$; j, removed; k, polysaccharides; l, starch (or glycogen or cellulose); m, hydrolysis.

Q12. In the liver.

Q13. They are isomers. An isomer is a chemical substance that has the same chemical formula but different structural formula. So, although glucose and galactose have the same number of carbon, hydrogen and oxygen atoms, they are arranged differently so as to give a different three dimensional structure. Since the shape is altered, the enzymatic function will be different. The analogy is a lock and key.

Q14. Lactose is digested by **lactase** and yields one molecule of glucose and one molecule of galactose.

Maltose is digested by **maltase** and yields two molecules of glucose.

Sucrose is digested by **sucrase** and yields one molecule of glucose and one molecule of fructose.

Q15. Glycogen.

Q16 The starches such as potatoes and bread; and cellulose.

Q17. Substrate-level phosphorylation and oxidative phosphorylation. (There is another mechanism known as photophosphorylation. It occurs in the photosynthetic cells of plants, and will not be discussed here.)

Q18. ATP production, amino acid synthesis, glycogenesis (conversion of glucose to glycogen), lipogenesis (glucose transformed into glycerol and fatty acids for the synthesis of glycerides) and excretion in the urine.

Glucose is not usually excreted in the urine, but if its level in the blood exceeds the renal threshold, it can then be excreted in the urine. This may occur for example, if a large amount of glucose has been consumed with very little protein or fats. You should remember, however, that glucose is present in the urine of diabetic individuals (especially if the individual is not well-controlled).

Q19. Insulin.

Q20. $C_6H_{12}O_6 + 6O_2 \longrightarrow 6CO_2 + 6H_2O + energy$

Q21. a. Anaerobic; b, glucose; c, phosphorylation; d, glucose 6–phosphate; e, hexokinase; f, two; g, four ATP; h, two; i, pyruvic; j, glyceraldehyde 3–phosphate; k, oxygen; l, lactic; m, lactic; n, pyruvic acid; o, coenzyme A.

Q22. a, Carbon dioxide; b, acetyl; c, coenzyme A; d, acetyl coenzyme A; e, oxaloacetic; f, citric.

Q23. Because its starting substance is oxaloacetic acid, which is regenerated again at the end of the process.

Q24. Loss of a molecule of carbon dioxide by a substance.

Q25. **Oxidation** means the removal of electrons or the loss of hydrogen atoms or ions. **Reduction** means the addition of electrons or the addition of hydrogen atoms or ions. The two terms are often used together, because in most chemical reactions in which they occur, one of the chemical substances is reduced whilst the other is oxidised. It is also known as a 'coupled reaction'.

Q26. Because the starting compound glucose contains **six** carbon atoms.

Q27. It is transported by the blood to the lungs and is exhaled with the expired air.

Q28. NAD (nicotinamide adenine dinucleotide) and FAD (flavin adenine dinucleotide). They are important carriers of hydrogen. When they pick up hydrogen atoms, they are said to be reduced. Reduced NAD may be represented as follows:

$NAD^+ + H_2 \longrightarrow NADH + H^+$

Q29. Flavine mononucleotide, cytochromes, copper atoms, ubiquinones, iron and sulphur.

Q30. a, FMN; b, reduced; c, FMNH$_2$; d, B$_2$ (Riboflavin); e, oxidised; f, FMN; g, iron; h, copper; i, sulphur; j, cytochrome a$_3$; k, oxygen; l, aerobic; m. inner; n, three; o, proton; p, outer; q, inner; r, proton; s, channels; t, mitochondrial; u, synthetase; v, chemiosmotic.

Q31. a, Glycogen; b, liver; c, insulin, d. approximately 400g; e, skeletal.

Q32. Splitting the glucose molecule from the branched glycogen to form glucose 1–phosphate. The enzyme involved in this process is phosphorylase (it is activated by the hormones glucagon or adrenaline). Glucose 1-phosphate is then converted to glucose 6-phosphate. Glucose 6-phosphate is then converted to glucose by the enzyme phosphatase.

Q33. Because muscles lack the enzyme phosphatase.

Q34. The process by which glucose is formed from noncarbohydrate sources. Glucose can be formed from the glycerol portion of triglycerides and also from amino acids.

Q35. Cortisol, thyroxine, adrenaline, glucagon and human growth hormone.

Q36. Lipids do not have a 2 : 1 ratio of hydrogen : oxygen. The amount of oxygen in lipids is usually less than in carbohydrates.

Q37. True.

Q38. See 📖 *Page 43, Exibit 2.3*

Q39. Neutral fats.

Q40. Saturated fat increases the level of cholesterol in the blood and can therefore give rise to the development of atherosclerosis. Atherosclerosis occludes blood vessels and can therefore lead to ischaemia (diminished blood supply to the tissues) and in time can lead to heart disease (myocardial infarction), stroke or cerebrovascular accident. The blood vessels in the legs may also be affected, thus causing intermittent claudication. In this condition, patients have severe pain in the calf muscles, when oxygen demand is increased, for example during exercise, walking uphill or climbing the stairs. The pain diminishes when the patient rests, but as the disease progresses, the pain may exist even when the patient is at rest. The pathology of this condition is very similar to that of angina pectoris.

Atherosclerosis can also give rise to hypertension (raised blood pressure). For more information, refer to the section on clinical application. 📖 *Page 44.*

Q41. Saturated – Triglycerides that contain only single covalent bonds between carbon atoms. Each carbon atom is fully bonded to the maximum number of hydrogen atoms. Therefore, it is more difficult for these molecules to enter into chemical reactions.

Monounsaturated – Fatty acids with one double covalent bond between two carbon atoms. They can therefore enter into chemical reactions more readily.

Polyunsaturated – Fatty acids that contain more than one double covalent bond between carbon atoms. It is more healthy to consume this type of fat than saturated fats.

Q42. In adipose tissue.

Q43. a. Molecule A is glycerol and molecule B is a fatty acid. b. Dehydration synthesis reaction. c. Monoglyceride.

Q44. Steroids, fat-soluble vitamins and eicosanoids. 📖 *Page 43.*

Q45. They store glycerides and act as insulation and protection. They contain the enzyme lipase, which is important for the hydrolysis of fats.

Q46. Lipid releases twice as much energy.

Q47. a, Fatty acid; b, glycerol; c, lipolysis. d. glyceraldehyde 3–phosphate; e, glucose; f, gluconeogenesis; g, mitochondria; h, beta-oxidation; i, acetic; j, coenzyme A; k, acetyl coenzyme A; l, Kreb's; m, acetoacetic acid; n, acetone; o, ketone; p, ketoacidosis. q. ketoacidosis.

Q48. Partly explained in question 47. In the absence of glucose for glycolysis, fats are used instead. The catabolic process gives rise to acetic acid and hence acetyl coenzyme A. Coenzyme A enters the Kreb's cycle only when it can react with oxaloacetic acid. In the absence of glucose as the main source of energy, the level of oxaloacetic acid is reduced. Therefore, two molecules of acetyl coenzyme A combine with each other to form acatoacetic acid. This also explains the reason why ketone appears in the urine of a diabetic patient. It is therefore important that diabetic patients are well controlled, so that their bodies do not utilise fats as the main source of energy.

Q49. Oxygen, carbon, hydrogen and nitrogen.

Q50. Sulphur.

Q51. a, Amino acids. (Please note that (a) throughout this section is amino acid); b, 20; c, amino; d, carboxyl; e, peptide; f, water; g, hydroxyl. h, amino.

Q52.

dehydration synthesis \ hydrolysis / peptide bond + H_2O

water molecule

Q53. A dipeptide contains two amino acids. A tripeptide contains three amino acids. A polypeptide contains from 100 to over 2000 amino acids.

Q54. Because in general they cannot be synthesised by the body. However, two of them can be synthesised, but in very small amounts.

Q55. Nonessential.

Q56. An enzyme is a biological catalyst. It can speed up chemical reactions. An enzyme is also a protein.

Q57. An enzyme's actions can be affected by pH, temperature and amount of substrate.

Q58. Pa, Pb, Pc, Ad, Ae, Af, Pg.

Q59. Liver glycogen or muscle glycogen, lactic acid during exercise, glycerol from fats, amino acids from tissue proteins.

Q60. No. Mammals cannot convert acetyl coenzyme A into pyruvic acid; therefore fatty acids cannot be used to form glucose. However, gluconeogenesis can occur and the glycerol portion of the triglycerides can be converted to glyceraldehyde 3–phosphate and hence to pyruvic acid.

Q61. Insulin, b. *Glucagon*, c. *Human growth hormone*, d. *Glucocorticoids*, e. *Thyroxine*, f. *Adrenaline, noradrenaline*, g. Beta cells of islets of langerhans in pancreas, h. Anterior lobe of pituitary, i. Adrenal cortex, j. Gluconeogensis, k. Lipolysis, protein breakdown, l. Lipolysis, protein synthesis, gluconegenesis, m. Lipolysis, protein synthesis, n. Glucogenolysis, lipolysis.

Q62. An inorganic substance needed in small quantities for proper functioning of the body.

Q63. 2a, 9b, 1c, 5d, 7e, 6f, 3g, 11h, 4i, 10j.

Q64. Organic substances that are required in minute amounts for growth and normal metabolism and the regulation of physiological processes. Most vitamins are used as coenzymes. 📖 *Pages 850–1, Exhibit 25.6.*

Q65. Water-soluble vitamins (B vitamins, vitamin C) and fat-soluble vitamins (A, D, E and K). Water-soluble vitamins are easily destroyed by heat and their storage is minimal. Fat-soluble vitamins are not easily destroyed by heat, and they are stored in sufficient amounts in the liver. They can only be absorbed in the presence of fats and bile. If fat digestion is affected, the fat soluble vitamins will not be absorbed.

Q66. 8a, 6b, 3c, 2d, 1e, 5f, 4g, 7h.

Q67. La, C and Lb, Cc, Ld.

Q68. 2a, 5b, 3c, 1d, 4e, 6f.

Q69. a, D; b, K; c, A; d, C.

Q70. 6a, 2b, 5c, 4d, 3e, 1f.

Q71. a, Nitrogen; b, monosaccharides; c, amino acids; d, removed; e, dehydration synthesis; f, peptide bond. g. protein.

Q72. 1a, 2b, 3c, 4d.

Q73. Insulin and human growth hormone.

Q74. a, Transamination; b, deamination; c, ammonia; d, urea; e, Kreb's cycle; f, glucose.

Q75. c.

Q76. d.

Q77. b.

Q78. a.

Q79. e.

Q80. e.

Q81. d.

Q82. a, b, d, c, f, e.

Q83. a. T. It is derived from the B vitamin.

    b.   F. Inner (cristae) membrane.

    c.   F. Oxidation is removal of hydrogen.

    d.   F. Can be synthetised by the body.

    e.   F. 36 to 38.

    f.   F. Not vitamins.

Q84. In the individual affected, the enzyme phenylalanine hydroxylase is missing. Therefore the metabolism of phenylalanine is affected and consequently the level of phenylalanine increases in the blood. The symptoms of this condition are a direct consequence of the increase in phenylalanine. If not treated promptly, the child could suffer from mental retardation. For more information, 📖 *Page 858.*

Q85. a, Soluble; b, gluten; c, grains; d, malabsorption; e, rice; f, maize.

Q86. The test is known as the Guthrie's test.

Q87. As explained in the 'overview' section, phenylalanine interferes with the metabolism of myelin and amines in the brain and if present in excess, it could lead to mental retardation. However, Carl still needs to have at least one-third to one-tenth of the protein in the diet, so that a certain amount of phenylalanine is obtained, since it is important for both mental and physical growth.

Q88. This is really a psychosocial question and you can give many examples of why you think school children could influence Carl's dietary habits. This is perhaps the first time that Carl is away from home and therefore not being directly supervised by his mother. He may therefore be open to suggestions and partake in the foods of his colleagues. Children do like to share many of their things at this age. Certainly many sweets may contain proteins and therefore phenylalanine; many drinks also contain aspartame as sweeteners and Carl may be given such drinks by his friends.

Q89. You should bear in mind Carl's age and therefore try to estimate how many kilocalories he should be entitled to. Carl is at an age where growth and development is taking place, and the diet should reflect this. The types of foods would depend on the likes and dislikes and fads for a child of this age. You should therefore think in terms of a balanced diet and one that is nutritionally acceptable. You should identify the types of carbohydrates and fats, but give careful consideration to the protein intake. Most proteins contain phenylalanine and it is therefore important to ensure that Carl receives a low-phenylalanine diet. Please refer to the section on 'overview of phenylketonuria' and also the reference of Smith (1990) in the *Archives of Disease of Childhood.*

Q90. The pancreas secretes digestive enzymes, such as amylase, trypsin, and lipase. All three enzymes play an important role in the process of digestion. In cystic fibrosis, due to the tenacious nature of pancreatic secretions, these enzymes are unable to reach the duodenum. Therefore, the digestion of proteins, fats and carbohydrates is affected. Fats cannot be digested and are therefore excreted, in many instances unchanged in the stools, and this is referred to as 'steatorrhoea'. Failure of fat digestion also affects absorption of fat-soluble vitamins. Thus, Debbie may suffer from lack of vitamins, especially A, D, E and K.

Failure of carbohydrate digestion may result in a low level of glucose, and therefore energy will be affected. Debbie may feel tired, lethargic and weak. She may not feel keen to participate in physical activities.

If proteins cannot be digested, there will be a reduction in available amino acids, which are important for growth, repair of tissues and formation of various chemicals that are necessary for the body.

Taking into consideration all of the above, Debbie's health may be affected in the following ways: loss of weight, possible anaemia, infections possibly due to reduced function of the immune system, physical growth possibly affected, energy malnutrition, fat soluble vitamin malabsorption which may result in night blindness (as a result of lack of vitamin A), or bleeding as a result of lack of vitamin K.

Q91. Any specific diet therapy would need to take into consideration Debbie's age, her activities, her food preferences and tolerances, and her general health status. Thus, as a growing child and on account of steatorrhoea and frequent pulmonary infection, Debbie's energy requirements should be increased. It is generally accepted that energy intake may have to be increased by up to 50%. This should include proteins, fats and carbohydrates. Supplements of vitamins and minerals may also need to be provided.

Since fat is the most concentrated source of energy in the diet, it is now generally accepted that it should provide at least 35–40% of the total energy intake. It is therefore appropriate to include in the diet energy-rich foods such as cheese, meat, full cream milk, milk puddings, butter, cakes and biscuits. Debbie should also be encouraged to have regular meals and frequent snacks. A variety of proteins foods should also be encouraged. Farrell and Hubbard (1983) have suggested that protein intake should provide at least 15–20% of the energy.

High calorie foods should also be encouraged. This is not difficult to achieve, since children usually like very sweet foods, such as chocolates, etc. Various glucose drinks should also be encouraged. It is suggested that glucose dietary supplement in a child of eight should be approximately 600kcal.

It may be prudent to avoid high fibre foods, as they are bulky and may therefore make the child feel full.

Depending on the child's condition, vitamins may be required. These may include vitamins A, D, E and K. In some cases iron may also be prescribed.

It should be noted that Debbie would be taking pancreatic enzyme preparations to assist with the digestion of her foods.

Q92. Pancreatic enzyme preparations contain a mixture of enzymes such as trypsin, amylase and lipase. Trypsin is important for the digestion of proteins; lipase digests fats and amylase continues the digestion of carbohydrates.

Such preparations should be given with every meal and should be increased with large snacks or milky drinks. Enzymes should not be given with lemonade, squash, fruit or boiled and jelly sweets. Enzymes can be mixed with a little jam or honey and thus makes it easier for the child to swallow them. Enteric-coated capsules such as Creon® and Pancrease® can be swallowed whole. If the child has difficulty in swallowing these, the capsules may be opened and the content mixed with honey or jam.

Loose or fatty stools indicate that digestion is incomplete, due perhaps to a low level of enzyme administration. It is therefore suggested in these cases that the amount of enzymes be increased. These enzyme preparations may cause excoriation of the mouth, lips and anus. Debbie should therefore be given this information.

Q93. The main cause of steatorrhoea is the lack or absence of the enzyme lipase for fat digestion, as the flow of pancreatic juice is obstructed and cannot reach the duodenum. As fat is not digested, it is therefore excreted in the stools unchanged.

Q94. Most of the explanations as to the cause and altered physiological changes in cystic fibrosis can be found in the section 'overview of cystic fibrosis'.

The symptoms usually appear in infancy and the mother may have noticed, for example, that the child was not putting on weight (one of the conditions giving rise to failure to thrive). The stools might be large and very offensive. The child might look unwell and not wanting his feeds. Respiratory tract infection may also occur and may be frequent.

In some cases, the indication of the disease may be detected from birth by the presence of meconium ileum. This is characterised by very sticky first stools.

Q95. It is important to understand the parents' dilemma, since it is true that the dietary advice is in contradiction of what is usually given for normal healthy eating recommendations. It is therefore imperative that the nurse is familiar with the rationale for this dietary treatment. The rationale is that to compensate for the steatorrhoea and for the frequency of respiratory tract infections, energy requirements are increased. Since fats provide more energy then proteins or carbohydrates, it is reasonable that they are increased in the diet.

There is also evidence that patients who consume normal fat intakes show better growth and this does not affect or increase fat malabsorption.

Q96. Most of the answers to this question may be found in the section on 'overview of coeliac disease'. Many of the symptoms are associated with malabsorption of various nutrients and vitamins and certain minerals, in particular iron. Thus, the tiredness may be due to iron deficiency anaemia or lack of folate and vitamin B_{12}. Malabsorption of digested fats leads to steatorrhoea and therefore to the nature of the stools. The weight loss occurs because the product of protein digestion is not absorbed and therefore physical growth is affected.

Q97. The problems are both psychosocial and biological. A change in dietary habit at this age may be very difficult. Tracy is by now used to types of foods that she likes and dislikes. To have to face a gluten-free diet may be very difficult. She is now more influenced by her peers and may want those types of food such as chocolates or various sweets that may contain gluten. So there is a need for a period of adjustment. It may be difficult for Tracy to go out to a restaurant or to parties, unless gluten-free foods are available. You can give many examples that relate to those mentioned above.

Q98. The reason for a gluten-free diet is abundantly explained in the section 'overview of coeliac disease'. Tracy should avoid any foods that may contain wheat, rye and barley. She should therefore avoid ordinary bread, biscuits, cakes, pies and pastries. It is also advisable not to eat processed foods, as they often contain wheat flour. To be on the safe side, Tracy should preferably consume products that she knows are gluten-free, and many of those products are available on prescription.

Tracy should be made aware that she is able to eat many types of foods without restriction and these are as follows: eggs, dairy products, fish, meat, fruits, vegetables, rice or maize.

Q99. Most of the relevant factors appertain to the dietary management. To avoid the problems of malabsorption and to maintain normal health, Tracy and her parents must understand the importance of taking a gluten-free diet. Tracy must be encouraged to adopt a positive attitude toward her health and therefore her diet. She must concentrate on the foods that she can eat as opposed to those that she cannot. She should also be very vigilant in making observations on the types of foods which may contain wheat flour, although this may not always be very apparent. If certain types of foods should upset her, she should abstain from them in the future.

One problem that Tracy and her parents should be aware of, is that of constipation. This can be managed by increasing fibre intake in the diet, and eating plenty of fruits and vegetables.

Excessive weight gain may be a problem, and therefore Tracy and her parents should be aware of this. It is prudent to advise Tracy to keep an eye on her weight, but at the same time she should not become obsessed with this, to the point that she mismanages her dietary regime.

Q100. The diet should contain sufficient protein so that a positive nitrogen balance is maintained. It is also important to maintain a good energy intake. Jonathan should therefore be given a diet that may be able to promote his appetite. He should be given foods that he can tolerate. To assist in the control of oedema, it is also advisable for Jonathan to be on a 'no added salt diet'. Glucose drinks may be encouraged, especially if Jonathan is very reluctant to eat his foods.

It is advisable to give some consideration to the amount of fat to be included in the diet, since hyperlipidaemia is present in most nephrotic patients and the cholesterol level may also be elevated. Jonathan should be given polyunsaturated fats with a reduction of saturated fats.

Q101. All fluid intake and output should be monitored. All fluids should be measured and recorded as accurately as possible. Jonathan should be encouraged to be involved in his management.

Weighing Jonathan may be another method of monitoring fluid balance. For accuracy, it is important that the scales are in good working order, and that Jonathan is weighed at approximately the same time every day. It is also important that his clothing is the same, or at least of similar weight.

Q102. Frusemide is a diuretic and its main role is in the control of oedema by promoting fluid loss in the urine.

Q103. He would need to lose 10 litres of fluid, since 1kg is equivalent to 1l.

Q104. The answer is 25g of protein per day. This is based on his weight (25kg) and his allowance, which is 1g protein/kg body weight.

Overview and key terms

Fluid, electrolyte, acid–base homeostasis

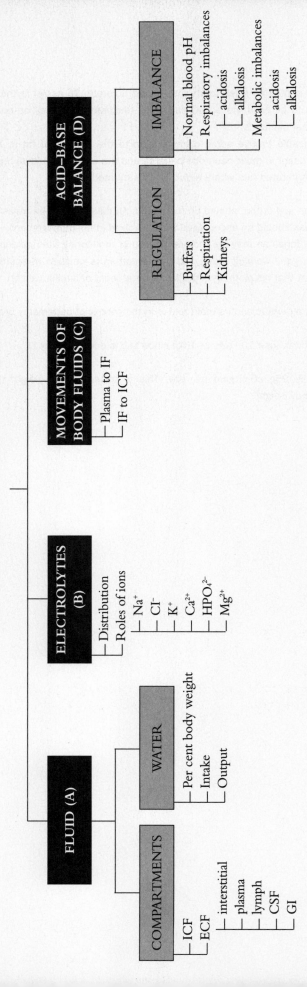

FLUID (A)

COMPARTMENTS
- ICF
- ECF
  - interstitial
  - plasma
  - lymph
  - CSF
  - GI

WATER
- Per cent body weight
- Intake
- Output

ELECTROLYTES (B)
- Distribution
- Roles of ions
  - Na^+
  - Cl^-
  - K^+
  - Ca^{2+}
  - HPO_4^{2-}
  - Mg^{2+}

MOVEMENTS OF BODY FLUIDS (C)
- Plasma to IF
- IF to ICF

ACID–BASE BALANCE (D)

REGULATION
- Buffers
- Respiration
- Kidneys

IMBALANCE
- Normal blood pH
- Respiratory imbalances
  - acidosis
  - alkalosis
- Metabolic imbalances
  - acidosis
  - alkalosis

18. Fluid, Electrolyte and Acid–base Homeostasis

Learning outcomes

1. To describe the various fluid compartments of the body.

2. To define the processes available for fluid intake and fluid output and how they are regulated.

3. To explain the functions of the following electrolytes: sodium, potassium, calcium, chloride, phosphate and magnesium.

4. To describe the factors involved in the movements of fluid between plasma and interstitial fluid, and between interstitial fluid and intracellular fluid.

5. To explain the role of buffers in maintaining pH of body fluids.

6. To define acid–base imbalances and describe their effects on the body and how they are treated.

Chapter 27

INTRODUCTION

You have met the term **homeostasis** in other chapters, and you should therefore be aware that fluids, electrolytes, acids and bases in the body need to be kept relatively constant. Any change from normal limits may give rise to various physiological problems, which may have serious consequences on the individual. For example, an excess of potassium ions may cause cardiac arrest; lack of calcium may result in tetany; excess fluid loss can lead to dehydration.

Many organs play a vital role in the maintenance of various homeostatic mechanisms, for example both the kidneys and the lungs assist in the control of blood pH.

It is hoped that through this study, you will become aware of the importance of the body's homeostatic mechanisms and why health problems may arise if there is failure in any of the homeostatic control mechanisms. As nurses you will be involved in many of the observations, or management of patients with homeostasis disturbances.

This study will commence by looking at fluid compartments and fluid balance.

FLUIDS COMPARTMENTS AND FLUID BALANCE 📖 *Pages 905–7*

Q1.   **What is the name given to fluid in the cells?**

_____

Q2.   **What is the name given to the fluids outside the cells?**

_____

Q3.   **What is the name given to the 80% of fluid forming part of the extracellular fluid?**

_____

Q4.   **Check your understanding of fluid compartments by circling all fluids that are considered extracellular fluids.**

a.   Blood plasma.

b.   Lymph.

c.   Synovial fluid.

d.   Pericardial fluid.

e.   Cerebrospinal fluid.

f.   Aqueous humour and vitreous of the eyes.

g.   Fluids within liver cells.

h.   Endolymph and perilymph of the ears.

i.   Fluid surrounding liver cells.

Q5.   **Complete the following exercise, which relates to intake and output of fluid.**

Daily intake and output of fluid is equal to (a) ——————— ml or (b) ———————
litres. Of the intake, about (c) ——————— ml is ingested in food and drink, and
(d) ——————— ml is a product of catabolism of foods (discussed in Chapter 17).

Q6. **List four systems of the body that eliminate water. Indicate the amounts lost by each system on an average day.**

a. Integument (skin): _____ ml/day.

b. _____ : _____ ml/day.

c. _____ : _____ ml/day.

d. _____ : _____ ml/day

On a day when you exercise vigorously, how would you expect these values to change?

_____

Q7. **Outline three mechanisms that can bring about the thirst reflex, to maintain homeostasis of body fluids.**

_____

_____

_____

Q8. **Circle the factors that can increase fluid output.**

a. ADH.

b. Aldosterone.

c. Diarrhoea.

d. Fever.

e. Hyperventilation.

f. Increase in blood pressure.

ELECTROLYTES *Pages 907–11*

Amongst some of the important substances dissolved in body fluids are the **electrolytes**.

Q9. **Define the term electrolyte.**

_____

_____

Q10. **Is glucose an electrolyte? Give the rationale for your answer.**

_____

Q11.   Circle the substances that are classified as electrolytes.

a.   Proteins in solutions.

b.   Potassium and sodium.

c.   Anions.

d.   Compounds containing at least one ionic bond.

e.   Lipids.

Q12.   List four general functions of electrolytes.

_____

_____

_____

_____

Q13.   a. On Figure 18.1 (a), write the chemical symbols for electrolytes that are found in greatest concentrations in each of the three compartments. Write one symbol on each line provided. Use the list of symbols in the box below. For assistance, 📖 *Page 909, Figure 27.4.*

Cl^-, Chloride HCO_3^-, Bicarbonate HPO_3^-, Phosphate K^+, Potassium Na^+, Sodium Mg^{2+}, Magnesium $Protein^-$, Protein

---

b. On Figure 18.1 (b), show the shift of fluid resulting from loss of Na^+, for example by excessive loss of sweat.

1.   Shift of fluid possibly leading to hypovolaemic shock.

2.   Shift of fluid leading to overhydration of H_2O intoxication of brain cells, possibly leading to convulsions and coma.

Figure 18.1.
Diagrams of fluid compartments. (a) Electrolytes; (b) Direction of fluid shift resulting from Na+ deficit.

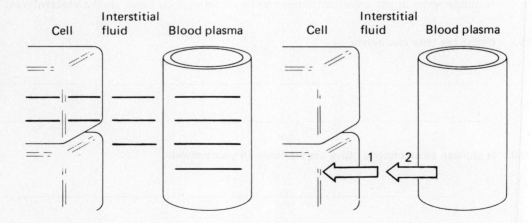

Q14.   Analyse the information in Figure 18.1 by answering these questions.

a.   Circle the **two** compartments that are most similar in electrolyte concentration: Cell Plasma
Interstitial fluid.

b.   List **two** major differences in electrolyte content of these two similar compartments.

_____

c.   Most body protein is located in which compartment?

_____

d.   Protein anions in intracellular fluid are more likely to be bound to the cation (sodium?
potassium?).

_____

**Q15.   Which hormone is responsible for the absorption of sodium from the distal convoluted tubule
of the kidney?**

_____

_____

**Q16.   Check your understanding of the functions and disorders related to major electrolytes by
completing the following table.**

Electrolytes	Main functions	Hyper-	Hypo-
a.	Important for bones and teeth, blood clotting, neurotransmitter release, maintenance of muscle tone		
b. Potassium		Irritability, diarrhoea, weakness, can cause atrial fibrillation of the heart; can lead to cardiac arrest	
c.	Necessary for conduction of action potentials in nervous and muscle tissue; creates most of the osmotic pressure		

MOVEMENTS OF BODY FLUIDS 📖 *Pages 911–12*

Q17. Four forces are involved in the movement of water between plasma and interstitial compartments and between interstitial and intracellular compartments. (They include the same types of forces involved in glomerular filtration.) Movement across capillary membranes due to these four forces is according to ———————— law of capillaries.

Q18. List the four main factors that influence the movement of fluid in the body.

———————————————————————————

———————————————————————————

———————————————————————————

———————————————————————————

Q19. Explain what happens to any excess of fluids and proteins that have not been reabsorbed by the venous capillaries.

———————————————————————————

———————————————————————————

———————————————————————————

ACID–BASE BALANCE AND IMBALANCE 📖 *Pages 912–7*

From earlier study, you will have gathered that one of the important electrolytes in the body's acid–base balance is the hydrogen ion (H^+). The study which follows should enable you to understand the importance of homeostasis of hydrogen ion concentration.

Q20. Apart from ingested foods, what is the main source of hydrogen ions?

———————————————————————————

Q21. What is the pH of extracellular fluid?

———————————————————————————

Q22. Name three major mechanisms that work together to maintain acid–base balance.

———————————————————————————

———————————————————————————

Figure 18.2.
Buffering action of carbonic acid–sodium carbonate system.

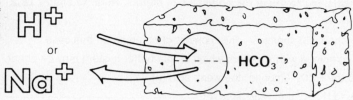

a. H^+ and Na^+: only one of you can join me at any one time.

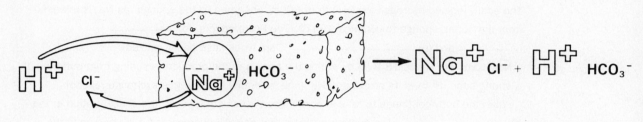

b. Na^+ is squeezed out as H^+ is drawn in.

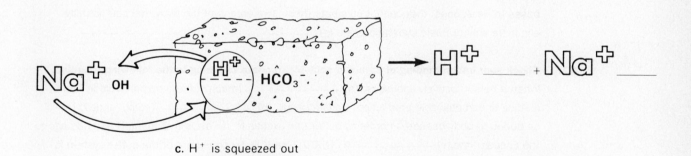

c. H^+ is squeezed out as Na^+ is drawn in.

○ H^+ and arrows showing movement of H^+

○ Na^+ and arrows showing movement of Na^+

Q23. List four important buffer systems in the body.

_____

_____

Q24. **The exercise below should enable you to grasp the principles of buffers. Refer to Figure 18.2 and complete this exercise.**

Buffers are sometimes called 'chemical sponges'. They consist of an anion (in this case bicarbonate, or HCO_3^-) that is combined with a cation, which in this buffer system may be either H^+ or Na^+. When H^+ is drawn to the HCO_3^- 'sponge' the weak acid (a) —————————— is formed. When sodium attaches to HCO_3^-, the weak base (b) —————————— —————————— is formed.

Buffers are chemicals that help the body to cope with (c) —————————— (strong? weak?) acids or bases that are easily ionised and can cause harm to the body. When a strong acid, such as hydrochloric acid, is added to body fluids, buffering occurs, as shown in Figure 18.2 (b). The easily ionised hydrogen ion ($H+$) from HCl is 'absorbed by the sponge' as Na^+ is released from the buffer/sponge to combine with Cl^-. The two products, (d) ——————— ——————— and (e) ——————— ———————, are weak (less easily ionized).

Now complete Figure 18.2 (c) by writing the names of the products resulting from buffering of a strong base, H^+ (and its arrow) and Na^+ (and its arrow) to show this exchange reaction.

When the body continues to take in or produce excess strong acid, the concentration of the (f) ——————— ——————— member of this buffer pair will decrease as it is used up in the attempt to maintain the homeostasis of pH.

Though buffer systems provide a rapid response to acid–base imbalance, they are limited, since one member of the buffer pair can be used up. They can convert only strong acids or bases to weak ones; they cannot eliminate them. Two organs of the body that can actually eliminate acid or basic substances are (g) —————————— and (h) ——————————.

Q25. **Check your understanding of carbonic acid–bicarbonate buffering in the following exercise.**

When a person actively exercises, (a) —————————— (much? little?) carbon dioxide forms, leading to carbonic acid production. Consequently, (b) —————————— (much? little?) H^+ will be added to body tissues. In order to buffer this excess H^+ (to avoid a drop in pH and damage to the tissues), the (c) —————————— (H_2CO_3? $NaHCO_3$?) component of the buffer system is called upon. The excess H^+ then replaces the (d) —————————— ions of $NaHCO_3$, in a sense 'tying up' the potentially harmful H^+.

Q26. Phosphates are more concentrated in (a) ——————— (ECF? ICF?). Name one type of cell in which the phosphate buffer system is most important: (b) ———————————.

Q27. **Which is the most abundant buffer system in the body?**

_____

Circle the part of the amino acid shown below that buffers acid. Draw a square around the part of the amino acid that buffers base.

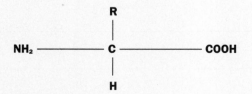

Q28. Explain how the haemoglobin buffer system buffers carbonic acid, so that an acid even weaker than carbonic acid (that is, haemoglobin) is formed.

_____

_____

Q29. Complete the exercise below, relating respiration and the kidneys to pH.

Hyperventilation will tend to (a) —————— (raise? lower?) blood pH, since as a person exhales CO_2, less CO_2 is available for formation of (b) —————— acid and free hydrogen ion.

A slight decrease in blood pH will tend to (c) —————— (stimulate? inhibit?) the respiratory centre and so will (d) —————— (increase? decrease?) respiration.

The kidneys regulate acid–base balance by altering their tubular secretion of (e) —————— or eliminating (f) —————— ion.

Q30. An acid–base imbalance caused by abnormal alteration of the respiratory system is classified as (a) —————— (metabolic? respiratory?) acidosis or alkalosis. Any other cause of acid–base imbalance, such as urinary or digestive tract disorder, is identified as (b) —————— (metabolic? respiratory?) acidosis or alkalosis.

Q31. Indicate which of the four categories of acid–base imbalance listed in the box is most likely to occur as a result of each condition described below.

---

1. Metabolic acidosis 2. Metabolic alkalosis 3. Respiratory acidosis 4. Respiratory alkalosis

---

☐ a. Decreased blood level of CO_2 as a result of hyperventilation.

☐ b. Decreased respiratory rate in a patient taking an overdose of morphine.

☐ c. Excessive intake of acids.

☐ d. Prolonged vomiting of stomach contents.

☐ e. Ketosis in uncontrolled diabetes mellitus.

☐ f. Decreased respiratory minute volume in a patient with emphysema or fractured rib.

☐ g. Excessive loss of bicarbonate from the body, as in prolonged diarrhoea or renal dysfunction.

Q32. Briefly outline the treatment for each of the following (📖 _Page 916)._

a. Respiratory acidosis.

_____

_____

b. Respiratory alkalosis.

_____

_____

c. Metabolic acidosis.

_____

_____

d. Metabolic alkalosis.

_____

_____

This completes the study on fluid, electrolyte and acid–base homeostasis. Well done! To check your progress, you may wish to do the Checkpoints Exercise below.

CHECKPOINTS EXERCISE

Q33. Circle 'T' (true) or 'F' (false) for the following statements.

T   F   a. Hyperventilation tends to raise pH.

T   F   b. Carbonic acid is a weaker acid than reduced haemoglobin.

T   F   c. Under normal circumstances, fluid intake each day is greater than fluid output.

T   F   d. During oedema, there is increased movement of fluid out of plasma and into interstitial fluid.

T   F   e. Parathyroid hormone causes an increase in the blood level of calcium.

T   F   f. When aldosterone is in high concentration, sodium is conserved (in blood) and potassium is excreted (in urine).

T   F   g. In general, electrolytes cause greater osmotic effects than nonelectrolytes.

T   F   h. The body of an infant contains a higher percentage of water than the body of an adult.

T   F   i. Starch, glucose, bicarbonates, sodium and potassium are all electrolytes.

T   F   j. Loss of blood via haemorrhage is likely to decrease hydrostatic pressure and also to decrease NFP.

T   F   k. Protein is the most abundant buffer system in the body.

T   F   l. The carbonic acid portion of the bicarbonate–carbonic acid system buffers base.

T   F   m. The pH of arterial blood should be higher than that of venous blood and should be about pH 7.40–7.45.

T   F   n. Hydrostatic pressure of blood and hydrostatic pressure of interstitial fluid tend to move substances in the same direction: out of blood and into interstitial fluid.

T   F   o. Interstitial fluid, blood plasma and lymph are all extracellular fluids.

Q34.   On an average day the greatest volume of fluid output is via :

a.   Faeces.

b.   Sweat.

c.   Lungs.

d.   Urine.

Q35.   Which term refers to a lower than normal blood level of sodium?

a.   Hyperkalaemia.

b.   Hypokalaemia.

c.   Hypernatraemia.

d.   Hypercalcaemia.

e.   Hyponatremia.

Q36.   Which one of the following is not likely to increase fluid output?

a.   Fever.

b.   Hyperventilation.

c.   Vomiting and diarrhoea.

d.   Decreased blood pressure.

e.   Increased glomerular filtration rate.

PATIENT SCENARIO 1

John Kensington, aged 3, has been admitted to the ward in a severe state of dehydration. His medical diagnosis is that he is suffering from bacterial gastroenteritis (a common infection in babies and young children). He has been vomiting several times and he also has diarrhoea. He has a slight elevation of temperature.

He is accompanied by his mother, who is extremely anxious. She is assisting with John's management by giving him Dioralyte® solution, which has been prescribed by the medical staff.

John's urine output is to be measured and recorded. Since admission, he has passed a small amount of dark urine. On planning the care for John, the nurse also observes that he has a dry mouth and flushed inelastic skin, and his eyes appear sunken.

Q37.   Study a sachet of Dioralyte and then briefly outline its main purpose in the management of fluid and electrolyte replacement therapy.

_____

_____

_____

Q38. Briefly explain the physiological effects of vomiting and diarrhoea on John.

_____

_____

_____

_____

_____

Q39. Why is it important for fluid intake and output to be measured and recorded?

_____

_____

Q40. Explain why John is passing a small amount of dark urine.

_____

_____

Q41. John's mother wants to know why her son's eyes appear sunken. If you were the nurse caring for John, what explanations should you give the mother to allay her anxiety?

_____

_____

_____

Q42. Why is dehydration a cause for concern in a child of three?

_____

_____

_____

Q43. Briefly outline the possible causes of gastroenteritis. What advice should you give to John's parents in order to reduce its occurrence.

_____

_____

_____

Acute gastroenteritis and food poisoning

Acute gastroenteritis is a very common infection (more common in children than adults) affecting the gastrointestinal tract, and resulting in nausea, vomiting, diarrhoea, abdominal pain and often a pyrexia. In babies and small chidren the severe vomiting and diarrhoea could lead to dehydration and severe loss of electrolytes and may thus be life-threatening. The severe dehydration may lead to hypovolaemic shock. Gastroenteritis is usually caused by bacteria (e.g salmonellae, streptococci, clostridia) and viruses. The sources of bacteria are usually the contamination of milk, meat and water.

Bacterial food poisoning is more prevalent in poor urban communities as a result of poor facilities for storage of foods, inadequate water and poor sanitary conditions. Bacterial food poisoning affects about 8000 – 12000 individuals each year in England and Wales (as indicated by the annual notification figure).

The commonest cause of gastroenteritis is *Salmonella typhimurium*, which may be found in milk, meat, poultry, raw eggs and egg powders. The organisms may enter the bloodstream and invade the tissues, causing an enteric fever like typhoid, which is confined to the intestines.

The transfer of these organisms is usually by human hands, foods and utensils. The infection is often called the **faecal–oral disease**.

Salmonella is the commonest cause of gastroenteritis, which is often associated with food poisoning (gastroenteritis following *Salmonella* infection accounts for 70% of reported cases). The incubation period is from 12 to 36 hours and the disease lasts for 1–7 days, obviously depending on the virulence of the organisms.

Many individuals with apparently no symptoms (subclinical disease) following an infection with *Salmonella* may become carriers and can pass the infection to others who are more susceptible.

Gastroenteritis in babies and children is often associated with poor hygiene conditions in the household, and this is often the result of lack of education. In babies, it could well be that the bottle and teat for feeding are not properly cleaned and sterilised. Preparation of the milk itself may be contaminated. Other kitchen equipment may be contaminated. Cooked foods in the refrigerator may become contaminated if they are in close proximity to raw food sources.

PATIENT SCENARIO 2

Robert Sullivan is aged 19 and weighs 90kg. He is spending his holiday in the tropics. After much sunbathing and walking in the sun, he has developed heat exhaustion. He is sweating profusely and has lost approximately 4 litres of fluids.

Q44. **What is Robert's new weight following the bout of sweating?**

_____

Q45. **Which main ions has Robert lost in the sweat?**

_____

Q46. **Suggest the possible symptoms that could have occurred in Robert and give the rationale for your answer.**

_____

_____

Q47. **Prior to heat exhaustion, calculate the amount of fluid in Robert's body. Hint: refer to the amount of fluid per body weight.**

_____

_____

Q48. **What sensible advice should Robert be given for his next trip to the tropics?**

_____

_____

_____

For more information on heat exhaustion, please refer to 📖 *Page 856.*

FURTHER UNDERSTANDING OF HOMEOSTATIC FLUID AND ELECTROLYTE BALANCE AND MANAGEMENT

Having completed the two case histories, you should by now be able to appreciate the importance of fluids and electrolytes in the body. Whilst the medical management in the two case histories was straightforward, there are many diseases in which drastic measures may have to be taken in order to correct the water and electrolyte balance of the patients. This can occur, for example, in patients suffering from kidney failure. In such patients, little or no urine is produced and therefore many of the waste products of the body (e.g urea and creatinine) cannot be excreted. Therefore, the blood urea level is increased. This increase in blood urea is responsible for many of the symptoms of kidney failure, such as nausea and vomiting, hiccups as a result of irritation of the gastrointestinal tract, and pruritus (intense skin itching). In addition, the electrolyte and acid–base balance are also impaired and both hydrogen and potassium ions are retained. Water and sodium are also retained, which can give rise to oedema. The oedema can affect both pulmonary functions (pulmonary oedema) and cardiovascular functions (heart failure). Pulmonary oedema may cause difficulty in breathing. The retention in fluid can also lead to hypertension.

The increased level in the blood of potassium (hyperkalaemia) can lead to cardiac arrhythmias (abnormal heart rhythm), whilst the increase in hydrogen ions can give rise to metabolic acidosis (this can also affect the respiratory system, leading to dyspnoea). Other symptoms include fits, confusion and coma which occur because of the accumulation of toxic waste products (may be referred to as uraemia). The management of the patients will include the control of water, electrolytes and protein in the diet.

The discussion to follow will only relate to fluid and electrolyte balance.

One of the measures in the control of water and electrolytes may be achieved by the use of either **peritoneal dialysis** or **haemodialysis**. In both procedures, the desired outcome can be achieved, although a quicker result is obtained through haemodialysis. The choice of one procedure as opposed to the other depends on the patient's condition, the cause of the illness and availability of equipment.

Both types of dialysis depend on two basic physical principles, that of water movement by **osmosis** and solute movement by **diffusion** across a selectively permeable membrane to produce a concentration equilibrium on either side of the membrane.

In haemodialysis, a synthetic membrane is employed and is part of what is referred to as the 'artificial kidney'. Peritoneal dialysis (the procedure to be described here) is made possible by the peritoneum acting as the selectively permeable membrane.

Peritoneal dialysis

Peritoneal dialysis is a life-saving medical procedure that is used in children and adults as a way of removing nitrogenous wastes such as urea and creatinine, excess water, excess potassium and sometimes sodium from the body, when the kidney's functions are impaired. When referring to kidney disease in which the kidney functions are sufficiently reduced, the term 'renal failure' is used. Renal failure may be acute or chronic.

Renal failure is often described as **prerenal**, **renal**, or **postrenal**. Prerenal failure occurs as a result of reduction in blood volume due to haemorrhage, severe burns, cardiac failure or dehydration. Renal failure includes ischaemia (reduced blood supply to the area) which causes a reduction in renal functions by causing **acute tubular necrosis**. The causes include toxins, drugs and certain types of glomerulonephritis. Postrenal failure occurs as a result of prostatic enlargement (the common cause is senile hypertrophy) which therefore includes obstruction of the urinary tract and bilateral calculi.

The procedure of peritoneal dialysis involves the insertion of a special catheter under aseptic conditions by a medical practitioner in between the two layers of the peritoneum (for more information on the peritoneum, please refer to 📖 *Pages 768–70*. A sealed system is used and clamps are employed to control the inflow and outflow of fluids to and from the peritoneum (refer to Figure 18.3).

Figure 18.3.
Peritoneal dialysis.

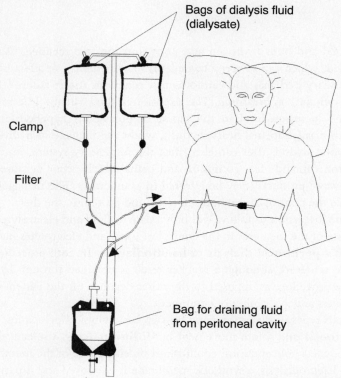

Bags of dialysis fluid
(dialysate)

Clamp

Filter

Bag for draining fluid
from peritoneal cavity

The catheter allows dialysate (contains no nitrogenous products or potassium and therefore allows the movement of these molecules from the blood to the dialysis fluid) to enter the peritoneal cavity and there it remains for at least 45 minutes. The length of time that fluid is allowed to remain in the peritoneal cavity depends on the patient's condition and the medical management. After the 45 minutes or so, the dialysis fluid from the peritoneal cavity is allowed to drain over approximately 20 to 30 minutes. The volume of fluid removed is measured and recorded. The drained fluid contains the waste products, such as urea, potassium and any excess of water.

The dialysis fluid to be used is usually administered at **body temperature** (this is usually achieved by the use of an incubator). The types of dialysis fluids to be used (that is, the chemical composition of the fluids) depends on the patient's condition, for example how much oedema or electrolyte imbalance is present.

Peritoneal dialysis may be short-term, but in many cases it is a long-term strategy, especially in patients who are awaiting kidney transplants. In children, dialysis is often undertaken as a continuous process and this is referred to as **continuous ambulatory peritoneal dialysis** (CAPD). Jerrum (1991) has reported that CAPD provides a more constant internal environment than does haemodialysis.

QUESTIONS FOR DISCUSSION

1. Giving the rationale for your answer, explain the physiological processes that make it possible for excess of electrolytes and water to be removed from the body in the procedure of peritoneal dialysis.

2. Giving reasons for your answer, suggest why excess fluids have to be removed from the body when the kidneys have failed.

3. If more water is to be removed from the patient undergoing peritoneal dialysis, suggest how this might be achieved.

4. Explain why fluid intake and output (in terms of urinary output and dialysate drainage) have to be measured and recorded.

5. Suggest the potential complications that may occur in an individual who is on long-term peritoneal dialysis.

6. What possible laboratory results could the nurse have at her disposal in order that she may assess the patient's progress during peritoneal dialysis?

7. Study two different types of dialysis fluid and then decide how each may influence the progress of peritoneal dialysis.

Answers to questions

Q1. Intracellular fluid.

Q2. Extracellular fluid.

Q3. Interstitial fluid.

Q4. All of the statements, except i.

Q5. a, 2500; b, 2.5; c, 2300; d, 200.

Q6. a, 500; b, kidneys, 1500; c, lungs, 300; d, GI tract, 200.

Order of the above answers does not matter.

Output of fluid increases greatly via sweat glands and also slightly through respiration. To compensate for this, urinary output decreases and intake increases.

Q7. Osmotic pressure increases and inhibits ADH secretion; release of renin leads to the production of angiotensin; blood volume decreases. The thirst centre is situated in the hypothalamus.

Q8. c, d, e and f.

Q9. Any chemical substance that can dissolve in water to form ions (cations and anions). The solution can usually conduct electricity.

Q10. No. Because it does not dissociate in water.

Q11. All except lipids.

Q12. Essential minerals; control the osmosis of water between body compartments; maintain the acid–base balance required for normal cellular activities; allow the production of action potentials.

Q13a. See diagram opposite.

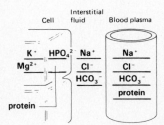

b   1. Shift of fluid leading to overdehydration or water intoxication of brain cells, possibly leading to convulsions and coma.

    2. Shift of fluid from plasma to replace IF that entered cells. This may lead to hypovolaemic shock.

Q14.   a. Plasma and interstitial fluid.

    b. Plasma contains more protein and slightly more sodium and less chloride than interstitial fluid.

    c. Intracellular.

    d. Potassium.

Q15.   Aldosterone. You should recall that aldosterone promotes the reabsorption of sodium but decreases the reabsorption of potassium.

Q16.   a. Calcium; b. Lethargy, weakness, anorexia, nausea, vomiting, polyuria, itching, bone pain, depression, paresthesia, stupor, coma; c. numbness and tingling of fingers, hyperactive reflexes, muscle cramps, tetany, convulsions; may cause spasms of laryngeal muscles that can cause death by asphyxiation; d. Plays an important role in establishing the resting membrane potential and in the repolarisation phase of action potentials in nervous and muscle tissue; e. Cramps and fatigue, flaccid paralysis, nausea, vomiting, mental confusion, increased urine output, shallow respirations, changes in electrocardiogram; f. Sodium; g. Intense thirst, fatigue, restlessness, agitation, coma; h. Muscular weakness, dizziness, headache, hypotension, tachycardia, shock; can lead to mental confusion, stupor and coma.

Q17.   Starling's law.

Q18.   Blood hydrostatic pressure; interstitial fluid hydrostatic pressure, blood colloid osmotic pressure and interstitial fluid colloid osmotic pressure.

Q19.   Fluids pass into lymphatic capillaries, where they then move through lymph vessels to the appropriate ducts and to the heart via the subclavian veins.

Q20.   Cellular metabolism of substances such as glucose, fatty acids and amino acids.

Q21.   7.35–7.45.

Q22.   Buffer systems, exhalation of carbon dioxide and kidney excretion. For more information 📖 *Page 913.*

Q23.   Carbonic acid, bicarbonate, phosphate and proteins.

Q24.   a, Carbonic acid; b, sodium bicarbonate; c, strong; d, sodium chloride; e, carbonic acid; f, sodium bicarbonate; g, lungs; h, kidneys. The order does not matter for answers to g and h.

Q25.   a, Much; b, much; c, $NaHCO_3$; d, sodium.

Q26.   a, ICF; b, kidney cells.

Q27.   Proteins.

Q28. Reduced haemoglobin carries a negative charge (Hb$^-$) and it combines with H$^+$ ions to form an acid (HbH) that is weaker than carbonic acid.

Q29. a, Raise; b, carbonic; c, stimulate; d, increase; e, H$^+$; f, HCO$_3^-$.

Q30. a, Respiratory; b, metabolic.

Q31. 4a, 3b, 2c, 2d, 1e, 3f, 1g.

Q32. Refer to page 916 of PAP.

Q33 Ta, Fb, Fc, Td, Te, Tf, Th, Fi, Tj, Tk, Tl, Tm, Fn, To.

Q34. d. Urine.

Q35. e. Hyponatraemia.

Q36. e. Increased glomerular filtration rate.

Q37. Dioralyte contains sodium chloride, potassium chloride, sodium bicarbonate and glucose. When reconstituted with boiled water, it provides all the necessary electrolytes that have been lost in vomiting and diarrhoea. It therefore can correct hypokalaemia and also replenish the important extracellular ions such as sodium. The bicarbonate can control any metabolic acidosis.

Q38. Both vomiting and diarrhoea will lead to the loss of electrolytes such as sodium, potassium and chlorides and also water. Severe vomiting causes loss of hydrogen ions, part of hydrochloric acid, and this can lead to metabolic alkalosis. Severe depletion of potassium ions may cause cardiac arrhythmias and even cardiac arrest.

Loss of water can lead to dehydration and therefore hypovolaemia, thus causing reduction in blood volume and a subsequent decrease in cardiac output. A decrease in cardiac output will result in low blood pressure (hypotension). This is also accompanied by a tachycardia at first.

Reduction in blood volume will affect blood flow to the kidneys and this can lead to oliguria (decrease in urine output) at first, but later can cause anuria (no urine formation) and eventually acute renal failure.

All of the symptoms are associated with the state of dehydration and these are as follows: dry mouth, inelastic and dry skin, sunken eyes and diminished urine output.

Q39. This is in order to assess fluid management, to ensure that John is adequately hydrated and also to reduce the incidence of overhydration.

Q40. This is explained in question 38 above.

Q41. The explanation should be given in a manner that John's mother will understand. It is important to let her know that as fluid replacement progresses, John will look much better. Much of your explanations should focus on water depletion and much of that information is to be found in the answer to question 38 above.

Q42. Dehydration is a cause for concern in anyone who has lost a large amount of fluid, but in a child of three, it is perhaps of more significance, since the proportion of body weight as fluids is much larger (75% to 80%) than in the adult (60%). This therefore implies that a child will become dehydrated much quicker than an adult and has a higher risk of developing complications sooner.

Q43. The section on 'overview of gastroenteritis' should help you to answer this question. Much of the advice should focus on aspects of hygiene in the home, such as the preparation of foods, washing up of cutlery and also cleanliness of both the parents and the child. It may be advisable to suggest the use of safe detergents in the washing of kitchen surfaces and also other areas in the home. The importance of hand washing should be emphasised.

Q44. His new weight will be 86kg. This is because **one** litre of fluid is equivalent to **one** kg. Robert has therefore lost 4kg in weight.

Q45. Mainly sodium and chlorides.

Q46. The body temperature may be normal, although the skin may be cool and clammy, as a result of profuse sweating. Severe loss of sodium ions may give rise to muscle cramps, dizziness, vomiting and fainting. Fluid loss may result in hypovolaemia and hence low blood pressure on account of reduced cardiac output.

Q47. If you assume that 65% of the body weight is fluid, then the amount of fluid in Robert's body would be approximately 58.5 litres.

$$\frac{65 \times 90}{100}$$

Q48. Obviously, the advice should focus on ways of preventing dehydration. He should take plenty of fluids if he is to engage in any physical activity. He should avoid walking or sunbathing when the sun is at its highest in the sky. Indeed, he should avoid staying in the sun for long periods of time. If he should sweat profusely, it may be advisable to take a bit more salt in the diet, or alternatively he can take salt tablets.

Overview and key terms

The male urinary and reproductive system

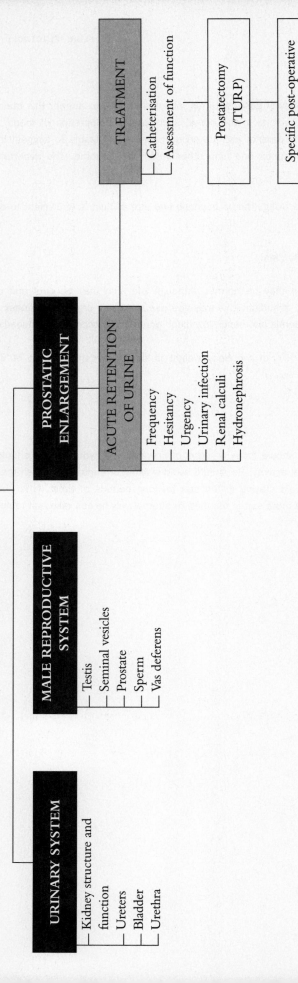

URINARY SYSTEM
- Kidney structure and function
- Ureters
- Bladder
- Urethra

MALE REPRODUCTIVE SYSTEM
- Testis
- Seminal vesicles
- Prostate
- Sperm
- Vas deferens

PROSTATIC ENLARGEMENT

ACUTE RETENTION OF URINE
- Frequency
- Hesitancy
- Urgency
- Urinary infection
- Renal calculi
- Hydronephrosis

TREATMENT
- Catheterisation
- Assessment of function

Prostatectomy (TURP)

Specific post-operative problems
- Haemorrhage
- Urinary incontinence
- Retrograde ejaculation
- Epididymitis
- Chronic renal failure

19. The Male Urinary and Reproductive System

Learning outcomes

1. To understand the structure and function(s) of the male urinary and reproductive system.

2. To relate this knowledge to an understanding of the patient problems that arise when the prostate gland enlarges.

3. To understand the long-term consequences that can arise when urine flow is chronically obstructed.

4. To relate the surgical treatment of an enlarged prostate gland to normal anatomy.

5. To explain some of the specific postoperative problems that may follow prostatectomy.

Chapters 26–28

INTRODUCTION

Although the male urinary and reproductive systems are functionally different, they are anatomical neighbours and share a common anatomical outflow – the urethra. For this reason, they are often considered together.

The scenario, though, will focus mainly on a urinary problem – that of difficulty in passing urine as a result of an enlarged prostate gland. Some of the problems and complications arising from this will be discussed. For example, urinary tract infection and kidney failure. Briefly, some of the likely effects of prostatic surgery on reproductive functioning will be considered.

In preparation for this, the chapter commences with questions that will help you to learn the necessary anatomical and physiological background knowledge. Questions that cover some topics on fluid and electrolyte balance (📖 *Chapter 27*) which relate to kidney function, will be brought in towards the end of the chapter.

Figure 19.1.
Organs of the
urinary system.

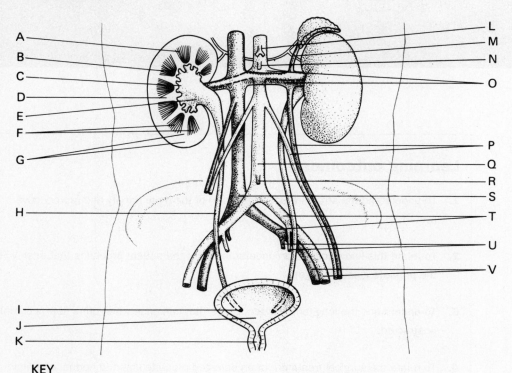

KEY

A. Pyramid
B. Papilla
C. Calyx
D. Renal column
O E. Pelvis
F. Medulla
O G. Cortex
O H. Ureter
I. Ureteral opening
J. Bladder
O K. Urethra

L. Celiac artery
M. Left adrenal (suprarenal vein
N. Superior mesenteric artery
O. Left renal artery and vein
P. Left spermatic or ovarian artery and vein
Q. Aorta
R. Inferior mesenteric artery
S. Inferior vena cava
T. Left common iliac artery and vein
U. Left internal iliac artery and vein
V. Left external iliac artery and vein

THE URINARY SYSTEM 📖 *Chapter 26*

Q1. **Describe the functions of the urinary system in this exercise.**

List the waste products eliminated through urine: (a) _____ . Which ion do kidneys excrete when blood pH is too low? (b) _____ . Kidneys produce (c) _____ , which regulates blood pressure, and (d) _____ , which is vital to normal red blood cell formation. Kidneys also activate vitamin (e) _____ .

Q2. **Look at the organs that make up the urinary system on Figure 19.1 and answer the following questions about them.**

The kidneys are located at about (a) _____ (waist? hip?) level, between (b) _____ and (c) _____ vertebrae. Each kidney is about (d) _____ cm ((e) _____ inches) long. Visualise the kidney location and size on yourself.

The kidneys are in an extreme (f) _____ (anterior? posterior?) position in the abdomen. They are described as (g) _____ since they are posterior to the peritoneum.

Figure 19.2.
Diagram of a nephron.

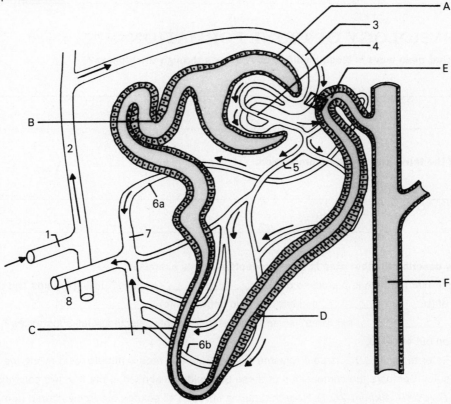

Q3. **Complete this exercise about the functional unit of the kidney, a nephron.**

a. On Figure 19.2, label parts A–F of the nephron, with letters arranged according to the flow of urine.

b. Which one of these structures forms part of the renal corpuscle?

c.   The other part of the renal corpuscle is a cluster of capillaries. What is it called, and what is its number in the figure (4? 6b?).

_____

d.   Arrange in order the layers that fluid and solutes pass through, as they move from blood into the formation of urine (filtrate).

1. Filtration slits between podocytes of visceral layer of globular capsule

2. Basement membrane of the glomerulus

3. Endothelial pores of capillary membrane.

_____ _____ _____

e.   List the functional advantages of endothelial pores and filtration slits.

_____

_____

PHYSIOLOGY OF URINE FORMATION 📖 *Pages 874–91*

Q4.   In what main ways is blood modified as it passes through the kidneys?

_____

_____

Q5.   List the three steps in urine production:

_____

_____

Q6.   Now describe the first step in urine production in this exercise.

Glomerular filtration is a process of (a) _____ (pushing? pulling?) fluids and solutes out of (b) _____ and into the fluid known as (c) _____ .

(d) _____ (all types? all small substances? only selected small substances?) are forced out of blood.

Refer to Figure 19.3, area A (plasma in glomeruli) and area B (filtrate just beyond the capsule). Compare the composition of these two fluids (described in the first two columns of 📖 *Page 880, Exhibit 26.1*). Note that during filtration all solutes are freely filtered from blood except (e) _____ .

Blood pressure (or hydrostatic pressure) in glomerular capillaries is about (f) _____ mmHg. This value is (g) _____ (higher? lower?) than that in other capillaries of the body. This extra pressure is accounted for by the fact that the diameter of the efferent arteriole is (h) _____ (larger? smaller?) than that of the afferent arteriole. Picture three garden hoses connected to each other, representing the afferent arteriole, glomerular capillaries and efferent arteriole. The third one (efferent arteriole) is extremely narrow; it creates such resistance that pressure builds up in the first two. Fluids will be forced out of pores in the middle (glomerular) hose.

List three structural features of renal corpuscles that enhance their filtration capacity:

(i) _____ _____ _____ .

Q7.   Blood hydrostatic pressure is not the only force determining the amount of filtration occurring in glomeruli.

a.   Name **two** other forces (shown on 📖 *Page 876, Figure 26.10*).

_____

_____

b.   Normal values for these three forces are given on *Page 876, Figure 26.10*. Write the formula for calculating net filtration pressure (NFP). Draw an arrow beneath each term to show the direction of the force in Figure 19.3. Then calculate a normal NFP, using the values given.

Figure 19.3.
Diagram of a nephron with renal tubule abbreviated.

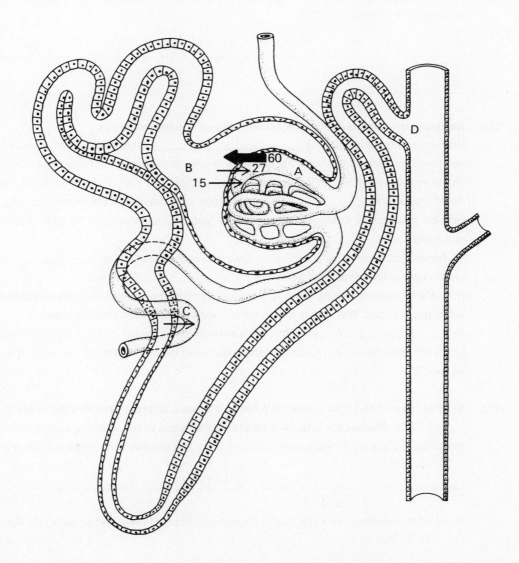

NFP = (glomerular blood hydrostatic pressure) – (_____ + _____)

Normal NFP = (_____ mmHg) – (_____ mmHg + _____ mmHg) = _____ mmHg

Q8. **A clinical challenge. Show the effects of alterations of these pressures in a pathological situation. Determine the NFP of the patient whose pressure values are shown below. Note which values are abnormal and suggest causes.**

Glomerular blood hydrostatic pressure = 42

Blood colloid osmotic pressure = 27

Capsular filtrate hydrostatic pressure = 15

NFP = _____

Q9. **Define GFR in this exercise.**

a. To what do the letters GFR refer? G _____ F _____ R _____ .

b. Write a normal value for GFR: _____ ml/min (_____ litres/day).

c. If NFP decreases, GFR _____ -creases. What consequences may be expected to accompany a decrease in GFR?

_____

_____

Q10. **Complete this exercise about the second step up of urine formation.**

Glomerular filtration is a(n) (a) _____(passive, nonselective? active, selective?) process. If this were the only step in urine formation, all of the substances in the filtrate would leave the body in the urine. Note from 📖 *Page 880, Exhibit 26.1*, that the body would produce (b) _____ litres of urine each day! And it would contain many valuable substances. Obviously, some of these 'good' substances must be drawn back into blood and saved.

Recall that blood in most capillaries flows into vessels named (c) _____ , but blood in glomerular capillaries flows into (d) _____ and (e) _____ . This unique arrangement permits blood to recapture some of the substances indiscriminately pushed out during filtration. This occurs during the second step of urine formation, called (f) _____ . This process moves substances in the (g) _____ (same? opposite?) direction as glomerular filtration, as shown by the direction of the arrow at area C of Figure 19.3.

Q11. **Refer to areas C and D on Figure 19.3 and to the two columns on the far right of** 📖 *Page 880, Exhibit 26.1*. **Discuss the effects of tubular reabsorption in this learning activity.**

a. Which solutes are 100% reabsorbed into area C, so that virtually none remains in urine (area D)?

_____

b. About what percentage of water that is filtered out of blood is reabsorbed back into blood?

_____

c.   Which chemicals are about 90% reabsorbed?

_____

d.   Which solute is about 50% reabsorbed?

_____

e.   Identify the solute that is filtered from blood and not reabsorbed. State the clinical significance of this fact.

_____

_____

Q12.   The third step in urine production is (a) _____ . It involves movement of substances from (b) _____ (blood to urine? urine to blood?). In other words, tubular secretion is movement of substances in (c) _____ (the same? the opposite?) direction as movement occurring in filtration. List four substances that are secreted by the process of tubular secretion: (d) _____ _____ _____ _____ .

URETERS, URINARY BLADDER, AND URETHRA 📖 *Pages 891–5*

Q13.   **Refer to Figure 19.1 as you complete the following exercise.**

Ureters connect (a) _____ to (b) _____ . Ureters are about (c) _____ cm ((d) _____ inches) long.

These tubes enter the urinary bladder at two of the three corners of the (e) _____ . The third corner marks the opening into the (f) _____ .

The bladder is lined with (g) _____ epithelium. Explain how the presence of this type of epithelium serves the primary function of the urinary bladder.

The urinary bladder is located in the (h) _____ (abdomen? true pelvis?). Two sphincters lie just inferior to it. The (i) _____ (internal? external?) sphincter is under voluntary control.

Urine leaves the bladder through the (j) _____ . In females the length of this tube is (k) _____ cm ((l) _____ inches); in males it is about (m) _____ cm ((n) _____ inches). Write in sequence (according to pathway of urine) the three portions of the male urethra: (o) _____ → (p) _____ → (q) _____ .

THE MALE REPRODUCTIVE SYSTEM 📖 *Pages 923–36, Chapter 28*

Figure 19.4.
Male organs of reproduction seen in sagittal section. Structures are numbered in order along the pathway taken by sperm.

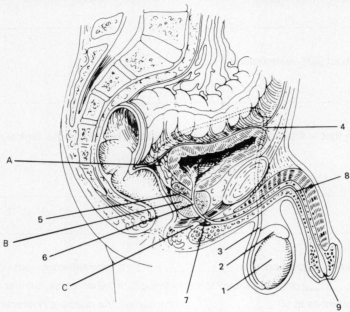

Q14. **Refer to Figure 19.4. Structures in the male reproductive system are numbered in order along the pathway that sperm take from their site of origin to the point where they exit from the body. Match the structures in the Figure (using numbers 1–9) with descriptions below.**

☐ a. Ejaculatory duct
☐ b. Epididymis
☐ c. Prostatic urethra
☐ d. Spongy (cavernous) urethra
☐ e. Membranous urethra
☐ f. Ductus (vas) deferens (portion within the abdomen)
☐ g. Ductus (vas) deferens (portion within the scrotum)
☐ h. Urethral orifice
☐ i. Testis

Q15. **Which structures numbered 1–9 in Figure 19.4 are paired? Circle their numbers:**

1   2   3   4   5   6   7   8   9

Which structures are single? Write their numbers:

_____

Q16. **Answer these questions about the ductus (vas) deferens.**

The ductus deferens is about (a) _____ cm ((b) _____ inches) long.

It is located (c) _____ (entirely? partially?) in the abdomen. It enters the abdomen

via the (d) _____ . Protrusion of abdominal contents through this weakened area is

known as (e) _____ .

What structure besides the vas composes the seminal cord? (f) _____ .

Q17.   Match the accessory sex glands with their descriptions.

> **B. Bulbourethral glands   P. Prostate gland   S. Seminal vesicles**

☐   a.   Paired pouches posterior to the urinary bladder.

☐   b.   Structures that empty secretions (along with contents of vas deferens) into ejaculatory duct.

☐   c.   Single doughnut – shaped gland located inferior to the bladder; surrounds and empties secretions into urethra.

☐   d.   Contribute about 60 per cent of seminal fluid.

☐   e.   Pair of pea-sized glands located in the urogenital diaphragm.

☐   f.   Produces clotting enzymes and fibrinolysin.

Q18.   Label the seminal vesicle, prostate gland, and bulbourethral gland on Figure 19.4.

Q19.   Complete the following exercise about semen.

The average amount per ejaculation is (a) _____ ml. The normal range of number of sperm is (b) _____ /ml. When the count falls below (c) _____ /ml, the male is likely to be sterile. Only one sperm fertilizes the ovum. Explain why such a high sperm count is required for fertility.

_____

_____

The pH of semen is slightly (d) _____ (acid? alkaline?). State the advantage of this fact.

_____

_____

(e) What is the function of seminal plasmin?

_____

_____

(f) What is the function of fibrinolysin in semen?

_____

_____

CHECKPOINTS EXERCISE

Q20.   Where is the glomerular capsule? What is its function?

_____

_____

Q21.   What is the average value for glomerular filtration?

_____

Q22.   What is the second stage of urine formation called?

_____

Q23.   What substances are reabsorbed by the tubules?

_____

_____

Q24.   Which hormones control water and sodium reabsorption?

_____

_____

Q25.   Where is urine stored prior to excretion from the body?

_____

Q26.   Where is the prostate gland situated?

_____

PATIENT SCENARIO

Mr Ewing is a 63-year-old headmaster of a comprehensive school. He is happily married, with a son and daughter aged 18 and 20, respectively. Mrs Ewing works part-time as a secretary.

Recently Mr Ewing has noticed that he has been experiencing some difficulty in starting to pass urine. It seems to take much longer to start – compared to when he was younger. Also, he appears to have to empty his bladder once or twice during the night.

He puts all these symptoms down to his advancing years. But whilst attending a careers evening at school he drinks a glass of wine and then subsequently finds he is unable to pass urine – despite an increasing desire to do so.

After a number of attempts he abandons his efforts and asks a colleague to drive him to the accident and emergency department of the local hospital.

Acute retention of urine

Mr Ewing's condition is due to an enlarged prostate gland (📖 *Page 935, Figure 28.10*) which has pressed on the urethra and made it gradually more difficult for Mr Ewing to pass urine. The prostate has now enlarged to the point where it has completely obstructed the urethra, from external pressure. The urethra is unable to open and thus allow urine to flow from the bladder. This is known as **acute retention of urine.** If urine is retained in the bladder, then it means that the kidneys are working and producing urine. When, and if, the kidneys stop working – possibly because of back pressure – this is known as **suppression of urine.**

The following questions are based on 📖 *Page 895.*

Q27.   How much urine will stimulate stretch receptors in the bladder wall?

_____

Q28.   What is the next stage in the process of micturition?

_____

_____

Q29.   What is a sphincter?

_____

Q30.   What is the next step in micturition, involving a sphincter?

_____

_____

Q31. **Imagine that you are having difficulty in passing urine. What can you do to assist the act?**

_____

_____

_____

_____

But Mr Ewing's bladder has not responded to any of this, and by now he must be suffering acute discomfort. As men grow older, so this condition becomes more common. An enlarged gland is said to be suffered by 50% of men aged 50 and 70% of men aged 70. Why the gland should enlarge is not fully understood – but it is probably linked to hormonal changes.

Q32. **What is the principal male hormone and what are its actions? (** 📖 _Page 552_ **)**

_____

The fact that this does not occur until about the age of 50 suggests that it is a very gradual process, and not something that happens overnight. As the bladder is now faced with an ever-narrowing outlet, it has to work harder to overcome this, and this leads to enlargement of the muscle wall. This can lead to small areas of the bladder wall becoming pushed out like balloons. These are called **diverticula.** Urine can stagnate in these, and as a result become infected.

The bladder wall can also become unstable and produce spontaneous contractions that are not under the control of higher centres. This is what leads to some of the major problems for Mr Ewing, for example, **frequency** of micturition and **urgency.**

Mr Ewing's problems

Because Mr Ewing's prostate has slowly enlarged over the years, his problems will also have developed slowly. The following questions will help you understand both these long-term problems and those of a more immediate nature. The questions then build on this and extend into aspects of Mr Ewing's care and treatment.

Q33. **Mr Ewing has, for a number of years, had to pass urine at increasingly frequent intervals. Why is this?**

_____

_____

_____

_____

Q34. During this time, Mr Ewing will also have been predisposed to develop urinary infections. Why is this?

_____

_____

_____

_____

_____

Q35. What form of treatment will Mr Ewing require to help him to pass urine?

_____

_____

_____

_____

_____

Q36. Mr Ewing's over-distended bladder will raise intra-abdominal pressure and this will affect venous return (_Page 634_). What may happen if his bladder is suddenly and rapidly emptied?

_____

_____

_____

_____

Q37. What is a major long-term problem that Mr Ewing may develop as a result of continuous bladder catheterisation?

_____

_____

_____

_____

_____

Q38. If Mr Ewing is suspected of developing a urinary infection, how will this be confirmed?

_____

_____

_____

_____

_____

Q39. Mr Ewing's other problems can stem from the fact that an enlarged prostate has chronically obstructed the free flow of urine in the urinary tract. What may be the effect of this on urine production in the kidneys?

_____

_____

_____

_____

_____

Q40. The treatment for Mr Ewing's condition is to surgically remove the prostate gland (prostatectomy). From your knowledge of its functions (📖 _Page 934_), how will Mr Ewing be disadvantaged by prostate removal?

_____

_____

_____

_____

_____

Q41. In the hours following surgery, haemorrhage can present a problem. What are the likely effects of this on Mr Ewing and how can they be recognised?

_____

_____

_____

_____

Q42. Because of the site of the operation, where is any blood likely to accumulate – and what may be the effect of this?

_____

_____

_____

_____

Q43. The epididymis (📖 _Page 925_) is likely to become inflamed following prostatectomy. How would you recognise this?

_____

_____

_____

_____

Q44. Following the removal of his bladder catheter some days after the operation, what problems are Mr Ewing likely to face?

_____

_____

_____

_____

Q45. The other long-term problem, that Mr Ewing may face stems from the problems of back

pressure on the kidneys (and hydronephrosis), that were discussed earlier. Can you suggest what these problems may lead to?

_____

_____

_____

_____

_____

QUESTIONS FOR DISCUSSION

1. What types of bladder catheters are there? What research evidence is there for specific practices in the good management of bladder catheters?

2. Devise a full pre- and postoperative care plan for Mr Ewing, showing the problems that are connected to bodily systems other than the urinary/reproductive system. How would these differ if Mr Ewing had undergone a retropubic prostatectomy?

3. Other than urine and blood tests, what investigations is Mr Ewing likely to undergo in assessing the function of his urinary tract? How should he be prepared – physically and psychologically – for these?

4. If Mr Ewing develops chronic renal failure, what problems will arise as a result of retained water, electrolytes and waste products?

5. Construct a health promotion teaching plan that can be used with Mr Ewing prior to his discharge.

Answers to questions

Q1.   a, Nitrogen-containing products of protein catabolism, such as ammonia and urea; also certain ions and excessive water; b, H^+; c, renin; d, erythropoietin; e, d.

Q2.   a, Waist; b, T12, c, L3; d, 10–12; e, 4–5; f, posterior; g, retroperitoneal.

Q3.   a. A, glomerular (Bowman's) capsule; B, proximal convoluted tubule (PCT); C, descending limb of the loop of the nephron (loop of Henle); D, ascending limb of the loop of the nephron (loop of Henle); E, distal convoluted tubule (DCT); F, collecting duct.
b. A, glomerular (Bowman's) capsule.
c. Glomerulus (4).
d. 3, 2, 1.
e. Their size restricts the passage of red blood cells and proteins from blood to urine.

Q4.   Its volume, electrolyte content and pH are adjusted; toxic wastes are removed.

Q5.   Glomerular filtration; tubular reabsorption; tubular secretion.

Q6.   a, Pushing; b, blood; c, filtrate; d, all small substances; e, protein molecules, (they are too large to pass through filtration slits of healthy endothelial–capsular membranes); f, 60; g, higher; h, smaller; i, glomerular capillaries are long, thin and porous, and have high blood pressure.

Q7.   a. Blood colloid osmotic pressure (BCOP) and capsular filtrate hydrostatic pressure (CHP)
b. NFP = (GBHP) – (CHP + BCOP)
NFP = (60) – (15 + 27) = 18

Q8.   NFP = 0 mmHg = (42) – (27+15)
Anuria due to low glomerular blood pressure could be related to haemorrhage or stress.

Q9.   a. Glomerular filtration rate.
b. 125 (180).
c. De; additional water and waste products (such as H^+ and urea) normally eliminated in urine are retained in blood, possibly resulting in hypertension and acidosis.

Q10.   a, Passive, nonselective; b, 180;
c, Venules; d, peritubular capillaries; e, vasa recta; f, tubular reabsorption; g, opposite.

Q11. a. Glucose and bicarbonate (HCO_3^-); b, 99; c, Protein, Na^+, Cl^-, K^+, and uric acid; d. Urea; e, Creatinine. Creatinine clearance is often used as a measure of glomerular filtration rate (GFR); 100% of the creatinine (a breakdown product of muscle protein) filtered or 'cleared' out of blood will show up in urine, since 0% is reabsorbed.

Q12. a, Tubular secretion; b, blood to urine; c, the same; d, K^+, H^+, ammonium (NH_4^+), creatinine, penicillin and para-aminohippuric acid.

Q13. a, Kidneys; b, bladder; c, 25–30; d, 10–12; e, trigone; f, urethra; g, transitional. This type of epithelium stretches and becomes thinner as the bladder fills; h, true pelvis; i, external; j, urethra; k, 3.8; l, 1.5; m, 20; n, 8; o, prostatic; p, membranous; q, spongy.

Q14. 5a, 2b, 6c, 8d, 7e, 4f, 3g, 9h, 1i.

Q15. Paired: 1–5.
Singular 6–9.

Q16. a, 45; b, 18; c, partially; d, inguinal canal and rings; e, inguinal hernia; f, testicular artery and veins, lymphatics, nerves and cremaster muscle.

Q17. Sa, Sb, Pc, Sd, Be, Pf.

Q18. A: Seminal vesicles.
B: Prostate.
C: Bulbourethral glands.

Q19. a, 2.5–5; b, 50–150 million; c, 20 million; a high sperm count increases the likelihood of fertilisation, since only a small percentage of sperm ever reaches the secondary oocyte; in addition, a large number of sperm are required to release sufficient enzyme to digest the barrier around the secondary oocyte; d, alkaline; protects sperm against acidity of the male urethra and the female vagina; e, serves as an antibiotic that destroys bacteria; f, it liquefies the clotted semen within 20 minutes of the entrance of semen to the vagina, thereby permitting the movement of sperm into the uterus.

Q20. It is the first part of the nephron, and it is involved in glomerular filtration.

Q21. 125 ml/min (180 l/day)

Q22. Selective reabsorption.

Q23. Most of the water and electrolytes and waste products such as urea, creatinine and uric acid. And thus they form 'urine'.

Q24. Water – ADH (anti-diuretic hormone).
Sodium – aldosterone.

Q25. The urinary bladder.

Q26. Wrapped around the first part of the urethra, at the base of the bladder.

Q27. A volume of 200 to 400 ml. This initiates a conscious desire to pass urine.

Q28. Parasympathetic impulses pass from spinal cord to urinary bladder wall (the detrusor muscle) and internal urethral sphincter.

Q29. A circular band of muscle. The urethral sphincters surround the urethra and either compress (close) the urethra or open it.

Q30. There is conscious relaxation of the external sphincter. Babies and toddlers have not yet learned to control this, so once the bladder fills, it will empty automatically – irrespective of time and place. The adult has essentially learned to consciously control a reflex action (for reflexes, 📖 *Page 382*).

Q31. You could 'push' or 'strain'. This involves raising the pressure inside the abdomen – and so pressing on the bladder in the pelvis – by contracting the muscles of the abdominal wall and forcing the diaphragm downwards. However, if the pressure is excessive, this can be dangerous, because the raised abdominal pressure will slow venous return from the legs – by 'pushing' it down into the legs. This means that the volume of blood returned to the heart is low and so cardiac output and blood (O_2) supply to the brain will be lowered. This is likely to produce fainting, which can be counteracted by deep breathing (the respiratory pump, 📖 *Page 634).*

Q32. Testosterone, which regulates sperm production and development and the maintenance of male sexual characteristics (bodily hair, enlarged muscles, deepening of the voice).

Q33. **Frequency of micturition** is a common sympton of prostate disease. The prostate is compressing the urethra, making it difficult to empty the bladder and so the bladder is only partially emptied each time. Consequently, it begins to fill again and very shortly reaches the point (above 200 ml) at which the stretch receptors in the wall of the bladder are stimulated.

Thus, the stimulus to micturition is frequently perceived, and each time the bladder is only partially emptied. When Mr Ewing is admitted to hospital, he will be questioned on his micturition pattern, which can be summarised as:

D (Day) = 9
N (Night) = 3

Frequency is often accompanied by a sense of **urgency** – a sudden desire to pass urine, and **hesitancy** – difficulty in starting to pass urine, because of urethral compression.

Both frequency and urgency are associated with conditions other than an enlarged prostate. For example, young women who develop an infection in the urinary bladder also suffer these symptoms. Bacteria can change the pH of urine (on average this is 6) and this can lead to a stimulation of the bladder wall receptors. In addition, this can cause a burning sensation when urine passes down the urethra.

Q34. Because Mr Ewing's bladder is only partially emptied, each time he passes urine, there is always a pool of urine in the bladder. This warm stagnant pool is an excellent breeding ground for bacteria.

Also, the passage of urine is something that regularly cleanses the urethra. The lower third of the urethra – in both men and women – is permanently colonised by bacteria which have gained entry from the external skin. It is only the passage of a good stream of urine that prevents these bacteria from travelling further along the urethra and colonising the bladder.

Mr Ewing has a poor stream of urine, because the prostate is compressing the urethra. If this should lead to a urinary infection, then his urine will turn **cloudy** and smell **fishy.** These would be important nursing observations, and should they be recognised then Mr Ewing would probably be prescribed a course of antibiotics.

A patient like Mr Ewing who develops these symptoms of frequency, hesitancy and urgency has two choices. He can either ignore them – which is very possible if they develop slowly over the years. The patient could pass them off as a part of the ageing process. Alternatively, the person could consult their doctor and be put on the waiting list for surgery.

For the patient who chooses to ignore the symptoms, one day – as with Mr Ewing – the urethral compression will reach the point at which it is no longer possible to pass urine. Emergency admission to hospital will then be necessary.

Q35. Mr Ewing will require **catheterisation** of the bladder. A bladder catheter is a narrow plastic or latex tube that is inserted into the urethra (under aseptic conditions). This bypasses the obstruction and allows the bladder to empty. The catheter can remain *in situ* or be removed following emptying.

The male urethra is about 20cm in length, (▥▥ *Page 935, Figure 28.10*) and catheterisation to bypass an enlarged prostate gland can be a tricky procedure. A metal introducer is sometimes used to make the catheter more rigid, and so facilitate its passage. However, great care must be taken not to damage the urethral lining and its transitional epithelium (▥▥ *Page 895*). A local anaesthetic gel is usually introduced into the urethra prior to catheterisation.

If Mr Ewing has not been circumcised then his foreskin (**prepuce**) will need to be retracted on the corona of the penis (*see* ▥▥ *Page 935, Figure 28.10*). Following insertion of the catheter, the foreskin should be put back into position. If this is not done, the foreskin can become swollen and painful, a condition known as **paraphimosis.** This will then require several (painful) days of treatment with saline packs to reduce it.

If urethral catheterisation is not possible then a **suprapubic** catheter may be inserted (see Figure 19.5).

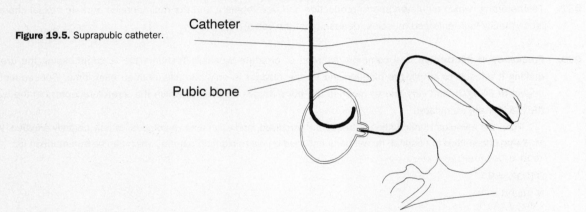

Figure 19.5. Suprapubic catheter.

Catheter

Pubic bone

This procedure would be performed under local anaesthetic and the catheter would be left in position to drain the bladder continuously.

Q36. The raised abdominal pressure will assist venous return to the heart – the so called abdominal pump. If this is suddenly released by rapidly draining the bladder, then venous return may fall. This means that blood would tend to settle in the abdomen and lower limbs – particularly if he is immobile in bed. There would then be less blood pumped to the brain, and as a result he may feel dizzy and faint.

To prevent this from happening, the bladder would be slowly drained – perhaps by about 200ml per hour. It would be an important part of Mr Ewing's care to carry this out and monitor it.

Q37. He will be prone to developing a urinary infection. It has already been noted that an enlarged prostate gland, and the consequent pooling of urine in the bladder, may predispose him to a urinary infection.

However, the effect of the catheter is to provide a channel for micro-organisms to gain entry. During insertion of the catheter, and subsequently, it is good practice to use aseptic technique to prevent infection. The catheter is connected to a drainage bag – the so-called closed drainage system – and disconnection should be rare. This will prevent micro-organisms gaining entry.

In addition, care is taken when emptying the bag (via a tap). However, bacteria may gain entry at the point where the catheter enters the urethra, and movements of the catheter can then push these organisms up the urethra – between the external wall of the catheter and the urethra. For this reason, it is recommended that catheters be anchored to the upper leg, to prevent in-out movement.

Despite these measures, people like Mr Ewing have a high incidence of developing urinary infections, for which antibiotics will then be prescribed. A good fluid intake will produce a good urine flow and wash out any organisms. This is also a good preventive measure.

Q38. A cloudy and smelly urine will raise the suspicion of urinary infection. A specimen of urine will then need to be taken for laboratory examination.

This needs to be taken from the drainage tube, because urine in the bag may be contaminated and contain micro-organisms that have gained entry during the emptying procedure.

However, disconnecting the catheter from the drainage tube – to collect a urine sample – may itself introduce micro-organisms into the catheter lumen.

To get around these problems, some drainage tubes have a sampling port built into the tube. This contains a rubber diaphragm, through which a needle (attached to a syringe) can be inserted. Urine can then be withdrawn and placed in a sterile container. On removing the needle, the diaphragm seals off and no hole is left.

The laboratory can then **culture** his urine and determine which, if any, organisms are present. Furthermore, the **sensitivity** of these to various antibiotics, can also be determined.

Q39. An enlarged prostate gland will, over the years, have caused back pressure up the bladder, ureter and kidneys, rather like the effect of a dam in a stream. The effect of this, is to oppose the **net filtration pressure** (📖 *Page 876*). This pressure is only of the order of 18mmHg. Once this pressure is opposed then glomerular filtration will stop and so there will be no urine formation – **kidney failure**.

It is probably the case that Mr Ewing will have some degree of kidney failure. How much, can be assessed by measuring the level of waste products (urea, creatinine) in the bloodstream. The kidneys normally clear these from the bloodstream; so any rise will indicate a reduction in kidney function. 📖 *Page 880, Exhibit 26.1,* shows the normal levels of these substances.

The anatomical changes that result from **obstruction** in the urinary tract are known as **hydronephrosis** (hydro = water, nephron = kidney). The kidneys become swollen and the renal pelvis distends. Then the kidney substance becomes thin and eventually a thin-walled functionless sac. Figure 19.6 shows the progressive changes associated with hydronephrosis.

Figure 19.6. Development of hydronephrosis.

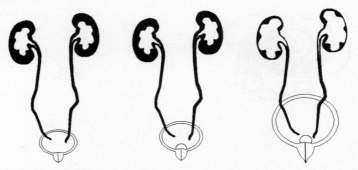

These changes can be seen by outlining the urinary tract with a dye that is opaque to X-rays (radio-opaque). This is injected into the bloodstream and then filtered by the kidneys. It is known as an intravenous pyelogram (IVP). (A pyelogram is an X-ray of the pelvis and kidney).

These changes can, of course, be halted by draining the urinary tract and operating to remove the obstruction. However, an operation may be dangerous on someone who has impending renal failure.

The other problem that Mr Ewing may develop, as a result of chronic obstruction to the free flow of urine, is that of **stones (calculi).** Slow movement of urine – coupled with infection – can easily lead to stone formation in the renal pelvis and/or ureters. The stones will themselves cause further obstruction and pain. However, they are usually detected fairly easily, by X-ray or ultrasound investigation.

Q40. The prostate produces prostatic fluid that contains enzymes, which have several roles. The first is to cause coagulation of the semen, and subsequently – when the semen is in the vagina – to dissolve the coagulation and thus allow the sperm to swim freely into the female reproductive tract. The other enzymes contribute to sperm mobility and viability.

Thus, it is possible to live without part or all of the gland. However, problems can arise after the operation because of damage to the **prostatic urethra** (📖 *Page 895*).

There are several types of operation that are used to remove or reduce the size of the prostate. The majority involve open surgery and their approaches are illustrated in Figure 19.7.

Figure 19.7. The types (routes) of Prostatectomy.

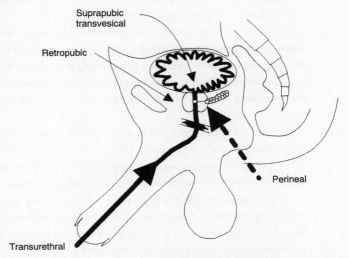

The transurethral operation does not involve open surgery and is performed via a long metal telescope called a **resectoscope**. This has a wire loop at the end which can shave off pieces of the gland.

Figure 19.8. Transurethral resection of the prostate gland.

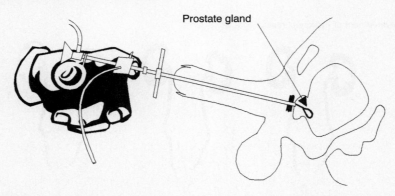

The transurethral resection of the prostate gland (TURP) has been the most favoured operation for many years, because it is the least traumatic and so usually involves less blood loss, and patients can go home sooner (five days usually). It also takes a shorter time, which is an advantage for elderly patients – like Mr Ewing – who may have a history of chest/heart disease, and who would not stand up well to a prolonged and deep anaesthetic. (A shorter time also means that a surgeon can perform more operations on a limited operating list.)

Open operations are not performed very often – and are usually reserved for very large glands, which cannot be shaved down.

Q41. Haemorrhage can occur at the time of the operation, when it is called **primary**. **Secondary** haemorrhage may occur in patients like Mr Ewing – in the hours following surgery – because of a rise in blood pressure. This is partly the effect of the anaesthetic wearing off. It means that blood vessels, which had previously been shut down are now beginning to open up (vasodilatation, 📖 *Page 631*), and the vessels may start to haemorrhage – if they were not sealed off at the time of the operation.

If Mr Ewing starts to haemorrhage, then his pulse will rise and the BP will fall. However, if the bleeding is slight, then the cardiovascular system may be able to maintain BP through a rise in **cardiac output** and **peripheral resistance** (📖 *Page 611*). Providing that the average-sized individual does not lose more than about one pint of blood, these mechanisms can act to maintain BP. Blood loss beyond this level will, however, lead to a fall in BP and a rise in pulse rate, as the **cardiovascular centre** (📖 *Page 611*) attempts to maintain BP. Thus, by the time a patient's BP recordings are falling, they are well on the way to significant blood loss.

Q42. An additional problem is that bleeding from the prostatic bed, (what remains of the prostate) will lead to blood accumulating in the bladder. This will tend to coagulate (clot formation, 📖 *Page 580*) and thus block the outlet from the bladder (a bladder catheter is normally *in situ* after the operation). This is known as **clot retention**, and can be prevented by continuously irrigating the bladder with a fluid such as normal saline. The apparatus for doing this is shown in Figure 19.9.

Figure 19.9. Continuous bladder irrigation.

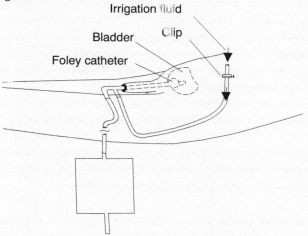

The fluid (from a 1- or 2 litre bag) flows into the bladder and is then drained out into a bag on the side of the bed. Note that this requires two channels (plus a channel through which to inflate the balloon, which keeps the catheter in place), and is commonly known as a three-way bladder catheter.

This would require a lot of nursing care and observation, to regulate the flow, measure the output, and note the colour of the urine. Is it getting darker? Is haemorrhaging increasing? The irrigation is usually stopped after 24–48 hours, when the urine is a pink colour. Without irrigation, **clot retention** can block urine output. Urine flow would then cease and the patient would experience increasing discomfort as the bladder became more full.

The clots could then be disrupted by using a large syringe, filled with normal saline, to wash out the bladder via the catheter – known as a **bladder washout.** If this fails, then the patient may need to be returned to theatre and the clots evacuated – under anaesthetic – by means of a telescope device similar to the TURP instrument.

Q43. The epididymis lies on the testis in the scrotum. This area can become inflamed and painful, and it is thought that this can be caused by infection spreading from the site of the prostate, along the ductus (vas) deferens (📖 *Page 923, Figure 28.1*) and down to the epididymis.

Cutting the vas (**vasectomy**) would prevent this happening. Some surgeons do this at the time of the operation. Vasectomy also sterilises the patient – something they may not want.

If Mr Ewing develops epididymitis, then his scrotum can be elevated on elastoplast, or bandages placed across the thighs. This prevents dragging – and pain – of the spermatic cord. Antibiotics can also be prescribed.

There is a danger that the infection will spread to the testis and produce inflammation (**orchitis**) and cause sterility.

Q44.   Mr Ewing is likely to face the problem of urinary incontinence. The internal sphincter (📖 *Page 935, Figure 28.10*), and the external sphincter (📖 *Page 893, Figure 26.23*), are both likely to be damaged at the time of the operation. The bladder catheter has put them 'at rest' for several days.

The sphincters are the 'doors' which allow urine to flow down the urethra; and as a result, Mr Ewing may now suffer dribbling and incontinence. Great tact and patience will need to be exerted in caring for him during this period.

A careful note is made of how much – and how often – he passes urine; both to monitor the situation and to try and encourage a pattern of regular voluntary micturition. He can also be given sphincter exercises to perform. For example, he can be instructed to stop passing urine in midstream and then start again. This is known as the **start–stop–start** exercise, and obviously involves contraction and relaxation of both sphincters and bladder muscle.

Psychological support and understanding are probably the best things that relatives, nurses and doctors can offer. If Mr Ewing is unable to pass urine following catheter removal, he may need re-catheterising.

Because of the damage to the prostatic urethra, Mr Ewing may find that he also suffers from **dry ejaculation**. Normally, during ejaculation, the sphincters close off and the semen (sperm and prostatic/seminal fluid) is propelled down the urethra. But the sphincter damage may now lead to the ejaculate being delivered into the bladder (**retrograde ejaculation**). As a result, Mr Ewing will have reduced fertility. The semen will, of course, appear in his urine some hours after ejaculation – giving it a 'thick' cloudy appearance. This is something that may worry him – unless he has been prepared for it.

This also raises the issue of when Mr Ewing should resume sexual intercourse. The general advice that is given, is that for the first few weeks following the operation it is unwise, for two reasons:

(a) He is likely to feel tired and requires rest to overcome the surgery and anaesthetic.
(b) Some bleeding is not uncommon in the 7-10 days following surgery. Sexual intercourse (ejaculation) is likely to make this worse – and so disrupt healing at the prostatic bed.

After a couple of weeks, normal sexual relations can be resumed. Mr Ewing may, once again, need reassurance that **impotence** (the inability to develop an erection) is not caused by this operation, but infertility – as discussed above – might be.

Q45.   It was earlier pointed out, that Mr Ewing's kidneys may have been damaged over the years by chronic obstruction – and back pressure – from an enlarged prostate gland. This pressure opposes the net filtration pressure in the kidneys, and thus **suppresses** the formation of urine. As a result, the kidneys can swell (hydronephrosis) and become stretched and permanently damaged. Once there is less than (roughly) the equivalent of one kidney's nephrons (50% of normal), then **renal failure** is said to have occurred.

Once urine volume falls below 400–500 ml, in 24 hours, then there is insufficient volume to excrete sufficient waste products (and electrolytes) to maintain life. Thus, the patient is now at risk of being poisoned from these waste products. Electrolytes, such as potassium (K^+) are finely balanced in the blood chemistry. High levels of K^+ in the bloodstream will interfere with heart muscle contraction, and can lead to **cardiac arrest** and death.

Thus, this is a serious condition and one that can only be treated by removing poisons, water and electrolytes from the body by dialysis (📖 *Page 891*) and at the same time, restricting the intake of these substances – particularly foods containing potassium, for example, bananas, oranges and grapes.

Figure 19.10 provides a summary of Mr Ewing's problems and his care and treatment.

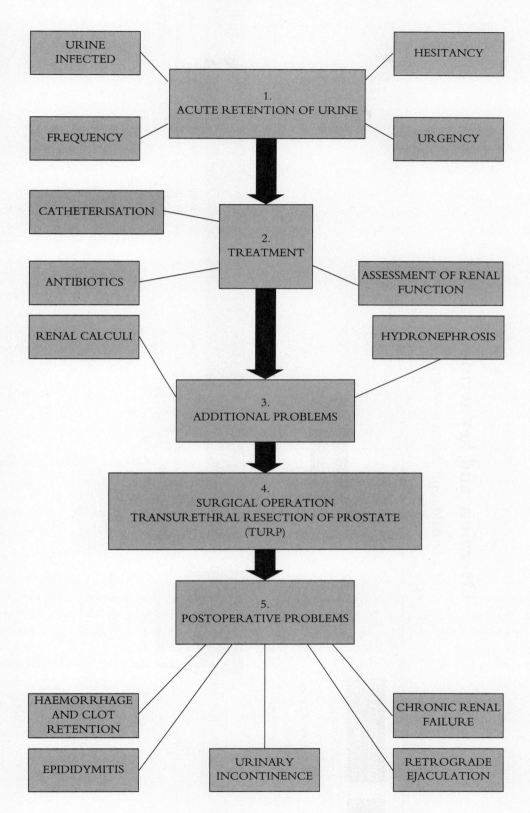

Figure 19.10.
A summary of the major stages and problems in Mr Ewing's illness.

Overview and key terms

The female reproductive system

ANATOMY
- Uterus
- Ovary
- Fallopian tubes
- Vagina
- Oogenesis
- Ovulation
- External genitalia
- Mammary glands

REPRODUCTIVE CYCLE
- Hypothalamus
- Ovarian hormones
- Menstrual cycle
- Estrogen
- Progesterone

PREGNANCY

EMBRYO AND FETAL DEVELOPMENT
- Fertilisation
- Blastocyst
- Embryo
- Placenta and umbilical cord

MATERNAL CHANGES
- BMR
- Circulatory volume
- Pigmentation
- Breast development
- Urinary infection
- Heartburn
- Pelvic joints

FETAL CHANGES
- Movements
- Heart rate

LABOUR
- Hormonal changes
- 1st, 2nd and 3rd stages
- Fetal changes

POSTNATAL CHANGES
- Puerperium
- Lactation
- Psychological changes

20. The Female Reproductive System

Learning outcomes

1. To relate the relevant anatomy and physiology of the female reproductive system to an understanding of the changes taking place in a woman's body during pregnancy.

2. To understand the growth and development of the embryo and fetus.

3. To be able to describe the stages of labour and some of their important changes.

4. To describe the changes taking place in a woman's body following the birth of a baby.

5. To understand the major changes that take place in the body of a newly born infant.

Chapters 28 & 29

INTRODUCTION

This chapter covers the female reproductive system, ovulation and the menstrual cycle, and also pregnancy.

Following the questions in the next few sections, a patient scenario related to pregnancy will be introduced. This will be followed by a review of embryo and fetal development. The three stages of pregnancy will then be dealt with, together with some of the problems that can arise. You will be prompted to reflect on the following, through the use of questions:

(1) The antenatal period.
(2) Birth and labour.
(3) The postnatal period.

The chapter will end with some discussion points. This chapter, unlike the others, deals with the normal processes of pregnancy, embryo and fetal development, labour and birth. These are all part of physiology – not pathology.

THE ANATOMY OF THE FEMALE REPRODUCTIVE SYSTEM (📖 *Pages 936–49*)

Q1. Refer to Figure 20.1 and match the structures numbered 1–5 with their descriptions. Note that structures are numbered in order along the pathway taken by ova from the site of formation to the point of exit from the body.

☐ a. Uterus (body)
☐ b. Uterus (cervix)
☐ c. Ovary
☐ d. Uterine (Fallopian) tube
☐ e. Vagina

Q2. Indicate which of the five structures in Figure 20.1 are paired.

_____

Which structures are singular?
Write their numbers

_____

1
2
3
4
5

Figure 20.1
Female organs of
reproduction

Figure 20.2.
Oogenesis.

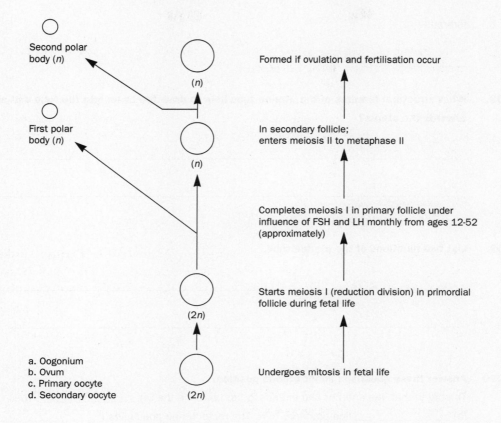

Second polar
body (*n*)

(*n*)

Formed if ovulation and fertilisation occur

First polar
body (*n*)

(*n*)

In secondary follicle;
enters meiosis II to metaphase II

Completes meiosis I in primary follicle under
influence of FSH and LH monthly from ages 12-52
(approximately)

(2*n*)

Starts meiosis I (reduction division) in primordial
follicle during fetal life

a. Oogonium
b. Ovum
c. Primary oocyte
d. Secondary oocyte

(2*n*)

Undergoes mitosis in fetal life

Q3.   Label the four large circles in Figure 20.2 with the names (a to d).

Q4.   Describe exactly what is expelled during ovulation.

_____

_____

Q5.   What determines whether the second meiotic (equatorial) division will occur?

_____

_____

Q6.   Complete this exercise about the uterine tubes.

Uterine tubes are also known as (a) _____ tubes. They are about

(b) _____ cm ((c) _____ inches) long.

Q7.   Arrange these parts of the uterine tubes in order from the most medial to the most lateral:

a.   Ampulla

b.   Infundibulum and fimbriae

c.   Isthmus

_____ _____ _____

Q8. **What structural features of the uterine tube help to draw the ovum into the tube and propel it towards the uterus?**

_____

_____

Q9. **List two functions of the uterine tube.**

_____

_____

Q10. **Answer these questions about uterine position.**
The organ that lies anterior and inferior to the uterus is the (a) _____. The
(b) _____ lies posterior to it. The rectouterine pouch lies (c) _____
(anterior? posterior?) to the uterus, whereas the (d) _____ -uterine pouch lies
between the urinary bladder and the uterus. The fundus of the uterus is normally tipped
(e) _____ (anteriorly? posteriorly?). If it is malpositioned posteriorly, it would be
(f) _____ (anteflexed? retroflexed?).
   The (g) _____ ligaments attach the uterus to the sacrum. The (h) _____
ligaments pass through the inguinal canal and anchor into external genitalia (labia majora). The
(i) _____ ligaments are broad, thin sheets of peritoneum extending laterally from
the uterus. Important ligaments in prevention of drooping (prolapse) of the uterus are the
(j) _____ ligaments, which attach the base of the uterus laterally to the pelvic wall.

Q11. **Refer to Figure 20.1 and complete this exercise about layers of the wall of the uterus.**
Most of the uterus consists of (a) _____ -metrium. This layer is (b) _____
(smooth muscle? epithelium?).
   Now colour the peritoneal covering over the uterus green. This is a (c) _____
(mucous? serous?) membrane.
   The innermost layer of the uterus is the (d) _____ -metrium. Which portion of it is
shed during menstruation? Stratum (e) _____ (basalis? functionalis?). Which
arteries supply the stratum functionalis? (f) _____ (spiral? straight?).

Q12.   Refer to Figure 20.1. In the normal position, at what angle does the uterus join the vagina?

_____

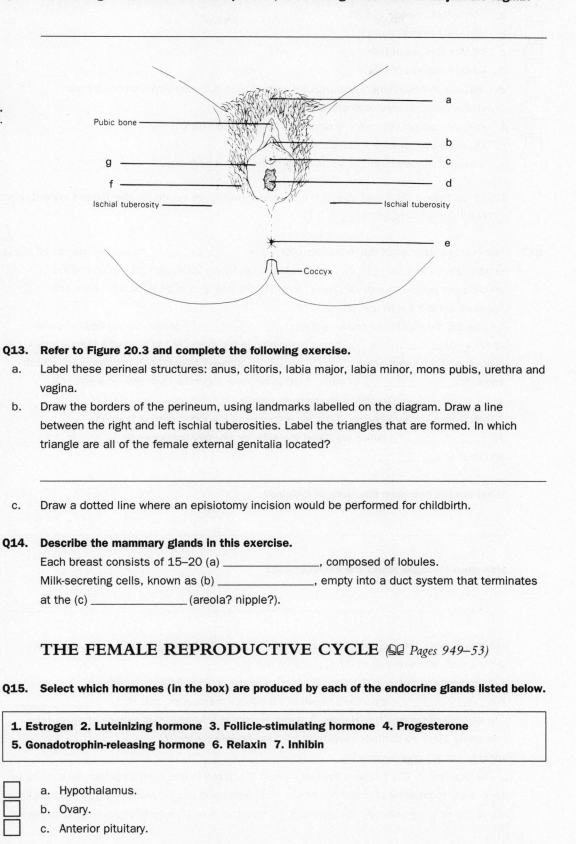

Figure 20.3.
The perineum.

Q13.   Refer to Figure 20.3 and complete the following exercise.

a.   Label these perineal structures: anus, clitoris, labia major, labia minor, mons pubis, urethra and vagina.

b.   Draw the borders of the perineum, using landmarks labelled on the diagram. Draw a line between the right and left ischial tuberosities. Label the triangles that are formed. In which triangle are all of the female external genitalia located?

_____

c.   Draw a dotted line where an episiotomy incision would be performed for childbirth.

Q14.   Describe the mammary glands in this exercise.

Each breast consists of 15–20 (a) _____, composed of lobules.

Milk-secreting cells, known as (b) _____, empty into a duct system that terminates at the (c) _____ (areola? nipple?).

THE FEMALE REPRODUCTIVE CYCLE _(Pages 949–53)_

Q15.   Select which hormones (in the box) are produced by each of the endocrine glands listed below.

> **1. Estrogen 2. Luteinizing hormone 3. Follicle-stimulating hormone 4. Progesterone**
> **5. Gonadotrophin-releasing hormone 6. Relaxin 7. Inhibin**

☐   a. Hypothalamus.
☐   b. Ovary.
☐   c. Anterior pituitary.

Q16. **Now select the hormones listed in question 15 that fit the descriptions below.**

☐ a. Stimulates release of FSH.

☐ b. Stimulates release of LH.

☐ c. Inhibits release of FSH.

☐ d. Inhibits release of LH.

☐ e. Stimulates development and maintenance of uterus, breasts and secondary sex characteristics; enhances protein anabolism.

☐ f. Prepares endometrium for implantation by fertilised ovum.

☐ g. Dilates cervix for labour and delivery.

☐ h. ß-oestradiol, oestrone and oestriol are forms of this hormone.

Refer to Figure 20.4 and check your understanding of events in the female reproductive cycle by completing questions 17–19.

Q17. The average duration of the menstrual cycle is (a) _____ days. The menstrual phase usually lasts about (b) _____ days. On Figure 20.4, part (d), colour red the endometrium in the menstrual phase, and note the changes in its thickness. Also write 'menses' on the line in that phase.

Following the menstrual phase is the (c) _____ phase. During both of these phases, (d) _____ begin to develop in the ovary. At the birth of a female infant, her ovaries contain numerous (e) _____ (primary? primordial?) follicles. Each month about (f) _____ of these follicles become secondary follicles, whereas only (g) _____ usually matures each month.

Follicle development occurs under the influence of the hypothalamic hormone (h) _____, which regulates the anterior pituitary hormones (i) _____ and later (j) _____ .

What are the two main functions of follicles?

_____

How does Estrogen affect the endometrium?

_____

For this reason, the preovulatary phase is also known as the (k) _____ phase. Write these labels on Figure 20.4, parts (b) and (d).

A moderate increase in estrogen production by the growing follicles initiates a (l) _____ (positive? negative?) feedback mechanism that (m) _____ (increases? decreases?) FSH level. It is this change in FSH level that causes atresia of the remaining 19 or so partially developed follicles. **Atresia** means (n) _____ (degeneration? regeneration?).

The principle of this negative feedback effect is utilised in oral contraceptives. By starting to take 'pills' (consisting of target hormones, oestrogen, and progesterone) early in the cycle (day 5), and continuing until day 25, a woman will maintain a very low level of the trophic hormone

(o) _____ . Without FSH, follicles and ova will not develop, and so the woman will not (p) _____ .

The second anterior pituitary hormone released during the cycle is (q) _____ at the end of the preovulatory phase. This is an example of a (r) _____ (positive? negative?) feedback mechanism. The LH surge causes the release of the ovum (actually secondary oocyte), the event known as (s) _____. The LH surge is the basis for a home test for (t) _____ (ovulation? pregnancy?).

Colour all stages of follicle development through ovulation on Figure 20.4b according to colour code ovals.

Following ovulation is the (u) _____ phase. It lasts until day (v) _____ of a 28-day cycle. Under the influence of trophic hormone (w) _____ , follicle cells are changed into the corpus (x) _____ . These cells secrete two hormones: (y) _____ _____ . Both prepare the endometrium for (z) _____ .

Q18. **a. What preparatory changes occur?**

_____

b. What effect do rising levels of the target hormones estrogen and progesterone have upon the GNRH and LH?

_____

Q19. **Continue with the description of the events in the female cycle by completing this exercise.**

One function of LH is to form and maintain the corpus luteum. As LH (a) _____ (increases? decreases?) the corpus luteum disintegrates, forming a white scar on the ovary known as the corpus (b) _____. The corpus luteum has been secreting (c)_____ and (d) _____. With the demise of the corpus luteum, the levels of these hormones rapidly (e)_____ (increase? decrease?). Since these hormones were maintaining the endometrium, endometrial tissue now deteriorates and will be shed during the next (f) _____ phase.

If fertilization should occur, estrogens and progesterone are needed to maintain the endometrial lining. The (g) _____ around the developing embryo secretes a hormone named (h) _____. It functions much like LH in that it maintains the corpus (i)_____, even though LH is inhibited (question 18). The corpus luteum continues to secrete estrogen and progesterone for several months until the placenta itself can secrete sufficient amounts. Incidentally, hCG is present in the urine of pregnant women only, and so is routinely used to detect (j) _____ .

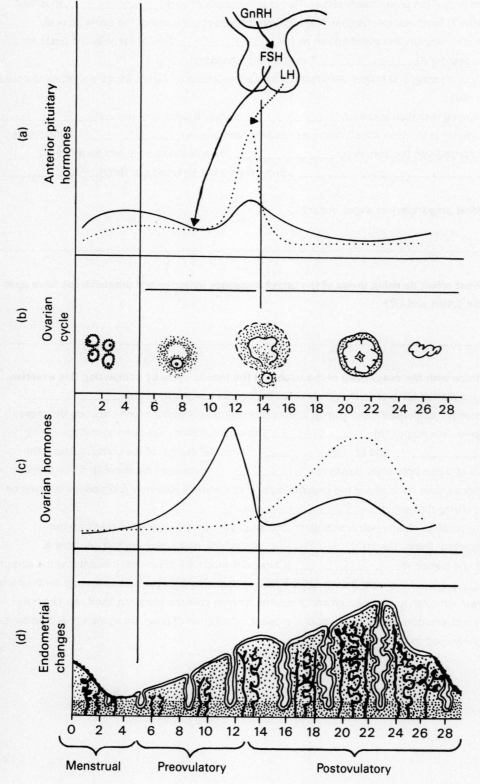

Figure 20.4.
Correlation of female cycles. (a) Anterior pituitary hormones; (b) ovarian changes: follicles and corpus luteum; (c) ovarian hormones; (d) uterine (endometrial) changes.

(a) Anterior pituitary hormones

GnRH

FSH

LH

(b) Ovarian cycle

2 4 6 8 10 12 14 16 18 20 22 24 26 28

(c) Ovarian hormones

(d) Endometrial changes

0 2 4 6 8 10 12 14 16 18 20 22 24 26 28

Menstrual   Preovulatory   Postovulatory

○ FSH
○ LH
○ Corpus albicans
○ Corpus luteum
○ Primary follicle
○ Secondary (graafian) follicle
○ Vesicular ovarian (Graafian follicle) rupturing
○ Estrogen
○ Progesterone

CHECKPOINTS EXERCISE

Q20. **From where does the ovum arise?**

_____

Q21. **For pregnancy to occur following sexual intercourse, where does the fertilised ovum need to embed?.**

_____

Q22. **Describe three signs of ovulation in this exercise.**

Ovulation is likely to occur during the 24-hour period after the basal temperature (a) _____ -creases by about 0.4–0.6°F. This temperature change is related to an increase in (b)_____ (estrogen? progesterone?). Under the influence of (c) _____ (estrogen? progesterone?), cervical mucus increases in quantity and becomes (d) _____ (more stretchy? thicker?) at midcycle. Some women experience a pain around the time of ovulation known as (e) _____.

Q23. **To check your understanding of the events of these cycles, list the letters of the major events below, in chronological order, beginning on day 1 of the cycle. To do this exercise it may help to list on a separate piece of paper days 1 to 28 and write each event next to the approximate day on which it occurs.**

  a.   Ovulation occurs.

  b.   Estrogen and progesterone levels drop.

  c.   FSH begins to stimulate follicles.

  d.   LH surge is stimulated by high estrogen levels.

  e.   High levels of oestrogens and progesterone inhibit LH.

  f.   Estrogens are secreted for the first time during the cycle.

  g.   Corpus luteum degenerates and becomes corpus albicans.

  h.   Endometrium begins to deteriorate, leading to next month's menses.

  i.   Follicle is converted into corpus luteum.

  j.   Rising level of estrogen inhibits FSH secretion.

  k.   Corpus luteum secretes estrogens and progesterone.

PATIENT SCENARIO

Mrs White is a happily married woman of 26 years. She is now pregnant and expecting her first child.

Mr White is a car salesman and he and his wife live in a mortgaged three-bedroom house. They have no next-of-kin in the locality, as both their parents live several hundred miles away.

Mrs White is only 1–2 months into her pregnancy and continues to work, part-time as a teacher. Her health is good and the pregnancy appears to be proceeding quite normally. The following section will provide you with an overview of the development of the fertilised ovum. There then follows a number of questions that will help you to understand the progression of Mrs White's pregnancy.

EMBRYO AND FETAL DEVELOPMENT

Fertilisation and implantation

Following sexual intercourse, sperm enter the vagina, uterus and uterine (Fallopian) tube, where a spermatozoon fertilises an ovum.

Q24. **How many chromosomes are there in the spermatozoon and in the ovum?** 📖 *Pages 927 & 941*

_____

Q25. **The fertilised ovum (zygote) starts to divide. What type of cell division is this?** (📖 *Page 971*)

_____

This means that, ultimately, every cell in the child's body has derived half its chromosomes from its mother, and half from its father.

Initially this ball of cells is called the **morula**, but at about four and a half days it moves into the uterine cavity and is called the **blastocyst**. At about six days, it implants itself into the uterine wall. This is accomplished by enzymes that 'eat' away at the uterus lining, and allow the blastocyst to embed itself (📖 *Pages 974–5, Figures 29.3 & 29.4*).

The embryonic period

This is the first two months following fertilisation. After this is the fetal period (**fetus**). The embryo develops very rapidly and individual clusters of cells soon become apparent. A membrane forms around the fetus (**the amnion**). This forms the **amniotic cavity** (📖 *Page 976, Figure. 29.5*). Eventually this cavity becomes filled with **amniotic fluid**.

Q26. **What are the functions of amniotic fluid?** (📖 *Page 977*).

_____

_____

This fluid, which contains fetal cells, can be sampled through a long needle. The sample can then be tested for such abnormalities as **Down's syndrome**, by microscopic examination of the fetal cells and their chromosomes. Sufferers from Down's syndrome have an extra chromosome and may be both physically and mentally handicapped. On the basis of this test, the parents may decide to seek a termination of the pregnancy known as a **therapeutic abortion**.

The three major layers of cells become visible during this period; the **endoderm, mesoderm** and **ectoderm**. These form the basis for all of the body's organs and systems. (📖 *Page 978, Exhibit 29.1*).

Placenta and umbilical cord

Placental development is accomplished by the third month of pregnancy. It is formed partly by the uterine wall and partly by the embryo's tissues. (📖 *Page 980, Figure 29.7*).

Q27. What is the function of the placenta?

_____

_____

Anything that Mrs White takes – drugs or alcohol – will also pass through the placenta and affect the baby. Viruses, such as HIV, German measles and chicken pox, can also cross the barrier, but most micro-organisms, such as bacteria, are too large to pass through.

The hormones of pregnancy

During the first three months of pregnancy, the **corpus luteum** continues to secrete estrogens and progesterone.

Q28. What is the corpus luteum? (📖 *Pages 952–3*)

_____

_____

Q29. LH stimulates the corpus luteum to secrete these hormones. What are the functions of these hormones?

_____

_____

From the third month of pregnancy the placenta secretes its own version of LH called **human chorionic gonadotrophin** (hCG).

This stimulates continued production of estrogens and progesterone. By the eighth day, after fertilisation, hCG can be detected in the woman's blood. It can be tested for, in urine, within a week of the first missed period. This is the basis for pregnancy testing kits – which Mrs White may have used at home following a missed period.

It is also thought that the high levels of hCG are the stimulus to **morning sickness**. The chorion of the placenta also begins to secrete estrogen at three to four weeks and progesterone by the sixth week.

Q30. **What are the other two hormones that are produced during pregnancy? And what are their functions?**

_____

_____

Mrs White's pregnancy

Over the forthcoming months Mrs White will experience various changes in her body. Some of these will be expected, and others could be quite hazardous and unexpected. The following questions will help you to explore and understand these events.

Q31. **During fetal development, the placenta may embed itself in the lower portion of the uterus. How can this be recognised?**

_____

_____

_____

Q32. **The sort of changes that take place in Mrs White's body include enlargement of some of the endocrine glands, for example the thyroid, and consequently more thyroxine is produced. What will be the effect of this on Mrs White?**

_____

_____

_____

_____

Q33. **One of the most noticable changes is enlargement of the breasts. In addition, the area around the nipple starts to darken. How is this related to hormonal changes?** (📖 _Pages 946–8)._

Q34. **What changes will take place in the following systems of Mrs. White's body?** 📖 *Pages 983–5)*

a.   Urinary system.

_____

_____

_____

b.   Gastrointestinal system.

_____

_____

_____

c.   Respiratory system.

_____

_____

d.   Cardiovascular system.

_____

_____

_____

e.   Skeletal System.

_____

_____

_____

Q35. In what ways could the health of the fetus be monitored during Mrs White's pregnancy?

_____

_____

Q36. In the light of the maternal changes, can you suggest how Mrs. White's health can be monitored during pregnancy?

_____

_____

_____

_____

Q37. What are the hormonal changes that are associated with the onset of labour (parturition)? (📖 *Pages 986–7*).

_____

_____

_____

Q38. What other signs of labour may Mrs White exhibit?

_____

_____

Q39. What are the names for the three stages of labour? Briefly describe them (📖 *Page 987*).

_____

_____

_____

_____

Q40. What methods of pain relief are likely to be used during Mrs White's labour?

_____

_____

_____

_____

_____

Q41. Following the birth, Mrs White's body will start to return to 'normal'. What are these changes? (📖 _Page 989)_

_____

_____

_____

_____

Q42. How is lactation controlled? (📖 _Pages 989–90)._

_____

_____

_____

_____

Q43. What would you expect Mrs White's psychological state to be, in the postnatal period?

_____

_____

_____

_____

Q44. Describe the changes that will take place in the heart and lungs of Mrs White's baby when it is born (📖 *Page 989*).

_____

_____

_____

_____

_____

Q45. Newly born babies are often jaundiced (the skin and eyes are a yellow colour). Why is this? (📖 *Page 794*).

_____

_____

_____

_____

QUESTIONS FOR DISCUSSION

1. Briefly summarise the developmental anatomy occurring in all bodily systems, throughout embryonic and fetal life.

2. What are the reasons – and how may they be overcome – why a couple may be unable to start a family?

3. List and discuss the advantages and disadvantages of breast feeding.

4. Make a list of the support services that are available to the parents of a newly born baby. (For example, family, friends, professionals, organisations).

5. Devise a care plan – with rationale – for Mrs White's baby, applicable to its first few days of life.

Answers to questions

Q1.   3a, 4b, 1c, 2d, 5e.

Q2.   Paired: 1, 2.

Singular: 3, 4, 5.

Q3.

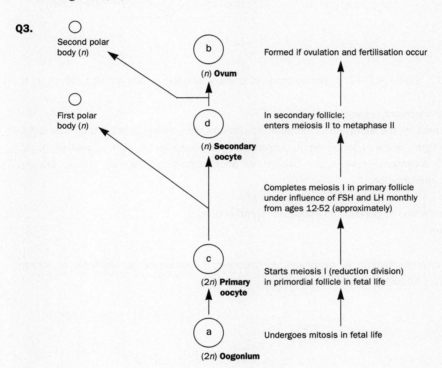

Q4.   The secondary oocyte, along with the first polar body and some surrounding supporting cells, are expelled.

Q5.   Meiosis II is completed only if the secondary oocyte is fertilised by a spermatozoon.

Q6.   a, Fallopian; b, 10; c, 4.

Q7.   c, a, b.

Q8.   Currents produced by movement of fimbriae, ciliary action of columnar epithelial cells lining the tubes, and peristalsis of the muscularis layer of the uterine tube wall.

Q9.   Passageway for secondary oocyte and sperm to move toward each other. Site of fertilisation.

Q10. a, Bladder; b, rectum; c, posterior; d, vesico; e, anteriorly; f, retroflexed; g, uterosacral; h, round; i, broad; j, cardinal.

Q11. a, Myo; b, smooth muscle; c, serous; d, endo; e, functionalis; f, spiral.

Q12. Close to a 90° angle.

Q13. a. See figure opposite.

b. Urogenital triangle

c. See figure opposite.

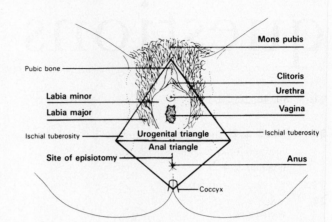

Q14. a, Lobes; b, alveoli; c, nipple.

Q15. 5a; 1, 4, 6, 7b; 2, 3c.

Q16. 5a, 5b, 7c, 7d, 1e, 4f, 6g, 1h.

Q17. a, 28; b, 5; *see* 📖 *Page 937, Figure 28.11*; c, preovulatory; d, primary follicles; e, primordial; f, 20; g, 1; h, GNRH; i, FSH; j, LH.
Secretion of estrogens and development of the ovum.
Estrogen stimulates replacement of the sloughed off stratum functionalis by growing (proliferating) new cells.
k, proliferative, follicular (see figure below); l, negative; m, decreases; n, degeneration; o, FSH; p, ovulate; q, LH; r, positive; s, ovulation; t, pregnancy; (see figure below); u, postovulatory; v, 28; w, LH; x, luteum; y, progesterone, estrogens; z, implantation.

Q18. a. Thickening by growth and secretion of glands, and increased retention of fluid.
b. Inhibition of these hormones.

Q19. a, Decreases; b, albicans; c, progesterone; d, estrogens; e, decrease; f, menstrual; g, placenta; h, human chorionic gonadotrophin (hCG); i, luteum; j, pregnancy.

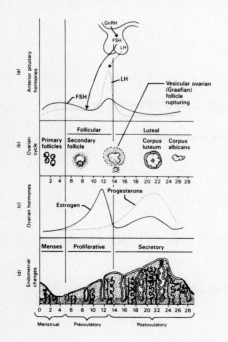

Q20. The ovary.

Q21. The lining of the uterus.

Q22. a, In; b, progesterone; c, oestrogen; d, more stretchy; e, mittelschmerz, or pains.

Q23. C, F, J, D, A, I, K, E, G, B, H.

Q24. 23 in each, so that following fertilisation, there are 23 pairs of chromosomes in the ovum.

Q25. Mitosis. So each new cell produced has an exact copy of the original chromosomes (23 pairs).

Q26. It acts as a shock absorber, regulates fetal temperature, receives fetal urine and prevents adhesions occurring between fetus and surrounding tissue.

Q27. It allows O_2 and nutrients to flow from maternal to fetal blood, via the umbilical cord. CO_2 and waste flows in the opposite direction (📖 *Page 978, Figure 29.6)*.

Q28. After ovulation, the graafian follicle, in the ovary, collapses and under the influence of luteinizing hormone (LH) it becomes the corpus luteum ('yellow body').

Q29. To maintain the lining of the uterus, and prepare the mammary glands to secrete milk.

Q30. **Relaxin** is produced by the placenta and ovaries. Its role is to relax the pubic symphysis and ligaments of the sacroiliac and sacrococcygeal joints (📖 *Page 214, Figure 8.15)*, and it also helps dilate the uterus (towards the end of pregnancy). These movements obviously help the pelvis (and uterus) to accommodate the developing Embryo.

　　Inhibin is produced by the ovaries and placenta. It inhibits secretion of FSH and helps to regulate hCG secretion.

Q31. This is the condition known as **placenta praevia**. It can be dangerous to the fetus, because it may cause both premature birth and a shortage of oxygen in the uterus, and this can lead to maternal haemorrhage and the risk of infection.

　　However, providing all goes well the fetus soon takes on a human form and the development of individual systems takes place (📖 *Page 981)*. 📖 *Page 982, Exhibit 29.2* provides a summary of embryonic and fetal growth.

Q32. It will increase her **basal metabolic rate** (📖 *Page 853)*. This will 'turn up' her metabolism so that it can cope with the increasing demands of a growing fetus.

　　The pituitary gland increases in size and subsequently there is increased production of trophic hormones (📖 *Pages 530–1)*.

　　These will, in turn, lead to increased production of adrenal gland hormones, which will further stimulate metabolism. **Aldosterone** will also lead to increased water and sodium retention, which will increase Mrs White's blood volume. This is another necessary development for sustained fetal growth.

　　The hormonal changes probably also cause enlargement of the uterus and painless contractions, called **Braxton–Hicks contractions**. It is thought that they assist in the flow of placental blood.

　　The enlarging uterus is assessed by the doctor or midwife, and by palpation its distance from the umbilicus is noted. Also, the vaginal wall softens and there is an increase in discharge due to increased vascularisation (from estrogen and progesterone activity).

Q33. The **areola** around the nipple becomes increasingly pigmented because of the effect of **melanocyte stimulating hormone**. This hormone leads to an increase in the number of **melanocytes** (📖 *Page 131*) cells in the skin that manufacture the dark pigment **melanin**.

This process can also lead to a dark line appearing between naval and pubis (the **linea nigra**), and for the same reason pigmentation on the face (the so-called **mask of pregnancy**).

Q34. a. The enlarged uterus displaces the bladder and this can lead to frequency – passing of urine in small, frequent amounts. Dilatation of the ureters can predispose to stagnation and subsequent infection of urine. It is only the free flow of urine that keeps the urinary tract free of bacteria (📖 *Pages 891–5)*

b. Because of muscle and cardiac sphincter relaxation (📖 *Pages 780–3)*, there is a tendency to **oesophageal reflux** of gastric acid contents. This causes heartburn.

Relaxation of the intestines (because of, again, hormonal changes) leads to difficulty emptying the bowel, and thus constipation. Taste and appetite changes are often a marked feature.

c. Oxygen requirements increase by 20% towards the end of pregnancy. The tidal volume (📖 *Page 742)* increases to supply this. But the respiratory rate does not change. There is upwards pressure from the uterus, pushing on the diaphragm and lower lobes of the lungs.

d. There is a 30–40% increase in blood volume. This is largely due to an increase in plasma (liquid), not cells. Heart rate and stroke volume increase to improve cardiac output (📖 *Page 608)*. However, blood pressure (📖 *Pages 630–1)* does not rise, because of a fall in peripheral resistance. This is due to haemodilution (increased plasma volume) and vasodilatation. Thus, overall, blood pressure remains stable.

One problem that can occur is **supine hypotension**. This is a fall in BP due to the mother lying flat on her back. Here the gravid uterus compresses the inferior vena cava (📖 *Page 629)*. This obstructs venous return to the heart and so cardiac output falls (and thus BP falls). Consequently, the mother can feel faint and the baby may have its circulation and oxygen compromised.

e. The pelvic joints loosen (as mentioned earlier), because of hormonal changes. The developing fetus uses a lot of calcium – which could deprive Mrs White's bones and teeth. Hence the importance of calcium and vitamin D (📖 *Pages 149–51)* intake.

The changes in maternal shape lead to a shift in the centre of gravity – which can lead to instability and possibly falls.

Because of the fetus and changes in blood volume, Mrs White is likely to weigh about 11 kg more at the end of pregnancy. The **period of gestation** for a human fetus is **266 days** from the day of conception.

The expected delivery date (EDD) is calculated from the first day of the last menstrual period (LMP). Pregnancy usually lasts for 280 days from the first day of LMP. Therefore, the EDD is calculated from this:

EDD = first day of LMP + 280 days.

Q35. Mrs White can be asked about any fetal movements that she may have felt. And the midwife/doctor can listen to the fetal heart beat, which is heard from the end of the third month. In addition, ultrasound examination will reveal a picture of the fetus – and may show any abnormalities.

Q36. Mrs White's cardiovascular system and increased blood volume can be monitored, by regularly recording her blood pressure, particularly when she attends the antenatal clinic. Also, anaemia – from lack of iron – is a common problem in pregnancy. It can be prevented by taking iron tablets.

Kidney function can be monitored by testing the urine for glucose and protein. The presence of these in the urine could indicate kidney or blood pressure problems.

Certain micro-organisms which Mrs White may come into contact with can harm the developing fetus. For this reason, it would be essential to perform blood tests for organisms that cause syphilis and for the HIV virus.

Generally, when Mrs White attends the antenatal clinic, she should be given health education advice on the following: sleep, rest, exercise, travel, alcohol and smoking. The last two are associated with causing damage to the developing fetus.

Figure 20.5.
summary of the
physiological
changes during
pregnancy.

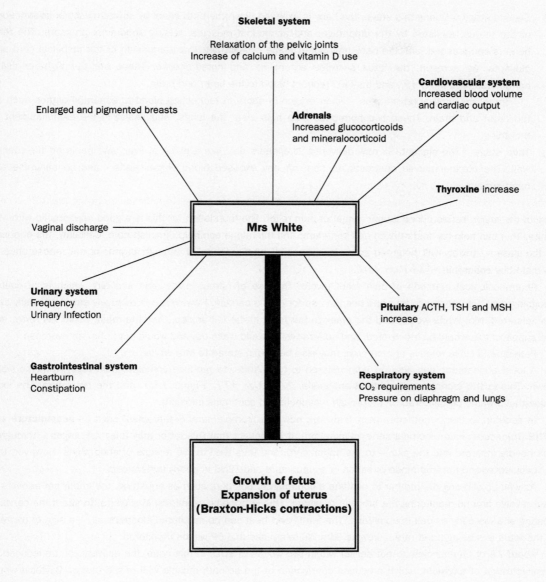

Skeletal system
Relaxation of the pelvic joints
Increase of calcium and vitamin D use

Cardiovascular system
Increased blood volume
and cardiac output

Enlarged and pigmented breasts

Adrenals
Increased glucocorticoids
and mineralocorticoid

Thyroxine increase

Vaginal discharge

Mrs White

Urinary system
Frequency
Urinary Infection

Pituitary ACTH, TSH and MSH
increase

Gastrointestinal system
Heartburn
Constipation

Respiratory system
CO₂ requirements
Pressure on diaphragm and lungs

**Growth of fetus
Expansion of uterus
(Braxton-Hicks contractions)**

Figure 20.5 provides a summary of the physiological changes during pregnancy.

Q37. There is a fall in progesterone levels – and thus a relative rise in oestrogen level. Cortisol and prostaglandins (📖 *Page 545)* are also thought to play a part in bringing about uterine contraction. Prostaglandins are used therapeutically, to produce a **termination of pregnancy**.

Oxytocin – from the pituitary gland – also stimulates uterine contractions. When these occur at regular intervals, Mrs White will be in labour.

Q38. There may be 'back' pain, a 'show' (a vaginal discharge of blood/mucus) and dilatation of the cervix – which can be seen via an internal examination.

Q39. Labour is divided into three stages:
(1) First stage   This is when the cervix dilates. The uterus contracts and usually the amniotic sac ruptures – or this can be done artificially.

(2) Second stage   During this stage, the baby is expelled down the birth canal by strong muscular contractions of the uterus; assisted by the diaphragm and abdominal muscles, raising abdominal pressure. The fetal head is compressed, and the baby may suffer some hypoxia due to compression of the umbilical cord and placenta. As a result, the fetus secretes adrenaline and noradrenaline. These are the 'fight or flight' hormones (📖 *Page 549),* and they will redirect blood to the heart and brain.

There are survival advantages – when oxygen is short- in redirecting blood to essential organs such as the heart and brain. These two hormones also help clear the lungs, and assist in the establishment of breathing.

(3) Third stage   The placenta is now delivered. It appears flat, like a piece of liver, and peels off the uterine wall. The uterine muscle contracts, to seal off any exposed blood vessel ends - and so minimise any haemorrhage.

Q40. One of the major issues during labour is that of pain relief. The foundation for this is a good relationship with Mrs White. This can help her feel relaxed and confident, and this alone can help diminish pain. Certainly, the opposite is the case – anxiety will heighten pain. It is possible that pain relief through psychological reassurance is mediated by **endorphins** (📖 *Page 430).*

Pharmacological methods of pain relief involve the use of nitrous oxide (gas and air), which is of course 'laughing gas' – a substance that has been in use for over a century. However, it is relatively safe and easily self-administered. Mrs White would hold the mask to her face. If she fell asleep, then the mask would fall away, and the supply of gas would be interrupted, and so Mrs White would wake up, and would not suffer an overdose.

Pethidine, a close relative of morphine, may also be administered to Mrs White.

A local anaesthetic can also be administered to Mrs White, to produce complete pain relief from the waist down. This is the technique of **epidural analgesia**. (📖 *Page 377, Figure 13.1,* and the note **dura**. The local anaesthetic would be delivered here, through a cannula and continous infusion).

In addition to these methods, many midwives now use 'complementary therapies' such as **acupuncture** and **TENS** (transcutaneous electrical nerve stimulation). It is thought that this latter may relay messages – through a fine needle inserted into the skin – to the spinal cord, and thus lead to the release of endorphins. However, this is speculative, and the true mode of action of acupuncture and TENS is poorly understood.

As well as allowing the mother to assume a comfortable position, such as squatting, the important aspects of care revolve around monitoring the process of labour. This is done by examining Mrs White, to see if the cervix is dilating and the baby's head is appearing. The fetal heart beat can be monitored electronically – a sign of distress in the fetus is a rising heart rate. Likewise, Mrs White's pulse and BP will be monitored.

About 7% of pregnancies do not deliver within two weeks of EDD. In this case, the delivery can be induced by administration of **oxytocin**, which produces contraction of the smooth muscle wall of the uterus. Oxytocin works via a **positive feedback mechanism** (📖 *Pages 11 & 533).* This is somewhat unusual, as most hormones are involved in negative feedback cycles. See 📖 *Page 533, Figure 18.11* which explains how this positive feedback is terminated. Following the baby's birth, oxytocin stimulates milk ejection from the **mammary gland** (📖 *Pages 989–90).*

Q41. The **puerperium** is a period of about six weeks following delivery, when Mrs White's reproductive anatomy and physiology will return to normal. Menstruation usually returns at the end of this period. The uterus undergoes a reduction in size, called **involution**. The vagina and pelvic floor muscles also return to normal. For several weeks, there is a uterine discharge called **lochia**. Other bodily systems also return to normal.

Perhaps the major feature of this period is **lactation** – the secretion and ejection of milk by the mammary glands.

Q42. Lactation is promoted by a hormone, **prolactin.** This is produced by the anterior pituitary gland. The main stimulus to prolactin release is the sucking reflex, which is initiated by the infant. This triggers nervous impulses, which are sent to the hypothalamus, which releases **prolactin releasing hormone**, and this in turn stimulates the pituitary to release prolactin. Hence, infant sucking turns on the milk supply. (Oxytocin, in its 'contracting' role, is also involved in ejecting milk from the breast). This whole process is an example of a **neuroendocrine reflex**. The nervous system, in the form of sensory neurones in the nipple, is communicating – via the hypothalamus – with the endocrine system. During the first few days following birth, the glands secrete a cloudy fluid called **colostrum**. It has less protein and fat than cows' milk, but still contains maternal antibodies. It is important for the baby to receive antibodies, because it takes 2–3 weeks (following birth) for its own immune system to begin to manufacture antibodies. During this time, the baby is dependent upon the mother's antibodies for protection against infection (📖 *Pages 702–3*).

Human milk is more nutritious than cows' milk, and there is less possibility of the nursing baby developing an allergy. In addition, breast feeding promotes a good mother–baby relationship, and helps develop the baby's facial muscles and teeth. The other effect of breast-feeding is that is usually renders the woman infertile. This is thought to occur because of endorphin release from the hypothalamus (due to the nipple-sucking reflex). This suppresses gonadotrophin release. However, this effect seems variable, and Mrs White would be advised not to rely upon it as a method of contraception.

Q43. Swings of mood are common after birth. Mrs White may be elated for a few days, and then depressed, possibly as a result of the stress of birth, and its associated anatomical and physiological changes. This can be coupled with anxiety about her role as a mother, and how she perceives her adequacy in fulfilling this.

It is vital that Mrs White receives support during this emotionally labile (unstable) period. Not only from her next-of-kin, but also from hospital staff. Understanding and listening to Mrs White can help her reach a stability, and provide feedback that can reassure her that she is a competent mother (and wife). This will help her gain confidence, which will further reinforce her positive behaviour. In this way, the whole experience can be – most of the time – joyous.

Within six to twelve weeks, Mrs. White should be established in a pattern, and feeling confident and capable. Sexual activity is possible at two to three weeks after delivery, but full libido may take some months to return.

Q44. Whilst in the uterus, the baby is dependent on the placenta, and mother, for its oxygen supply and CO_2 removal. Following birth this must all change. The amniotic fluid that fills its lungs, is emptied out at birth, and a rise in blood CO_2 level will trigger the baby's respiratory centre. Thus, the baby takes its first breath. Substances like **surfactant** (📖 *Page 740)*, help maintain the alveoli and prevent their collapse. Breathing rate is usually at 45/minute for the first few weeks of life.

The heart must make several adjustments, when the first inspiration occurs. The **foramen ovale** between the atria closes (see 📖 *Page 674, Figure 21.32)*. Thus, deoxygenated blood is diverted to the lungs for the first time, where it can now take up O_2 and release CO_2. The ductus arteriosus (📖 *Page 675, Figure 21.32)* closes – it may take some months – and this prevents blood from by-passing the lungs. When the umbilical cord is cut at birth this directs venous blood directly into the vena cava and to the right side of the heart (📖 *Page 675, Figure 21.32)*. Pulse rates for infants can be quite high at birth (120+ beats per minute).

Q45. Jaundice is a common problem following birth, and is usually described as 'physiological' – to distinguish it from pathological, (or disease) jaundice. It is due to the large numbers of red blood cells that the infant requires – in the uterus – to obtain sufficient O_2 from the placenta. Following birth, these are broken down (haemolysis). This releases bilirubin into the circulation (📖 *Page 794)*.

The newly born may suffer an overload of its liver (which may be physiologically immature) by this large amount of bilirubin, and this holds bilirubin back in the bloodstream. From there, it spills over into the skin, producing a yellow colour. The problem can partly be managed by using phototherapy (a blue and white lamp that delivers light of wavelength of 400–500nm). This will help the bilirubin to be dispersed, by converting it to a water-soluble form that can then be excreted by the kidneys.

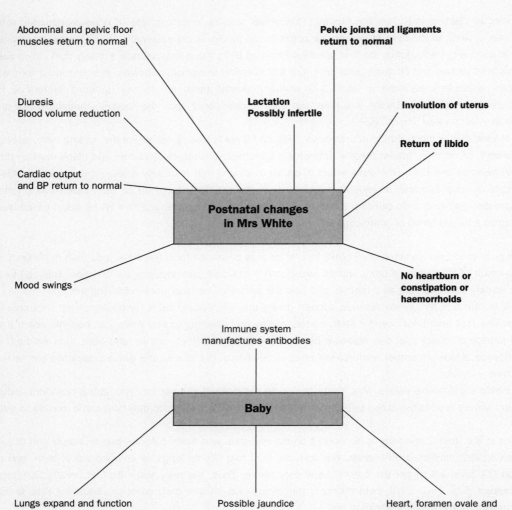

Figure 20.6.
A summary of the postnatal changes in Mrs White and her baby.

Overview and key terms

Cells

FUNCTIONS

INHERITANCE
MEDICAL TERMS (D)

- Genotype
- Phenotype
- Dominant
- Recessive
- Sex-linked
- Teratogens

GENE ACTION;
PROTEIN SYNTHESIS (E)

- Transcription
  Translation

- Recombinant
  DNA

NORMAL CELL
DIVISION (F)

Somatic

- Mitosis
- Cytokinesis

Reproductive

- Meiosis
- Cytokinesis

21. Understanding Mitosis, Meiosis and Inheritance

Learning outcomes

1. To describe the basic structure and function of DNA and RNA.

2. To outline the significance of meiosis and mitosis.

3. To define the following terms: chromosome, sex chromosome, autosome, diploid, haploid, homologous chromosome, homozygous, heterozygous, allele, genotype, phenotype, dominant and recessive alleles .

4. To outline the events that take place in protein synthesis in relation to transcription and translation, and the role of ribosomes.

5. To explain incomplete dominance, multiple-allele inheritance and polygenic inheritance.

6. To differentiate between autosomal recessive and sex-linked inheritance.

7. To discuss potential hazards to an embryo and fetus associated with chemicals and drugs, irradiation, alcohol and cigarette smoking.

8. To briefly describe the following genetic disorders: Down's syndrome, Turner's syndrome, Klinefelter's syndrome and fragile X syndrome.

Chapters 3 & 29

INTRODUCTION

If you have already studied the cell, this chapter is an extension of the function of the nucleus. You will be introduced to the nucleic acids, deoxyribonucleic acid (DNA) and ribonucleic acid (RNA). In the study of DNA and RNA, you will also meet various terms which you will need to understand if you are to grasp the essentials of genetic inheritance. These are chromosomes, dominant and recessive alleles, homologous, homozygous, heterozygous, gene, genotype, phenotype, mitosis and meiosis.

This study should also enable you to understand the principles of genetic inheritance – for example, how a particular genetic condition can be transmitted from parents to offspring. As a nurse, you may be called upon to give advice or to explain to patients the problems of a genetic nature, so as to allay their fear and anxiety. It is therefore imperative that you are aware of the basic principles of genetics.

This study will begin with an overview of gene action.

OVERVIEW OF GENE ACTION

Cells synthesise many chemicals to maintain homeostasis, but much of what is produced is in fact **proteins**. These proteins are essential for life. They may function as **enzymes**, **hormones** or **antibodies**. How much and what type of proteins are produced is dictated by the **genes**. Genes can perform such functions because they contain the **coding** information which is in fact found in a segment of DNA on the chromosome. The chromosomes themselves are found in the **nucleus**.

At this point, it is perhaps appropriate to review the structure of a **chromosome**.

For questions 1–6, *Page 86.*

Q1.   How many pairs of chromosomes are there in a somatic cell ?

_____

Q2.   How many chromosomes are there in the gamete cells ?

_____

Q3.   Define the terms haploid and diploid.

_____

_____

Q4.   Differentiate between the chromosomes in the male and the chromosomes in the female.

_____

_____

Q5.   **What are autosomes ?**

_____

Q6.   **What is the name given to the two chromosomes that make up a pair (one from the mother and one from the father) in a somatic cell?**

_____

Chromosomes are not usually visible in a non-dividing cell, but are observed when the cell is actively dividing. Question 7 will assist you in understanding the structure of chromosome.

Q7.   **Complete the exercise below which relates to chromosomal structure** (📖 *Pages 70–1*).
Chromosomes consist of bead-like subunits known as (a) _____, which are made of double-stranded (b) _____ wrapped around core proteins called (c) _____.
Nucleosome 'beads' are held together, necklace fashion, by (d) _____.
Nucleosomes are then held into chromatin fibres and folded into (e) _____.
  Before cell division, DNA duplicates and forms compact, coiled conformations known as (f) _____ that may be more easily moved around the cell during the division process.
  Chromosomes consist of DNA, and DNA is made up of nucleic acids. The basic units of nucleic acids are the nucleotides.

Q8.   **What are the three components of a nucleotide?**

_____

Q9.   **Name the four nitrogenous bases in DNA.**

_____

Q10.   **List the four types of atoms present in the bases.**

_____

Q11.   **Figure 21.1 below shows a schematic representation of DNA structure. Study it and then complete the following exercise.**

Figure 21.1.
Structure of DNA. P, phosphate; S, sugar (deoxyribose); A, adenine; T, thymine; G, guanine; C, cytosine.

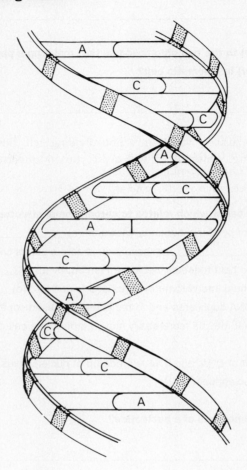

Circle one nucleotide. Label the complementary set of bases in the figure to produce the double-stranded structure of DNA. Bases are paired adenine to (a) _____ and
(b) _____ to (c) _____.

   DNA structure, like that of proteins, depends on sequence. Proteins differ from one another by their specific sequence of (d) _____.

Q12.   **What type of bond holds the bases together?**

_____

If you have grasped the basics of chromosomes and DNA, it is perhaps appropriate to look at ribonucleic acid (RNA), of which there are three main types.

Q13.   **Name the three types of RNA.**

_____

Q14.   Briefly differentiate between DNA and RNA.

_____

_____

GENE ACTION IN DETAIL 📖 *Pages 77–81*

In the introduction, it was mentioned that one of the main functions of the gene is that of directing the production of proteins. In the following study, you will discover how **genes** dictates protein synthesis (remember that genes are in fact groups of **nucleotides** on the DNA molecule of the chromosome).

There are two main processes involved in protein synthesis, and they are called **transcription** and **translation**. Transcription takes place in the nucleus, whilst translation occurs in the cytoplasm.

The instructions for making proteins are encoded in a sequence of three consecutive **bases** on either strand of **DNA** and are referred to as **codons**. Each **codon** is associated with a particular amino acid. Information from the codon is transcribed on the **messenger RNA (mRNA)**. The mRNA moves out of the nucleus and meets **transfer RNA (tRNA)** in the cytoplasm, the next step in protein synthesis which is referred to as **translation**. Each tRNA carries one of the 20 amino acids. The sequence of protein to be produced depends on the sequence of codons as dictated by the DNA molecule.

The exercise below should help you to understand the step–by–step synthesis of proteins.

Q15.   Study Figure 21.2, which shows various steps in protein synthesis in the cell, and then complete the exercise that follows.

Step 1 in the diagram indicates the process of (a) _____, which takes place in the (b) _____ with the help of the enzyme called (c) _____. In this process, a portion of one side of a double-stranded DNA molecule serves as a mould or (d) _____ and is called the (e) _____ strand. Nucleotides of (f) _____ line up in a complementary fashion next to DNA nucleotides.

In the diagram, the two mRNA contain (g) _____ and (h) _____ (write the letters of the complementary bases). You can also write them on your diagram.

The second step of protein synthesis is known as (i) _____, since it involves translation of one 'language' (the nucleotide base of (j) _____ RNA) into another language (the correct sequence of the 20 (k) _____ _____ to form a specific protein).

Translation occurs in the (l) _____ of the cell, specifically at a (m) _____ to which mRNA attaches. The (n) _____ ribosomal subunit binds to one end of the mRNA and finds the point where translation will begin, known as the (o) _____.

Each amino acid is transported to this site by a particular (p) _____ RNA, characterised by a specific three-base unit or (q) _____. For example, in your diagram, the amino acid **AA1** is transported by the three-base unit (r) _____ (write the letters of the bases). Fill in the bases for AA1 and AA2 in your diagram. These are in fact the anticodons.

As the ribosome moves along each mRNA codon, additional amino acids are transferred into

Figure 21.2.
Protein synthesis.

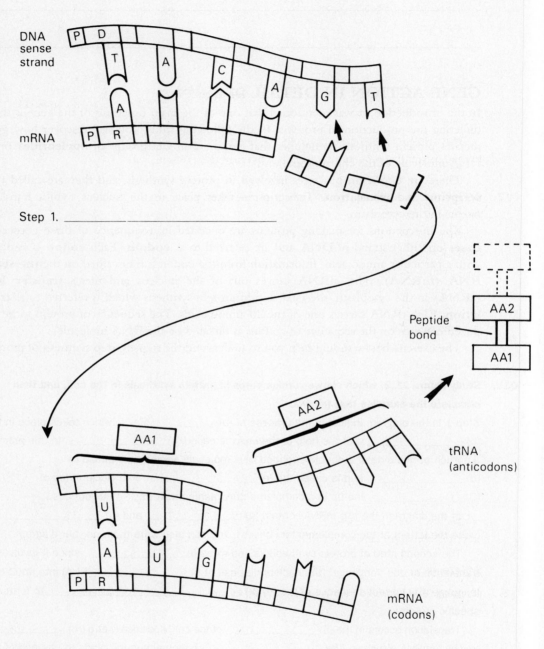

Step 1. _____

Step 2. _____

place by (s) _____ RNA. (t) _____ bonds form between adjacent amino acids with the help of enzymes from the (u) _____ subunit of the ribosome. Energy for the bond formation is provided by (v) _____ attached to the amino acid that is bound to tRNA.

One of the peptide bonds is shown on your diagram. Place an arrow against the other peptide bond.

When the protein is complete, synthesis is stopped by the (w) _____ codon. As the protein is released, the ribosome may be (x) _____ (indicate what happens to the ribosome).

When several ribosomes attach to the same strand of mRNA, a (y) _____ is formed, permitting repeated synthesis of the identical protein.

Q16. **Complete this additional activity about protein synthesis.**

Sections of DNA that do code for parts of proteins are known as (a) _____ whereas sections of DNA that do not code for parts of proteins are called (b) _____. The mRNA formed initially by transcription contains (c) _____ (only exons? only introns? both extrons and introns?).

RNA splicing is the process of removal of (d) _____, making up over 75% of the initial mRNA. This process occurs (e) _____ (before? after?) mRNA moves into the cytoplasm. In fact, variations of RNA splicing result in changes in function of a single gene to form different proteins as cells undergo the process of (f) _____.

The exon portion of a typical gene contains about (g) _____ to (h) _____ nucleotides that code for a protein containing (i) _____ to (j) _____ amino acids.

MITOSIS AND MEIOSIS 📖 *Pages 81–8.*

Before moving on to inheritance, it is as well to review **mitosis** and **meiosis**. In the study to follow, you will first be introduced to mitosis and then we will proceed on with meiosis. When you have worked through some of the exercises, you should be able to explain many of the processes that occur in both mitosis and meiosis – for example, interphase, replication, prophase, metaphase, anaphase, telophase, synapsis, tetrad formation and crossing-over.

Mitosis

Q17. **Complete the exercise below, which relates to some aspects of cell division.**

Division of any cell in the body consists of two processes: division of the (a) _____ and division of the (b) _____. In the formation of mature spermatozoa and ova, nuclear division is known as (c) _____. In the formation of all other body cells, that is **somatic** cells, nuclear division is called (d) _____.

Cytoplasmic division in both somatic and reproductive division is known as (e) _____. In (f) _____ the two daughter cells have the same hereditary material and genetic potential as the parent cell.

Q18. **Describe interphase in this exercise.**

Interphase occurs (a) _____ (during? between?) cell division. During the

(b) _____ phase of interphase, chromosomes are replicated. During this

phase, the DNA helix partially uncoils and the double DNA strand separates at the point where

(c) _____ connect so that the new complementary nucleotides can attach here. In

this manner, the DNA of a single chromosome is doubled to form two identical

(d) _____.

    Two periods of growth occur during interphase, preparing the cell for cell division. The

(e) _____ phase immediately precedes the S phase, whereas the (f) _____

phase follows the S portion of interphase. Two types of chemicals formed during G phases

are (g) _____ and (h) _____ ; organelles formed then include

(i) _____. The 'G' of these two phases also refers to 'gaps' since these periods are

gaps in (j) _____.

Q19. **Carefully study the phases of the cell cycle shown in** 📖 *Page 84, Figure 3.24.* **Then check**
your understanding of the process, by completing the matching exercise below. Place the
appropriate number against the letter of the correct statement. You may have to use some
letters more than once.

1. Anaphase 2. Interphase 3. Metaphase 4. Prophase 5. Telophase

☐ a. This phase immediately follows interphase.

☐ b. Chromosomes condense into distinct chromosomes (chromatids) each held together by a
centromere complexed with a kinetochore.

☐ c. Nucleoli and nuclear envelope break up; the two centrioles move to opposite poles of the
cell, and formation of the mitotic spindle begins.

☐ d. Chromatids line up with their centromeres along the equatorial plate.

☐ e. Centromeres divide; chromatids (now called daughter chromosomes) are dragged by
microtubules to opposite poles of the cell. Cytokinesis begins.

☐ f. Events of this phase are essentially a reversal of prophase; cytokinesis is completed.

☐ g. This phase of cell division is longest.

Now that you have completed the study on mitosis, you can proceed to meiosis.

Meiosis

Q20. **Read the section on meiosis** (📖 *Pages 86–7)* **in your text and then complete the exercise**
below.

Meiosis is a special type of nuclear division that occurs only in (a) _____ and is one

process in the production of sex cells or (b) _____. Fusion of gametes during the

process of (c) _____ results in formation of a (d) _____.

    Cells that begin the process of meiosis are ovarian or testicular cells that have been

undergoing mitosis up to this point. Each cell initially contains (e) _____

chromosomes, which is the (f) _____ number for humans. These chromosomes

consist of (g) _____ homologous pairs. One pair is known as the

(h) _____ chromosomes, and in the female this pair consists of two
(i) _____ chromosomes. The remaining 22 pairs are known as (j) _____.

By the time that cells complete meiosis, they will contain (k) _____ chromosomes, the (l) _____ (2n? n?) number.

Meiosis differs from mitosis in that meiosis involves (m) _____ divisions with replication of DNA only (n) _____ (once? twice?). The first division is known as the (o) _____ division, whereas the second division is the (p) _____ division.

Replication of DNA occurs (q) _____ (before? after?) reduction division, resulting in doubling of chromosome number in humans from 46 chromosomes to (r) _____ 'chromatids'. Chromatids are held together by means of (s) _____.

A unique event that occurs in prophase I is the lining up of chromosomes in homologous pairs, a process called (t) _____. This process **does not** occur in mitosis. The four chromatids of the homologous pair are known as a (u) _____. The proximity of chromatids permits the exchange or (v) _____ between maternal and paternal chromatids. The advantage of crossing-over in sexual reproduction is to (w) _____ _____ (just give an explanation).

Q21. **This question will provide you with more information as to the reason for the increased possibilities of variety among spermatozoa and ova.**

Another factor that increases possibilities for variety among spermatozoa and ova production is the random assortment of chromosomes as they line up on either side of the equator in metaphase (a) _____ (I? II?).

Division I reduces the chromosome number to (b) _____ chromatids. Division II results in the separation of double chromatids by the splitting of (c) _____ so that resulting cells contain only (d) _____ chromosomes.

Meiosis is only one part of the process in the production of spermatozoa and ova. Each original diploid cell in a testis will lead to the production of (e) _____ spermatozoa, while each diploid ovary cell produces (f) _____ mature ova plus three small cells known as (g) _____.

INHERITANCE 📖 *Pages 991–7.*

From your answer to question 20, you will have discovered the importance of **crossing-over**. This allows for an exchange of genes amongst **homologous** chromosomes. Hence, the great genetic variation amongst humans and other organisms.

In the study to follow, you will be exploring more about genes, how they are inherited and their significance in diseases.

Q22. **Define the terms inheritance and genome.**

_____

_____

Q23. **Briefly outline what you understand by the term homologous chromosomes.**

_____

_____

Q24. **Define the term alleles.**

_____

_____

Figure 21.3 below represents a schematic diagram of a pair of homologous chromosomes and the alleles.

Figure 21.3

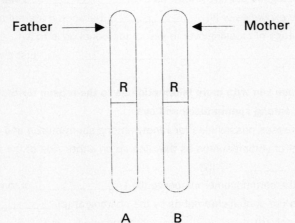

Explanation for diagram: A and B are a pair of homologous chromosomes and R, R are the two alleles for the same trait. A is the chromosome from the father and B is the chromosome from the mother.

To understand how genes are inherited, and especially if one is trying to explain to someone whether he/she may be at risk of inheriting a particular gene that may be the cause of a disorder, in genetics it is conventional to denote **genes** by the use of letters of the alphabet. A capital letter is used when referring to a **dominant** gene/allele and a lower case letter is used when referring to recessive gene/allele.

Q25. **Differentiate between a dominant and a recessive allele with reference to a particular trait.**

_____

_____

Q26.   Define the terms genotype and phenotype.

_____

_____

If you have understood the terms dominant and recessive, you will have established that there only three ways in which an individual may inherit his/her genes.

The exercise below should demonstrate to you whether or not you have grasped the significance of **dominant** and **recessive** and also the terms **homozygous** and **heterozygous**.

Q27.   Study Figure 21.4, which shows the three possible ways in which genes are inherited within a homologous pair of chromosomes (remember that in a homologous pair of chromosomes, there is a maternal and a paternal gene in an individual). Capital C represents a dominant gene/allele (coding for black hair colour) and lower case c is the recessive gene/allele (coding for brown hair colour).

a.   Write the genotype for each individual in the space beside the numbers 1, 2 and 3.

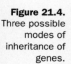

Figure 21.4.
Three possible modes of inheritance of genes.

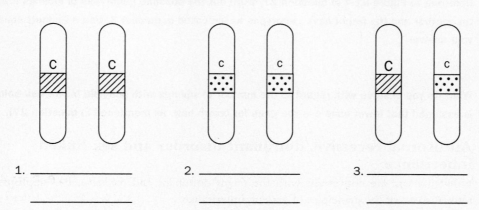

1. _____   2. _____   3. _____

   _____   _____   _____

b.   What will be the hair colour for individuals 2 and 3? Give the rationale for your answer.

_____

_____

Understanding the use of the Punnett square

In question 27 you specified three genotypes which are possible in an individual. Suppose you wanted to predict possible hair colour of the offsprings in a marital relationship where the **mother's** genotype was **Cc** and the **father's** genotype was **CC** as indicated in Figure 21.4. For this purpose, you would need to use a special chart, referred to as a **Punnett square**. The male gametes are usually placed at the side of the chart and the female gametes at the top as indicated in Figure 21.5.

Figure 21.5.
Example of a
Punnett square.

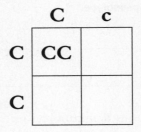

In working out the possible genotypes, one would make the assumption that there is a 50:50 chance that in the mother, some ova will be carrying gene C, whilst the others will be carrying gene c. In the father all the spermatozoa will be carrying gene C. Thus, it is easy to determine the possible genotypes – for example, if the spermatozoon with C meets the ovum with gene C, the genotype will be CC (as indicated in the top left-hand corner of the Punnett square).

Q28. Fill in the rest of the Punnett square in Figure 21.5. Suggest possible phenotypes for all the offsprings (refer to queston 27 for the genotype for hair colour).

Q29. Referring to Figure 21.4 in question 27, work out the possible genotypes of siblings if both the mother and the father have genotypes as indicated in number 3. Use a Punnett square for your answer.

What do you observe with regard to the number of siblings with possible brown hair colour (it is assumed that lower case c is the gene for brown hair, as mentioned in question 27).

Autosomal recessive/dominant disorder and sex linked inheritance

Now that you are conversant with the terms dominant and recessive, it is appropriate to look at some of the principles of genetic inheritance.

Genetic disorders are inherited as autosomal dominant or recessive, or through sex-linked inheritance. The discussion here will focus on **autosomal recessive**, since some of the common genetic disorders are inherited in this way.

What do we understand by the term autosomal inheritance? This simply means that the gene for the particular trait is carried on one of the **autosome** and not the **sex** chromosomes. For many genetic disorders, the particular chromosome has been identified. For example, in the disorder known as **cystic fibrosis**, the abnormal gene is found on chromosome number 7. Another example of an autosomal disorder is **phenylketonuria**. In an autosomal recessive disorder, the individual is affected because he/she has both recessive genes (double dose).

Q30. What is the genotype referred to for an individual who has an autosomal recessive disorder?

Q31.   In a family in which a child has an autosomal recessive disorder, both parents must be carrying the abnormal gene. True or false? (Give the rationale for your answer.)

_____

_____

Q32.   Autosomal recessive disorders only occur in boys. True or false? (Give the rationale for your answer.)

_____

_____

Q33.   Complete the exercise below, which refers to phenylketonuria.

The dominant gene for PKU is represented by (a) _____ (P? p?). The dominant gene is for the (b) _____ condition.

The letters PP are an example of a genetic makeup or (c) _____. A person with such a genotype is said to be (d) _____. The phenotype of that individual would be (e) _____.

The genotype for a heterozygous individual is (f) _____. The phenotype is (g) _____ , but a (h) _____ of PKU.

Incomplete dominance

Although in most autosomal recessive inheritance only the siblings with both recessive genes are affected, there is an exception in some disorders (for example, in **sickle–cell anaemia**). The type of inheritance in this case is referred to as **incomplete inheritance**.

Q34   Match the following genotype :

1. Homozygous recessive 2. Homozygous dominant 3. Heterozygous

☐   a.   Genotype present in persons who have the sickle-cell trait.

☐   b.   Genotypes present in persons who have sickle-cell anaemia.

Q35.   Using a Punnett square, work out the genotypes of the siblings for a couple who are both homozygous recessive for sickle cell anaemia. ▧ *Page 993, Figure 29.14.*

Q36. Using a Punnett square, work out the genotypes of the siblings for a couple, where the male is heterozygous and the female is homozygous recessive for sickle-cell anaemia.

Sex-linked inheritance 📖 *Pages 995–6*

In sex-linked inheritance the genes for the particular traits are usually only found on the **X chromosome**. This therefore suggests that the **Y chromosome** is not involved in this type of inheritance, which is why in sex-linked inheritance the females are carriers.

Q37. Explain why a female who is a carrier for a sex-linked disorder does not have the signs or symptoms of the disorder.

_____

_____

Q38. Name two disorders that are inherited in sex-linked fashion.

_____

Q39. Complete this exercise about sex-linked inheritance.

Sex chromosomes contain other genes besides those determining the sex of an individual. Such traits are called (a) _____ traits. Y chromosomes are shorter than X chromosomes and lack some genes. One of these is the gene controlling the ability to (b) _____ red from green colours. This ability is therefore controlled entirely by the (c) _____ gene.

The genotype for females who are colour blind may be written as (d) _____; the genotype for females who are carriers may be written as (e) _____; and the genotype for normal females is (f) _____.

The genotype for males who are colour blind may be written as (g) _____; the genotype for males who are normal is (h) _____.

Q40. Using a Punnett square, work out the genotypes of the children of a couple in which the male is colour blind and the female is normal but is carrying the recessive gene. 📖 *Page 996, Figure 29.19.*

Multiple-allele inheritance 📖 *Pages 992–3.*

So far, it has been shown that phenotypic traits are dependent on the genotypes (remember there are three types of genotype, example PP, Pp and pp). Thus for **homozygous dominant** and **heterozygous**, the dominant trait is expressed, whilst in the **homozygous recessive**, this is not so. This suggests that only one of the genes, in the pair of alleles (i.e. the dominant gene) is responsible for expression of the trait. However, in **multiple-allele** inheritance (for example, in the ABO blood groups) three different alleles are present.

Q41. Name the four main blood groups.

_____

Q42. List the three possible alleles for inheritance of the ABO group.

_____

Q43. List the possible genotypes of persons who produce A antigens (agglutinogens) on red blood cells.

_____

List the possible genotypes of persons who produce B antigens (agglutinogens) on red blood cells.

_____

Q44. Explain what you understand by the term codominant in relation to blood groups.

_____

_____

Q45. Using Punnett squares, explain how couples could produce children with blood group **O**. Hint: identify the genotypes and phenotypes of the couples.

Q46. List two examples of characteristics governed by polygenic inheritance.

Genes and the environment 📖 *Pages 993–4.*

When you have studied this section, you will understand that a given phenotype is the product of the genotype and the environment.

Q47. Complete the exercise about the potential hazards to the embryo and fetus. Match the term in the box with the appropriate statement.

1. Cigarette smoking 2. Fetal alcohol syndrome 3. Teratogen

☐ a. An agent or influence that causes defects in the developing embryo.
☐ b. May cause defects, such as small head, facial irregularities, defective heart and retardation.
☐ c. Linked to a variety of abnormalities, such as lower infant birth weight, higher mortality rate, gastrointestinal disturbances and sudden infant death syndrome.

Sex inheritance 📖 *Page 994*

When you have answered question 48, you should be able to explain sex inheritance.

Q48. Complete this exercise about sex inheritance.

All (a) _____ contain the X chromosome. About half of the spermatozoa produced by a male contain the (b) _____ chromosome, and half contain the

(c) _____ chromosome.

Every cell (except those forming ova) in a normal female contains (d) _____ sex chromosomes and (e) _____ pairs of (f) _____ (name given to chromosomes other than the sex chromosomes).

All male cells (except those forming spermatozoa) contain the (g) _____ sex chromosomes. It can be said that it is the (h) _____ who determine the sex of the child.

Q49. **Name the gene on the Y chromosome which determines that a developing individual will be male.**

_____

Aneuploidy 📖 *Pages 991 & 996–7.*

Aneuploidy can give rise to many types of genetic disorders, the majority of which are compatible with life.

Q50. **Define the term aneuploid and give three suitable examples.**

_____

_____

This concludes the study on mitosis, meiosis and genetic inheritance. We hope that you have enjoyed this study. Well done!

Answers to questions

Q1.   23 pairs.

Q2.   23.

Q3.   *Haploid* – the number of chromosomes in the gametes (ova and spermatozoa). This is half the number found in somatic cells.

Diploid – the full complement of chromosomes in the somatic cells. This is 46, or 23 pairs.

Q4.   Both have 22 pairs of autosomes, but in the male there are the X and Y chromosomes, whilst in the female there are the XX sex chromosomes.

Q5.   Autosomes are all the chromosomes found in the cell, excluding the sex chromosomes.

Q6.   Homologous chromosomes.

Q7.   a, Nucleosomes; b, DNA; c, histones; d, linker DNA; e, loops; f, chromatids.

Q8.   A sugar (deoxyribose in DNA), a base and a phosphate.

Q9.   Adenine, guanine, cytosine and thymine.

Q10.   Oxygen, carbon, nitrogen and hydrogen.

Q11.   See figure opposite.

a, Thymine; b, cytosine; c, guanine; d, amino acids.

Q12.   Hydrogen bonds.

Q13.   Messenger RNA, transfer RNA, ribosomal RNA.

Q14.   DNA is double-stranded, whilst RNA is single stranded. The sugar in DNA is deoxyribose, whilst in RNA it is ribose. In RNA, thymine is replaced by uracil.

Q15.   a, Transcription; b, nucleus; c, RNA polymerase; d, template; e, sense; f, messenger RNA; g, AUG;

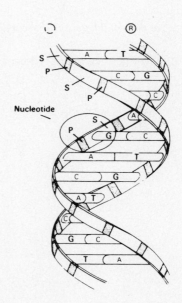

Nucleotide

h, UAC; i, translation; j, messenger RNA; k, amino acids; l, cytoplasm; m, ribosome; n, small; o, start codon; p, transfer; q, anticodon; r, UAC; s, transfer; t, peptide; u, large; v, ATP; w, stop; x, released and may be recycled to transfer another amino acid. y. polyribosome.

Q16.   a, Exons; b, introns; c, both exons and introns; d, introns; e, before; f, differentiation; g, 300; h, 3000; i, 100; j, 1000.

Q17.   a, Nucleus; b, cytoplasm; c, meiosis; d, mitosis; e, cytokinesis; f, mitosis.

Q18.   a, between cell division; b, S; c, nitrogenous bases; d, chromatids; e, G1; f, G2; g, RNA; h, proteins; i, centrosomes containing centrioles; j, DNA synthesis.

Q19.   4a, 4b, 4c, 3d, 1e, 5f, 4g.

Q20.   a, gonads (ovaries and testes); b, gametes; c, fertilisation; d, zygote; e, 46; f, diploid; g, 23; h, sex; i, XX; j, autosomes; k, 23; l, n; m, two; n, once; o, reduction; p, equatorial; q, before; r, 92; s, centromeres; t, synapsis; u, tetrad; v, cross-over of DNA; w, permit exchange of DNA between chromatids and greatly increase the possibility for variety amongst ova and spermatozoa and therefore the offsprings.

Q21.   a, II; b, 23 doubled; c, centromeres; d, 23; e, 4; f, one; g, polar bodies.

Q22.   *Genome* – complete genetic make up of an organism.
Inheritance – the acquisition of body characteristics and qualities by transmission of genetic information from parents to offspring.

Q23.   The two chromosomes in a cell that make up a pair (one from the mother and one from the father). Also known as *homologues.*

Q24.   The two genes that code for the same trait and are at the same location on homologous chromosomes.

Q25.   In the individual who is carrying the dominant gene, the particular trait is expressed, whilst for the individual carrying the recessive gene, the trait is not expressed. A word of caution: the individual carrying the dominant gene may be homozygous dominant or heterozygous (see question 27).

Q26.   Genotype means the genetic make up of an individual, that is the genes that are inherited. Phenotype refers to the expression of the genetic make up, for example in the colour of the hair.

Q27.   a. 1, Homozygous dominant; 2, Homozygous recessive; 3, Heterozygous.

   b. Individual 2 will have brown hair, since she has inherited both recessive genes. Individual 3 will have black hair, since he is heterozygous. The dominant gene will be expressed.

Q28.

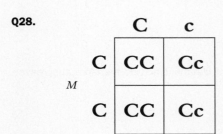

CC, black hair; and Cc, black hair.

Q29.

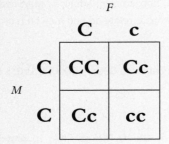

Only one sibling, cc, will have brown hair.

Q30. Homozygous recessive.

Q31. True. The child inherits one gene from each parent. If he is affected, he must therefore have inherited the double dose of the recessive genes. Both parents must be heterozygous.

Q32. False. Autosomes are not sex chromosomes, and therefore boys and girls may be equally affected.

Q33. a, P; b, normal; c, genotype; d, homozygous dominant; e, normal; f, Pp; g, carrier.

Q34. 3a, 1b.

Q35.

	Hb'	Hb'
Hb'	Hb'Hb'	Hb'Hb'
Hb'	Hb'Hb'	Hb'Hb'

Q36.

	Hb'	Hb'
Hb'	Hb'Hb'	Hb'Hb'
Hb^A	Hb^AHb'	Hb^AHb'

Q37. Because she has a normal X chromosome, which acts as the dominant chromosome and therefore suppresses the recessive trait.

Q38. Haemophilia and fragile X syndrome.

Q39. a, Sex-linked; b, differentiate; c, X gene; d, X^cX^c; e, X^cX^c; f, X^cX^c; g, X^cy; h, X^cy.

Q40.

	X^c	X^c
X^c	X^cX^c	X^cX^c
Y	X^cY	X^cY

X^cX^c, X^cX^c, X^cy, X^cy.

Q41. A, B, AB and O.

Q42. A, B and O.

Q43. AO and AA.
BO and BB.

Q44. When both genes are expressed, for example in the heterozygous state. An example is an individual with blood group AB.

Q45. O is recessive and if the child is blood group O, his/her genotype will be OO. The child can only be OO if the O genes have been inherited from each parent. Three possible combination of parental genotypes may produce individuals with blood group O. For example, if both parents have genotypes BO, if both parents have genotypes AO and if one parent is BO and the other AO.

	B	**O**
B	**BB**	**BO**
O	**BO**	**OO**

	A	**O**
A	**AA**	**AO**
O	**AO**	**OO**

	A	**O**
B	**AB**	**BO**
O	**AO**	**OO**

Q46. Skin colour and eye colour.

Q47. 3a, 2b, 1c.

Q48. a, gametes; b, X; c, Y; d, XX; e, 22; f, autosomes; g, XY; h, males.

Q49. Sex determining region of the Y chromosome.

Q50. A cell that has one or more chromosomes of a set added or deleted is referred to as *aneuploid*. Three examples are: Down's syndrome, Turner's syndrome and Klinefelter's syndrome.

Overview and key terms

Introduction to pharmacology

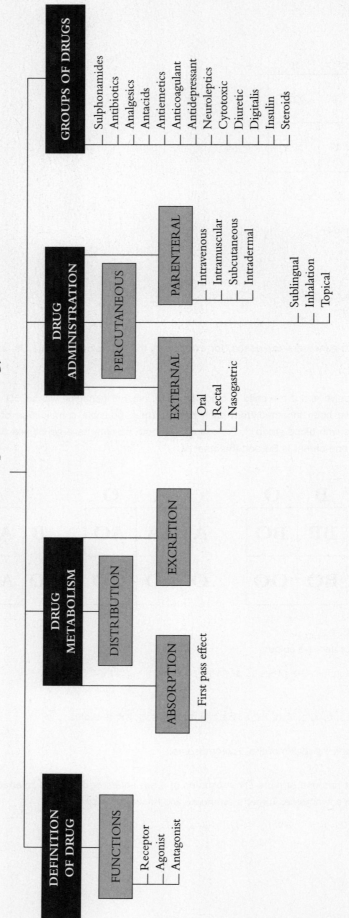

22. An Introduction to Pharmacology

Learning outcomes

1. To define the term drug.

2. To describe the terms: receptor, agonist, antagonist and half-life in relation to drugs.

3. To identify the five basic principles of drug action.

4. To list three categories of drug administration, and state the routes of administration of each category.

5. To explain the process of first pass effect in relation to drug action.

6. To describe nursing interventions that can enhance drug absorption.

7. To outline the reasons why a drug is metabolised differently in the infant, the adult and the elderly.

8. To apply basic principles of drug action and interactions to make sound judgements when administering medications to patients.

INTRODUCTION

Pharmacology is the study of the effects of drugs on the body. This short section on pharmacology is an attempt to introduce you to some of the basic principles of pharmacology and will include, for example: the definition of a drug, and drug interaction, absorption, distribution and excretion in the body.

It is not intended here to give details of the various groups of drugs and their functions, but only to mention some of the main groups to assist you in your nursing practice.

In previous study, you met various terms such as receptors, plasma membrane and cytosol, and if you have grasped their meanings, they should assist you in understanding how drugs interact with the tissues in the body.

DEFINITION AND OVERVIEW OF DRUG FUNCTION

A simple definition of a drug is that it is a chemical that alters body functions. This is achieved in several ways. For example, a drug may replace a missing substance from the body, allowing a reaction to take place, by interfering with enzyme action, inhibiting bacterial growth, altering existing physiological activity, acting as a metabolite or acting as a cytoxic substance that kills certain cells. When it acts as a metabolite, the drug chemistry is similar to that of a natural chemical that usually exists in the body. For example, in the case of a drug such as sulphonamide, the drug behaves as if it was folic acid. Thus, the bacteria which need folic acid for growth ingest the sulphonamide, having mistaken it for folic acid, and are therefore destroyed in the process. Cytotoxic drugs are usually administered to patients with cancer. Most drugs are either weak acids or weak bases.

Figure 22.1.
Schematic diagrams showing drug interacting with the receptor.

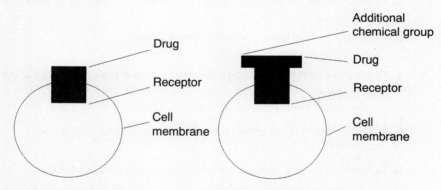

A Schematic diagram showing drug interacting with the receptor. A 'good fit' and therefore acts as an agonist.

B Schematic diagram showing drug interacting with the receptor, but in this case acts as antagonist as there are additional chemical groups which interfere with the 'receptor drug interaction'.

Drug receptors, agonist and antagonist

Drugs interact in the body in several ways. The most common way is by the formation of a **chemical bond** with specific **receptors**. A receptor is a large macromolecule, usually a protein, which is located on a cell membrane or within a cell. They are specific in that they have a specific shape (as a result of their three-dimensional structure) which only allows drugs with a specific chemical shape to interact. The interaction between a drug and a receptor is similar to the mechanism of a lock and key. The better the 'fit' between the receptor and the drug, the better the response. The maximum response of the drug also depends on the number of receptors that are occupied.

If the interaction between the drug and the receptor causes a response to occur, the drug is said to be an **agonist**. If the interaction does not stimulate a response, the drug is said to be an **antagonist**. Figure 22.1 illustrates agonist and antagonist by using the lock and key analogy.

Drugs that interact with a receptor to stimulate a response, but inhibit other responses, are called **partial agonists**.

In order for any drug to cause a response, it must first be **absorbed** and **distributed.** It must then be **metabolised** (broken down) and **excreted**.

ABSORPTION

Absorption is the process by which a drug is made available to the body fluids for distribution. However, before absorption, the drug needs to be introduced into the body. There are three main ways that drugs can be administered: **parenteral**, **enteral** and **percutaneous** (also called insufflated) routes.

Enteral route

The enteral route is administration of the drug directly into the gastrointestinal tract by the oral, rectal or nasogastric route. The oral route is the easiest route of administration of drugs. They may be taken in solutions, suspensions, capsules, compressed and coated tablets or sustained release tablets.

Nursing applications

It is important for nurses to understand the meaning of 'enteric coated' tablets. Nurses should therefore at no time (often supposed to be in the interest of the patient) crush the tablet before administering it to the patient. Enteric coated tablets are especially prepared to be protected from the stomach acid. The coating on the tablet is acid resistant.

It is also important for nurses to understand why some medications should be taken on an empty stomach. The presence of food in the stomach increases the time a drug is held in the stomach, so drugs that are unstable in acid should not be taken with food. On the other hand, drugs that irritate the gastric mucosa *should* be taken with food . One example of such a drug is **ibuprofen**. It can cause gastric irritation, which could in time give rise to an ulcer.

Rectal route

Rectal drug administration is useful for young children or babies. The drug dissolves and is absorbed by the mucous membrane of the large intestine. Most rectal medication is given as **suppositories**. Certain medications may need to be administered via a large amount of fluid contained in a clear plastic bag. This is then referred to as an **enema**.

Some of the medications that can be administered via this route are aminophylline (which is a bronchodilator, making breathing easier), analgesics (for the relief of pain) and laxatives.

Nursing applications

The nurse should provide privacy and respect the dignity of the patient at all times. The patient must be placed in the left lateral position, with the knees reaching as far as possible towards the chin (fetal position). A disposable glove or finger cot should be used. For ease of inserting the suppository, plain water or a water soluble lubricant should be used. To divert the patient's attention and to reduce contraction of the rectal muscle, the patient should be asked to take a deep breath, just prior to the insertion of the suppository. The suppository must be inserted gently, about 2.5cm beyond the orifice past the internal sphincter.

To allow for maximum absorption, the patient must be advised to remain lying on the side for about 15–20 minutes. It is advisable in children to compress the buttocks gently but firmly to prevent the medication from being expelled.

If an enema or a laxative is given, the nurse must ensure that a bed pan/commode and paper tissues are within easy reach of the patient. It is essential that the patient is made as comfortable as possible after the procedure, and strict hygiene is adhered to. The nurse must note the efficacy of the treatment.

Parenteral route

The parenteral routes include intravenous (IV), intramuscular (IM), subcutaneous (SC) and intradermal injections. Drug absorption is immediate via the intravenous route. This route is preferred for administering medications to patients in shock, those who are unconscious, and where quick action is needed.

Nursing applications

An intravenous drug should not be administered rapidly as a high concentration of the drug reaching the heart may interfere with cardiac functions. It may give rise to arrhythmias (irregular heart rhythm). A drug such as **potassium chloride** could cause cardiac arrest if it was administered too quickly. If the drug was administered via a large amount of fluids (i.e. if the patient is on a drip) and the fluid is running very fast in the patient's vein, this could cause circulatory overload and give rise to pulmonary oedema. The patient affected would experience breathing difficulty and might cough up frothy blood stained sputum (this is also seen in patients suffering from left ventricular failure).

Nurses should always ensure that the correct dose is calculated, for a mistake could be fatal. Nurses should also be aware of **drug interaction**, especially if the patient is receiving different medications by the intravenous route. Advice should be sought from the pharmacist. The nurse should check the hospital/ward's policy with regard to the **mixing** of IV drugs.

Nurses should also be aware of medications that would necessitate the wearing of disposable gloves – for example, when preparing cytotoxic drugs.

Nurses should also observe local signs of infection at the site of the cannula (can lead to phlebitis), extravasation of fluids, or haematoma.

Intramuscular injection

The intramuscular route is the administration of a drug into the muscles. The muscles of choice are vastus lateralis and rectus femoris muscles (both found in the thigh), the gluteal muscles (the buttocks) and the deltoid muscles (found in the upper arm). Figure 22.2 shows the locations of the various muscles and the position of the needle.

Figure 22.2.
ations of various
muscles and the
position of the
needle.

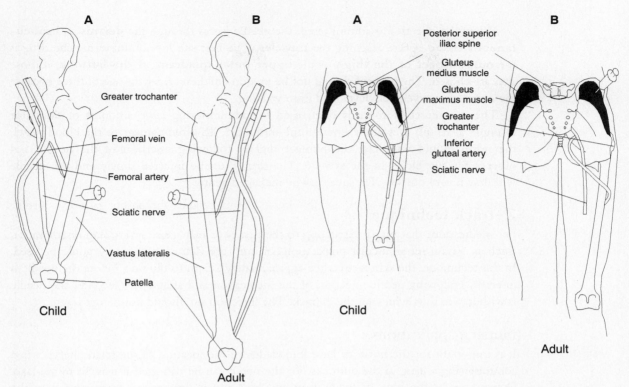

Vastus lateralis muscle. **A**, Child/infant. **B**, Adult.

Dorsal gluteal site. **A**, Child/infant. **B**, Adult.

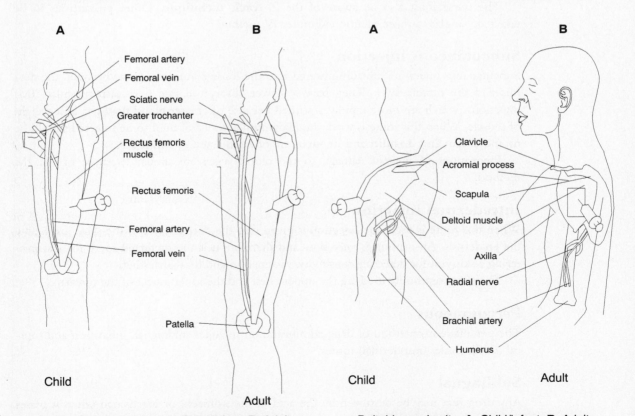

Rectus femoris muscle. **A**, Child/infant. **B**, Adult.

Deltoid muscle site. **A**, Child/infant. **B**, Adult.

When the injection is administered, the needle passes through the **dermis** and **subcutaneous tissue** before reaching the **muscles**. The best site for administering the drug is the **outer aspect of the thigh** or the **upper outer quadrant of the buttock**, if those sites are chosen. The **gluteal** should not be used in children under the age of three because the muscle is not yet well developed from walking.

The intramuscular route is often used for administering large amounts of fluid (for example 5–10 ml) as is often required for antibiotics. To avoid damage to the blood vessel, the nurse should withdraw the plunger slightly following insertion of the needle and observe for any blood in the syringe. The drug must be injected slowly and the needle withdrawn very quickly. The area may be massaged gently.

Z–track technique

For medications that may be irritating to the tissues or may cause severe skin discoloration (such as certain intramuscular preparations of iron) the Z-track technique should be used. In this technique, the skin is stretched approximately 2.5cm to the side, before the needle is inserted. Following gentle injection of the medication and after a few seconds, the needle is withdrawn, thus achieving the Z track. The injection site should not be massaged.

Nursing applications

It is important for the nurse to have knowledge of the location of the sciatic nerve when administering a drug in the buttocks, for the nerve can be damaged if it is hit by mistake. Depending on the type of medication and how much damage has been caused to the nerve, this could result in paralysis, numbness or a tingling sensation in the affected limb.

The nurse must also be aware of the **Z-track technique**. Other precautions to be taken are similar to those mentioned under IV method.

Subcutaneous injection

Subcutaneous injections are administered into the loose connective tissue between the dermis and the muscle layer. They have a slower absorption rate than intramuscular (IM) injections, which are more rapidly absorbed because of greater blood flow per unit weight of muscle. When this route is used, the maximum amount of fluid to be injected should be no more than 2ml. **Insulin** and **heparin** are often injected by this route.

Precautions to prevent damage to the blood vessel are similar to those of the IM method.

Intradermal injection

When this route is used, the injection is given into the dermal layer of the skin, just below the epidermis. Absorption is very slow and therefore it is the preferred route for administering a skin test for detecting sensitivity, vaccination and local anaesthetic.

The sites commonly used are the upper chest and the inner aspect of the forearm.

Percutaneous

The percutaneous method of drug administration includes sublingual, inhalation and topical (this includes transdermal) routes.

Sublingual

Any drug that may be destroyed by the acid in the stomach, or inactivated when it passes through the liver for the first time, should be given lingually. An example of a common sublingual medication is **glyceryl trinitrate**, which is given to ease the pain of angina.

Inhalation

This is quite an effective way of administering certain drugs, especially those for relieving bronchospasm in asthma sufferers. The drug may be given in pressurised aerosol inhalers, or nebulisers.

Nursing applications

Patients should be given clear instructions on how to use the inhaler to gain maximum benefit from the medication. They should not have more puffs than the prescribed dose ,in the hope that their spasm will be relieved quicker. It is important that the inhaler is shaken before use. The cap is removed and the mouthpiece is placed in the mouth and the lips are closed around it. The patient should breathe slowly and be delivered the required dose by depressing the plunger. The breath should be held for a few seconds, provided it does not cause any distress to the patient. The patient should wait at least 60 seconds for any subsequent delivery.

Transdermal

Some drugs (usually as patches) may be given by the transdermal route, as they can be absorbed effectively via the skin, especially where there is good skin permeability and capillary distribution. Such areas are, for example, behind the ears and on the trunk region. Examples of drugs that can be administered by this route are estrogen for hormone replacement therapy, and glyceryl trinitrate, which is used to ease the pain of angina.

Although this route may be preferred by some individuals, there may be adverse effects, such as skin reactions or variations in rate of absorption of the medication. It is also advisable for individuals wearing patches not to be exposed to the sun, especially for women with patches of estrogen for hormone replacement therapy.

First pass effect

To reach their target tissues, drugs when absorbed from the gastrointestinal tract, are transported via the hepatic portal vein to the liver and then into the blood circulation. Many drugs when entering the liver are broken down immediately by liver enzymes and therefore only a small amount of the drug is available for their specific action. The removal of drugs as they pass through the liver is called the **first pass effect**. Drugs that exhibit a large first pass effect may not be very active if they are taken orally and swallowed. It is for this reason that certain drugs (for example, glyceryl trinitrate) are given sublingually.

DISTRIBUTION

Distribution of drugs to the various tissues depends on blood flow. For example, organs that have an extensive blood supply, such as the liver and the kidney, will receive the drug much quicker. Two factors that influence drug distribution are protein binding and lipid solubility. Drug molecules bind mainly to plasma albumin, which acts as a carrier. When a drug is transported in the blood in that state, it is pharmacologically inactive. For the drug to be active, it needs to be in the unbound form. It is only then that the drug can diffuse into tissues and interact with receptors. Lipid soluble drugs cross cell membranes easily. Some drugs cannot pass the blood–brain barrier or the placental barrier.

Nursing applications

On account of the blood–brain barrier, antibiotics in the treatment of meningitis are often given intrathecally (introduced into the cerebrospinal fluid via a lumbar puncture). Any drug that is able to pass the placental barrier can harm the fetus. An example of such a drug is thalidomide (not available in the UK).

METABOLISM

Metabolism of a drug simply means the process by which the body breaks down or inactivates the drug. This is also referred to as 'biotransformation'. Most drugs are metabolised by enzymes in the liver.

Both the young (babies and children) and the elderly metabolise drugs more slowly. In the young, this is due to the immaturity of the liver, whilst in the elderly, it is as a result of the ageing process, whereby liver cells that are dying are not replaced.

Elimination

Most drugs are eliminated by the kidneys. Again, in both the young and the elderly, for the same reasons given above, excretion may be affected. In the elderly, renal blood flow falls, and there is also a reduced glomerular filtration rate. It is for this reason that in the elderly, a lower dose of drug is often prescribed.

Half life

The half life of a drug is a measure of the time required for a drug to be eliminated. In other words, the half life is defined as the amount of time required for 50% of the drug to be eliminated from the body. The serum drug level may be measured to assess the elimination of the drug.

Some of the factors that can influence drug action

As already mentioned, age, whether old or young, can have an effect on how drugs are distributed, metabolised and excreted in the body.

In infants, other factors that can affect drug action may include the percentage of total body water, the lower fat stores, different levels of circulatory plasma proteins and immature enzyme systems in the liver and the lungs.

Body weight can also affect drug action. For example, an overweight individual may require a larger dose of a drug for it to be of therapeutic value. Metabolic rate could also affect the metabolism of the drug. For example, any condition that increases the metabolic action of the body will also cause the drug to be metabolised much more rapidly.

Illnesses affecting the gastrointestinal tract will obviously interfere with the ingestion and absorption of a medication.

Adverse effects of drugs

Whilst most drugs are beneficial to the host, many drugs may also give rise to what are known as side effects or adverse effects. There are many reasons why these occur and they may include, for example, a patient's inability to metabolise a drug, due to a genetic deficiency of certain enzymes.

Whatever the reasons, many signs and symptoms can manifest in the affected individual and they will vary according to the types of medication taken. For example, various allergic reactions may present themselves as rashes, itching, urticaria and elevated temperature. The most severe form of allergic reaction is anaphylactic shock (explained in Chapter 14).

Other common side effects are nausea, vomiting and diarrhoea. Some drugs, such as the immunosuppressants, can cause alopecia (loss of hair), thrombocytopenia (decrease in the number of thrombocytes) or agranulocytosis (decrease in the number of granulocytes).

Another severe adverse effect is when the drug is a **teratogen**, and can therefore give rise to birth defects.

THE NURSE'S RESPONSIBILITY IN DRUG ADMINISTRATION

Drugs play an important part in the management of patients and their illnesses. The nurse often has the responsibility of administering drugs to the patients, whether in the community or in the hospital. It is therefore imperative that the nurse is aware of his/her responsibilities in giving drugs which are legislated in the UK by the **Misuse of Drugs Act 1971** for controlled drugs, and the **Medicines Act 1968** for prescription-only medicines. As of April 1994, new legislation has enabled district nurses and health visitors to prescribe a limited range of drugs (undertaken as a pilot study).

The nurse should also be familiar with the policies of the health authority where he/she is practising.

What follows is just a few of the **do's** and **don'ts** in relation to the nurse's responsibility in administering drugs so that the patient's safety and well-being are maintained at all times.

Do's

(1) Always give explanations to the patients as to the reason why particular medications are prescribed. Explain the importance of taking the drug at a regular time, and also whether the drug should be taken on an empty stomach or not. Whenever appropriate, advise as to the possible adverse effects of the particular drug. If in the community, the individual should report any severe adverse effects to the general practitioner.

(2) Before preparation and administration of the drug, wash and dry your hands thoroughly.

(3) Always check the prescription sheet and ensure that you can decipher the drug name and the dose clearly. The checking is usually undertaken with a trained member of staff (e.g. a first level nurse).

(4) Read the patient's full name from the prescription chart, and also check the identity bracelet.

(5) Prepare the patient to receive the medications – e.g. ensure that a glass of water, juice or milk is available (this depends on the drug and the patient's preference). Drinking straws and other aids should be made available if they are required.

(6) Always try to persuade patients to take the drug immediately.

(7) Record accurately the time that drugs are given and sign and date the record. Make notes if the patient refuses or does not take all the medications.

(8) Assess for efficacy of the drug administered, and note any adverse effects.

(9) Check and read the label of the container or vial for name, strength and dose of the drug, and when appropriate the expiry date.

(10) When giving suspensions, always shake the bottle and measure the drug correctly, using an accurate calibrated measure.

(11) Wear gloves for drugs where these are recommended (see the sections on cytotoxic drugs and antibiotics).

(12) Special precautions should be taken when additives are to be given via an intravenous infusion set. Ensure that the drug is thoroughly mixed and that it is not administered too quickly. If more than one additive is to be given, check that these drugs can be mixed.

(13) When giving injections, ensure that the correct type of syringe and needle are used.

(14) When giving an intramuscular injection, select the most appropriate site and rotate the choice of site if the patient is receiving frequent injections.

(15) For the injection of iron, use the Z-track method.

(16) Ensure the proper disposal of syringes and needles, according to agreed hospital policy.

Don'ts

(1) Do not administer drugs that you have not checked yourself.

(2) Do not administer drugs if you cannot decipher the name of the drug or patient.

(3) Do not administer drugs by other routes. Use only the one that has been prescribed.

(4) Do not ignore the adverse effects of drugs. They should be reported, and the medication may need to be changed.

(5) Do not use the colour of tablets as a means of recognising drugs.

(6) Do not administer drug unless there is the correct dose (for example, when giving suspensions).

SOME COMMON DRUG GROUPS

Having established some of the basic principles of pharmacology, it is now appropriate to review some of the common groups of drugs, their actions and possible adverse effects in the individual.

The groups of drugs mentioned here are not given in any particular order, but rather according to their common usage. They are the drugs that you are likely to come across when caring for patients in the hospital or community.

Wherever appropriate, essential nursing applications have been included.

Antimicrobial agents

This is a large group of drugs, which includes the **antibiotics** and the **sulphonamides**. They destroy bacterial growth either by killing the bacteria (**bactericidal effect**) or by preventing them from multiplying (**bacteriostatic effect**).

Sulphonamides

Sulphonamides are synthetic (man-made) and work because they mimic **folic acid**, a growth factor that is essential for bacterial growth. Sulphonamide chemical structure resembles that of folic acid and is known as *para*-**aminobenzoic acid** (**PABA**). When a patient receives sulphonamide medication, the bacteria in his body mistake PABA for folic acid. They take in PABA, but cannot use it for growth, and hence cannot multiply. Examples of sulphonamides are sulphadimidine and sulphasalazine. Sulphadimidine is often used in treating urinary tract infection. Sulphasalazine is used in the management of patients with Crohn's disease or ulcerative colitis.

Nursing applications

Observe patients for signs of nausea and rash, as these are common adverse effects of the sulphonamides. Patients should be encouraged to drink plenty of fluids as sulphonamides may cause precipitation in the kidney tubules, thus giving rise to stone formation (calculus). This is important in the elderly as they often tend to drink less fluid.

Antibiotics

Antibiotics are derived from natural sources (for example, **penicillin**) which is derived from the mould known as *Penicillium notatum*. However, many antibiotics these days are semisynthetic. They all contain the β lactam ring. The group contains the penicillins, the cephalosporins and many others. Examples of antibiotics are gentamicin, benzylpenicillin, streptomycin and rifampicin. Streptomycin and rifampicin are used in the treatment of patients with tuberculosis.

Adverse effects

All of the antibiotics can give rise to adverse effects. These may manifest as nausea, vomiting, diarrhoea and sometimes rashes. Some of them, especially gentamicin, can cause kidney damage (nephrotoxic effect). When patients are on gentamicin, the blood serum level for the drug is monitored regularly. The worst adverse effect with the penicillins is that of **anaphylactic shock**.

Nursing applications

Before administering patients any antibiotic, especially penicillin for the first time, it is always prudent to ask them if they have had any reactions previously when taking antibiotics. If so, this should be reported immediately and the treatment should be reassessed. This is obviously very important if the drug is to be administered intravenously.

Analgesics

Analgesics are drugs that relieve pain. These drugs may act at various sites along the pain pathways.

(1) They may reduce pain sensation by acting on the brain and spinal cord.

(2) They may suppress the release of various chemical mediators that trigger inflammation, and in so doing reduce the pain. Most of the nonsteroidal drugs work at this level.

(3) They may interfere with conduction in nerves carrying impulses from a painful area. Local anaesthetics work at this level.

Opioids (also called narcotics)

The opioid analgesics may be natural or synthetic. The natural opioids are opium (morphine) and codeine. The synthetic opioids are diamorphine, methadone, pethidine, phenazocine, dihydrocodeine, buprenorphine and oxycodeine.

Morphine is a powerful analgesic. It relieves most types of pain. Morphine does have many adverse effects, including: causing euphoria, depressing respiration and the cough centre, and causing constipation. One of the worst adverse effects is that of drug dependence.

Methadone is also a powerful analgesic, and is commonly used in the treatment of drug dependence.

Buprenorphine is a widely used analgesic, but it does not depress respiration. It can also be given sublingually. It is often used in the management of pain following surgery.

Oxycodeine is useful for patients who require an analgesic especially for a long period of time, during the night for example. It can be administered as suppositories.

Nonsteroidal anti-inflammatory agents

Most of these drugs act by interfering with the formation of prostaglandins. They block the action of the enzyme cyclo-oxygenase and therefore reduce the formation of prostaglandins from arachidonic acid. Examples of nonsteroidal anti-inflammatory drugs (NSAI) are aspirin, benorylate and indomethacin.

Both aspirin and indomethacin are widely used, especially for their anti-inflammatory and analgesic properties. Indomethacin is used in the treatment of rheumatoid arthritis and gout. One of the side effects of indomethacin is gastric bleeding and it should therefore be taken with caution. Patients should be advised about this adverse effect and should report this immediately to the general practitioner, should it occur.

Antacids

Antacids are used widely for neutralising the effects of hydrochloric acid in the stomach. Too much secretion of acid gives rise to indigestion (dyspepsia) and affected individuals complain of heartburn or a burning sensation in the stomach. Antacids can also reduce pepsin activity. They can relieve the pain of an ulcer. There are many preparations, but those commonly used in the hospital are magnesium trisilicate and magnesium hydroxide.

Anti-emetics

These are drugs that are administered in order to prevent vomiting. Examples are: metoclopramide, prochlorperazine and domperidone. They can also be used to prevent motion sickness. They are used regularly in the management of surgical patients. The usual route is intramuscular, although it can be given orally when appropriate.

Anticoagulants

These drugs affect the clotting mechanisms and are used in many diseases in which venous and arterial blood vessels are affected by thrombosis. The main effect of the drug is to prevent or reduce the formation of thrombi.

Anticoagulant therapy is always started with heparin, and it can be given intramuscularly, intravenously or subcutaneously. This is followed by an oral medication, of which the most popular is warfarin.

Both heparin and warfarin can cause haemorrhage from any part of the body – for example, haematuria (blood in the urine) may occur. The antidote for heparin is protamine sulphate, and the antidote for warfarin is vitamin K.

Nursing applications

The nurse should understand the adverse effects of anticoagulant therapy and therefore be in a position to give appropriate advice. Patients should be informed, for example, that their urine may be cloudy, pink or red and this could be an indication of haematuria. Patients should also report any dark brown vomitus, which may be the cause of haematemesis, and also red or black stools (melaena). There may also be bleeding of the gums or oral mucosa, or nose bleed (epistaxis). Patients should be advised to avoid alcohol consumption and also use of aspirin as they both may potentiate the effects of the anticoagulant. They should also avoid smoking and not take antihistamines. They should be advised to carry an identity card on their person at all times, indicating the dose of anticoagulant they are taking. Appointments to the hospital for estimation of prothrombin time and other tests must be kept.

The nurse must remember that in order to minimise tissue injury and haematoma, she/he **must not withdraw the plunger of the syringe to check the entry into a blood vessel**. He/she should also wait a few seconds before the needle is withdrawn, to prevent any leakage of the drug into the tissues. Injection sites should also be rotated

Antidepressant drugs

These drugs are used in the management of endogenous depression (no obvious cause). It is thought that these drugs work because they interfere with the various levels of neurotransmitters in the brain. The groups of drugs in the relief of depression are as follows:

(1) Tricyclic antidepressants.
(2) Tricyclic anxiolytics.
(3) 5 Hydroxytryptamine (5 HT) inhibitors.
(4) Monoamine oxidase inhibitors (MAOI).
(5) Lithium.

Trycyclic and anxiolytic tricyclic antidepressants

Most of these drugs produce their therapeutic effects by interfering with the re-uptake of the amines (dopamine, adrenaline, noradrenaline) at presynaptic nerve endings in the brain. In so doing, they prolong the activity and concentration of the various amines in the brain. Examples of some of the tricyclic antidepressants are imipramine and amitriptyline. Two examples of anxiolytic tricyclic antidepressants are doxepin and dothiepin.

Some patients may develop adverse effects, such as dryness of the mouth. Male individuals may also experience difficulty with micturition. Some patients may feel faint on account of a reduction in the blood pressure. Patients should be strongly advised not to take alcohol when they are taking tricyclic antidepressants, as alcohol may potentiate the effects of the drug.

5-HT re-uptake inhibitors

It is believed that the level of 5-HT in the brain is important for the modulation of an individual's behaviour and mood. When there is a deficiency of 5-HT, this may lead to depression. Therefore, administration of 5-HT is an attempt to raise the level of the neurotransmitters in the brain by interefering with the 5-HT re-uptake mechanism at nerve junctions. The therapeutic effects are similar to those of the tricyclic antidepressants and they have fewer side effects.

Examples of 5-HT re-uptake inhibitors are fluvoxamine, sertraline, paroxetine and fluoxetine.

Monoamine oxidase inhibitors

Monoamine oxidase is an enzyme that breaks down adrenaline, noradrenaline and 5-HT after their re-uptake at a presynaptic terminal in the brain, and thus regulates the level of these neurotransmitters in the brain. MAOI interferes with the activity of the enzyme MAO, and therefore allows the increase of neurotransmitters mentioned above. One example of a MAOI is phenelzine.

MAOI have many adverse effects such as insomnia, difficulties with micturition or increase in blood pressure. One very serious adverse effect is the so called **'cheese effect'**, which occurs if the individual consumes foods that contain substances called **tyramine** (a vasopressor). Tyramine is usually broken down by the enzyme MAO, but in its absence the level will rise, thus causing vasopressor effects, which may include a rise in blood pressure, headaches, flushing of the face, coma and even death.

Some of the foods containing tyramine are cheese, yeast extracts, Chianti wine, broad bean pods and pickled herrings.

It is important for individuals who are taking MAOI to carry some form of identification, listing the drug that they are taking. This may be required in an emergency, such as a surgical procedure that needs to be undertaken. Caution also needs to be taken in the use of analgesics, since the administration of morphine or pethidine may potentiate the effects of MAOI. Individuals should also be advised of the foods that they should avoid, and also perhaps be issued with some printed information.

Lithium

Lithium is given to patients suffering from what is known as bipolar depression (defined as periods of depression and mania). Lithium is used by nerve cells in a similar way to sodium ions, since it is a cation and it decreases nerve excitability.

It is important that the blood level of lithium is measured regularly, as lithium is excreted slowly and can therefore cause kidney damage.

NEUROLEPTICS

Following the antidepressant drugs, it is appropriate to discuss here the large group of drugs known as **neuroleptics**, since they are also widely used in the management of patients with behavioural problems such as schizophrenia, mania, delirium and paranoia.

Neuroleptic drugs can be classified into several groups according to their modes of action. They may be regarded as antipsychotic, anti-emetic and anxiolytic.

The antipsychotics are used widely in the treatment of patients with schizophrenia or mania, whilst the anxiolytic drugs are used in the management of patients with various types of anxiety reactions.

The neuroleptic drugs used principally for their antipsychotic properties fall into three groups: the phenothiazines, the butyrophenones and the thioxanthenes. Most of these drugs act on the central nervous system, but potencies of the various specific properties may differ according to the drugs being used. They interfere with the reticular formation and also with the basal ganglia, and they can therefore block both dopamine and acetylcholine receptors. Because of the blocking of dopamine receptors, these drugs have proved useful in the management of schizophrenia. It is widely recognised that the symptoms of schizophrenia may be attributed to an increase in the brain level of dopamine.

Phenothiazines

These drugs have antipsychotic effects and can therefore be used in the treatment of schizophrenia; they can produce sedation and they also have anti-emetic actions.

Examples of phenothiazines are: chlorpromazine (Largactil®), thioridazine (Melleril®), promazine (Sparine®), prochlorperazine (Stemetil®), trifluoperazine (Stelazine®) and fluphenazine decanoate (Modecate®).

Adverse effects are very common and are dose-dependent and also dependent on the types of drugs used. Various disorders of movement may occur, and these are due mainly to the blocking action of dopamine in the brain. The following may occur:

(1) Akathisia, where the patient feels restless and is unable to stand still.
(2) Dystonia, which is uncontrolled movement.
(3) Tardive dyskinesia, where patients develop abnormal movements of the mouth and tongue, and the upper limbs may also be affected.
(4) A Parkinson-like syndrome, which many patients may also develop.

Jaundice may also occur, and this is thought to be attributed to the blockage of the bile canaliculi in the liver. Skin rashes may occur and, especially with chlorpromazine, a photosensitivity reaction may occur. This manifests itself as cutaneous pigmentation, producing blue-grey coloration of exposed skin surfaces. Also associated with chlorpromazine, on account of its depressing action on the vasomotor centre, is hypotension, and there may also be depression of temperature regulation (in the elderly this could lead to hypothermia). Patients on chlorpromazine should therefore be advised not to expose themselves to extreme heat. Dry mouth may also be a problem.

Thioxanthenes

These drugs are very similar to the phenothiazines and are used in the management of schizophrenic individuals. An example of a thioxanthene is flupenthixol. Many of the side effects are similar to those of the phenothiazines.

Butyrophenones

These drugs have similar properties to those of the phenothiazines and they are less sedative. They are often used in patients with manic depressive symptoms. Examples of butyrophenones are haloperidol and droperidol.

Other neuroleptics

When patients do not respond to the common neuroleptics, they are then prescribed the newer types of drugs, examples of which are sulpiride, clozapine and pimozide.

These drugs may severely reduce the number of leukocytes, and if this reduction is not detected, patients will be at risk to various opportunistic infections. The drugs can also cause excessive salivation and hypotension.

Nursing implications

The patient's education is important, and in many individuals, especially schizophrenics, compliance may be a problem. The nurse should be aware of this and when appropriate should make sure that patients do take their drugs. Careful supervision is essential. The nurse should also be very vigilant in monitoring any adverse effect of the drugs being used, as some patients may be unable to recognise or report any of these side effects. Appropriate advice should also be given with regard to exposure to the sun (especially when patients are on chlorpromazine).

Special precautions may need to be taken when preparing solutions such as chlorpromazine for administration. Always follow the appropriate procedure.

CYTOTOXIC DRUGS

Cytotoxic drugs are given in the treatment of malignant diseases. They work by interfering with DNA or RNA and therefore have a negative effect on growth of the cells. There are different types of cytotoxic drugs: alkylating agents, antimetabolites and vinca alkaloids.

Alkylating agents

Some examples of alkylating agents are mustine, cyclophosphamide, chlorambucil, busulphan and mephalan. These drugs combine with DNA in the cell and they therefore damage or kill the cell. They are not selective and they therefore also damage 'good' cells, especially those of the gastrointestinal tract and the bone marrow. They all have unpleasant side effects.

Mustine

Mustine is administered intravenously and is usually given via a drip of saline.

Mustine can cause nausea, vomiting and leukopenia (decrease in the number of white blood cells).

Cyclophosphamide

Cyclophosphamide may be given orally or intravenously.

The adverse effects include alopecia (hair loss), bone marrow depression and cystitis. Cystitis is the result of a byproduct (acrolein) of cyclophosphamide metabolism.

Nursing applications

The nurse can assist in the prevention of cystitis by encouraging the patient to drink large amounts of fluids (at least 4 litres per day). Any persistent cystitis can be relieved by the administration of a cytotoxic antagonist (mesna, also known as Uromitexan®).

Chlorambucil

Chlorambucil is given orally and, though it does not usually cause vomiting, it can cause bone marrow depression.

Antimetabolites

These drugs are mistaken for the normal metabolic chemicals (usually folic acid) that are usually used by the cells. When taken in by malignant cells, they cannot be metabolised. Consequently, the malignant cells are killed.

Examples of antimetabolites are methotrexate, 6-mercaptopurine, cytarabine and 5-fluorouracil.

Methotrexate

Methotrexate can be given orally, intravenously or intrathecally. It can be used in the treatment of leukaemia and also in the management of patients with psoriasis.

Because the drug is largely excreted by the kidneys, it can cause kidney damage.

6-Mercaptopurine

6-Mercaptopurine can be given orally in the management of acute and chronic myeloid leukaemia.

5-Fluorouracil

5-Fluorouracil can be used in the treatment of various tumuors, including those of the gastrointestinal tract.

It can cause ulceration of the mouth.

Cytarabine

Cytarabine is also used in the treatment of acute leukaemia.

Nursing applications

All the antimetabolites can cause depression of the bone marrow. It is important that the nurse remembers this, since patients in their care are liable to develop infections. The nurse should understand why these patients may be particularly at risk to infections, and should take any necessary precaution that would minimise this risk. Patients should be advised to report any signs and symptoms that may suggest an infection.

Vinca alkaloids

Vinblastine and vincristine are examples of alkaloids. Vinblastine is an extract of periwinkle. Vincristine is related to vinblastine. Both drugs interfere with the metaphase of mitotic division. Both drugs can be administered by single weekly intravenous injection.

Vinblastine may be given in the treatment of Hodgkin's disease, lymphosarcoma and other malignancies. Vincristine may be given in the treatment of Hodgkin's disease, acute lymphoblastic leukaemia and other types of leukaemia.

Both vinblastine and vincristine may give rise to similar adverse effects, although those of vinblastine are usually more severe. The adverse effects may include the following:

leukopenia, peripheral neuropathy, paraesthesias of the hands and feet, loss of deep tendon reflexes, stomatitis, nausea, vomiting and diarrhoea.

Specific nursing applications relating to cytotoxic drugs

Apart from the usual precautions that should be taken when administering any medication, it is essential that the following be adhered to when administering cytotoxic medications:

(1) Only staff who have received certification of competency (as agreed by the local hospital policy/procedure) should prepare the drug for administration.

(2) Disposable gloves and plastic aprons should be worn when preparing the solutions to be administered.

(3) Special precautions should be taken to avoid the drug getting into the eyes.

(4) Inhalation of the drug should be avoided.

(5) Staff who are pregnant should not prepare cytotoxic drugs.

(6) Any spillage should be dealt with as per hospital policy/procedure.

(7) Staff should be aware of the use of the **vesicant** drugs, as they can cause severe tissue necrosis if they extravasate into the tissues. It is therefore important to monitor and check the sites of the cannula carefully, if the drug is being administered intravenously.

(8) Precautions for the disposal of used syringes and needles should be adhered to.

DIURETICS

The diuretics are a large group of drugs that have beneficial effects in patients who have oedema, which may be as a result of congestive cardiac failure, or hepatic or renal diseases, including nephrotic syndrome. Their main action is to increase urinary output and this is achieved by decreasing reabsorption of water and electrolytes, such as sodium, by the renal tubules. In getting rid of excess water, the blood volume is reduced and therefore in the case of heart failure, the heart is able to maintain the cardiac output with much less effort.

The most common diuretics may be classified into three main groups. They are the osmotic diuretics, the thiazides and the loop diuretics.

Mannitol – osmotic diuretic

Mannitol is an osmotic diuretic and its main function is to prevent the reabsorption of water and salt from the tubule. In so doing, it causes a diuresis. Its main use today is in the management of patients with intracranial pressure following head injury.

The thiazides

Two of the commonly used thiazides are bendrofluazide and chlorothiazide. They can be given orally and their main function is to cause a diuresis by reducing the reabsorption of sodium, chlorides and water.

Loop diuretics

The loop diuretics are more powerful than the thiazides, and they inhibit the reabsorption of sodium and chloride primarily in the loop of Henle and also in the proximal and distal tubules. Three of the loop diuretics are bumetanide, frusemide and ethacrynic acid.

Adverse effects of the thiazides and loop diuretics

Both group of drugs enhance the excretion of potassium, and there is therefore the danger of hypokalaemia. The blood level of potassium and sodium should be regularly monitored.

Potassium replacement is often given when patients are prescribed the above drugs. Because patients may lose a large volume of fluids, they may be at risk to dehydration. Also, they may suffer from postural hypotension as a result of low blood pressure. In the elderly, anorexia, nausea, vomiting, thirst and a dry mouth can occur.

Nursing applications

Patients on diuretics should be carefully monitored in the early stage, and the nurse should record the intake and output of fluids. The patient may need to be weighed once daily. Patients should therefore be given explanations of the importance of monitoring their own fluids if they are able to do so. The nurse should also ensure that for the patient who is not ambulant, a clean urinary bottle is provided, especially at night.

Blood pressure may need to be monitored in those patients who are at risk of developing postural hypotension. The nurse should monitor the mouth's hygiene and mouth care should be given if necessary. The nurse should also observe for signs of dehydration.

Other diuretics

Two diuretics that are frequently used are triamterene and spironolactone. They both possess anti-aldosterone activity and therefore reduce potassium excretion, but promote the excretion of sodium and chloride.

DIGITALIS

Digitalis is a common group of drugs that is used in the treatment of patients with heart failure. There are two types of digitalis: digoxin, which is obtained from the white foxglove and digitoxin, which is obtained from the purple foxglove. Digoxin is the one commonly used. Digoxin has a direct action on the heart muscle. It increases the activity of the vagus nerve by interfering with the sinoatrial node, thereby slowing the heart rate. It also increases the force of contraction of the ventricular muscles by promoting the movement of calcium ions into the heart muscle cells. It decreases the number of impulses reaching the ventricles and this may be beneficial in the management of atrial fibrillation, because it causes a decrease in the rate of ventricular contraction.

The main function of digoxin is to make the heart more efficient, by maintaining a sufficient cardiac output. Digoxin can be given orally or intravenously.

Adverse effects are very common, but are more frequent in the elderly. They may include nausea, vomiting, confusion, slowing of the heart rate (pulse rate below 60 per minute) or coupled beats.

Nursing applications

The patient's pulse rate and apex beat should be monitored and recorded. The drug may be omitted if the pulse rate is below 60 per minute. The nurse should observe for any signs of toxicity. This is more likely when the patient is taking a diuretic, which promotes the excretion of potassium.

INSULIN

You have already met the hormone insulin, when you studied the endocrine and the digestive systems. You should therefore recall that insulin is a protein and that its main function is to lower the concentration of glucose in the blood. This is achieved mainly by:

(1) Converting excess glucose into glycogen in the liver.

(2) Promoting the uptake of glucose by the tissues.

(3) Increasing the production of fat and protein.

Why some individuals may require insulin

Deficiency of insulin, especially in young people, gives rise to a type of diabetes mellitus which is known as **insulin-dependent diabetes of Type I**. In this condition carbohydrate metabolism is affected and the cells of the body are unable to use glucose effectively. As a result, a large amount of glucose is lost in the urine (glycosuria) and if the condition is not treated, fats are also metabolised and produce ketoacids. Proteins may also be metabolised, to provide energy in the early stage of the disease. This often results in severe weight loss in the affected child or young adult.

Individuals with Type I diabetes mellitus will require insulin in order that their bodies can effectively utilise carbohydrates to provide the main source of energy.

Use of insulin

Insulin is given according to the individual's energy requirements, and this should also take into account the diet, type of work or school activities and life style.

The main aim of treatment is the control of the blood glucose level, to reduce glycosuria and ketones presence in the urine.

There are many typres of insulin and they vary in strength and mode of actions (i.e. short-term or long-term acting). Some of the common insulin preparations are as follows: **short-acting** – Human Actrapid®, Humulin S®); **intermediate acting** – Humulin 1®, Human Monotard®); **long-acting** – Humulin Znc®, Hypurine Protamine Zinc®).

Insulin used in the UK is supplied in **100 units/ml** concentration (U 100 insulin).

Insulin may be given subcutaneously, intramuscularly or intravenously. The most common method of administration is the subcutaneous route, and it is the method that the patient will need to learn for self-administration of the drug. Individuals who require insulin may need to receive the medication three times a day (at least 15–30 minutes before meals, i.e. breakfast, lunch and supper).

Many of the adverse effects of insulin are as a result of severe reduction in blood sugar (hypoglycaemia). Some of the following symptoms may be experienced by individuals suffering from hypoglycaemia: profuse sweating, hunger, tremors, palpitations, weakness, fatigue, blurred vision, numbness of the mouth and tongue and other paraesthesias.

Nursing applications

Self-administration of insulin and its adverse effects should be carefully explained to the patient. Patients should be informed of the importance of carrying lumps of sugar or glucose, which they can have access to, should they develop hypoglycaemia. Patients should understand the importance of taking their diets as soon as possible following their insulin injection. Patients should also be advised to carry some form of identification indicating the nature of their illness.

The nurse should give instructions to the patient as to the best sites for injection (i.e. the abdomen, outer side of the upper arm and front of the thigh). Choice of injection sites should be rotated so as to reduce the risk of lipodystrophy. The needs of hygiene with regard to the patient's self-administration of insulin should also be emphasised. The patient should be given information on the storage of insulin and also on how to check that the drug has not expired. Advice should also be given on the testing of urine for the presence of glucose and ketones. Patients may need to be given instructions on how to keep an up-to-date urinalysis chart.

Young children and adolescents should be given appropriate advice with regard to insulin adjustment before exercise. Parents should also be given instructions on the management of their child. Patients should be advised to continue taking insulin even if there is an illness. They should drink copious amounts of fluids. Any illness should be reported to the general practitioner.

STEROIDS

This is an important group of drugs, which may be life-saving in some life-threatening situations. Steroids are hormones produced by the adrenal cortex and, as you should recall from previous study on the endocrine system, they may be classified into three main groups: the mineralocorticoids, the glucocorticoids and the sex corticoids. Please review the sections on the adrenal cortex if you wish to remind yourself of the functions of the three groups mentioned above.

Steroids are used as medications on account of their pharmacological properties which are similar to those of the natural steroids in the body. Steroids combine with cytoplasmic receptors to form complexes, which then enter the nucleus of the cells and bind to DNA, thereby initiating cytoplasmic synthesis of enzymes responsible for systemic effects of the corticoids. Because of their glucocorticoid properties, steroids promote gluconeogenesis, but decrease the peripheral utilisation of glucose.

In the main, the actions of steroids fall broadly into four categories and they are as follows: anti-inflammatory, anti-allergic, anti-tumour actions and immunological effects.

Anti-inflammatory effects

Many patients with inflammatory conditions (e.g. rheumatoid arthritis, dermatitis) are often prescribed steroids. Examples of some of the steroids that can be used as anti-inflammatory medications are prednisolone, betamethasone, prednisone and methyl prednisolone.

Steroids suppress inflammation as they interfere with histamine activity. They reduce proliferation of fibroblasts and collagen depositions. Thus, they also suppress healing.

Anti-allergic effects

Steroids decrease the number of lymphocytes (important for the production of antibodies) and can therefore suppress allergic reactions, such as hay fever, asthma and eczema and many other skin conditions.

A common steroid used in the management of individuals with hay fever and asthma is beclomethasone diproprionate (Becotide® or Beconase®).

Immunological effects

Many of the steroids have immunological effects, as they decrease the number of circulating neutrophils and lymphocytes. They can also suppress cell-mediated hypersensitivity reactions. They are therefore often used in the management of individuals with transplants, to reduce the risk of rejection. They are frequently used in the management of patients with autoimmune disorders, such as systemic lupus erythematosus.

Anti-tumour effects

Steroids can be used in combination with cytotoxic drugs to treat certain types of tumour, for example leukaemias and lymphomas.

Steroids can also be given as palliative treatment in patients with cerebral tumours. In this case, the drug of choice is dexamethasone.

Other uses of steroids

In patients in whom the adrenal glands have been surgically removed or destroyed by disease, steroids are administered as replacement therapy.

Adverse effects

All steroids, when used over a period of time, will give rise to adverse effects, although these depend on the specific properties (i.e. mineralocorticoid, glucocorticoid, sex corticoid or a mixture) of the steroids being administered. On the whole, the diverse effects are similar and are dose dependent.

One very serious side effect is that of the suppression of the adrenal cortex, which is due to the interference of the feedback mechanism, thereby affecting the release of hypothalamic and pituitary hormones that usually control the release of adrenal corticoids. Therfore, adrenocorticotrophic hormone secretion may be affected.

Long-term use of steroids can cause atrophy of the adrenal cortex and these individuals will be dependent on those drugs. Any change of circumstance that may give rise to various stressors (for example, a surgical emergency) could affect these individuals. For this reason, it is imperative that all individuals on long-term steroid treatment should carry appropriate identification, indicating the drug that they are taking and also the dose. In fact, such individuals may need to receive steroid cover if they are to have surgery.

On account of the mineralocorticoid properties of many steroids, sodium retention is likely, whilst potassium loss can be marked. Sodium retention also increases water retention and this may lead to oedema. The oedema can manifest itself in what is often referred to as 'moon face appearance' and 'buffalo hump', which is oedema around the back of the neck.

The increase in fluid volume can give rise to high blood pressure. The loss of potassium can cause weakness and fatigue, and can also give rise to cardiovascular problems.

The glucocorticoid activities of some steroids can disturb the carbohydrate metabolism and give rise to glycosuria and symptoms of diabetes. Many of the steroids can also cause gastric irritation, and this can lead to development of an ulcer or aggravate an existing peptic ulcer. It is advisable that such steroids are taken with meals to reduce the gastric irritation.

Due to their anti-inflammatory effects, steroids can mask the symptoms of infection and also inhibit the healing process. Decalcification of bones can occur and, if patients are taking large doses of steroids, this can lead to potential fractures.

Because of their immunologically suppressive effects, steroids can cause a severe decrease in the number of neutrophils and lymphocytes, thus making the patients more prone to infection. This can be more serious in patients who are receiving immunosuppressive therapy following transplant.

Other adverse effects of steroids are those of hirsutism affecting the face and the trunk; there may be muscle wasting and weakness; the skin can be susceptible to bruising.

Nursing applications

The patient's education is important, both in terms of the reason for taking the steroids and the possible adverse effects. Advice should be given in a mannner that does not cause any undue anxiety in the patient. Patients should be advised to take medications as prescribed and not to reduce or increase the dose. A patient who is on long-term steroid treatment should be advised to carry an identity card indicating the type of steroid taken and the dose. Explanations should be given as to the side effects – for example, weight gain and gastric disturbances (heartburn and indigestion). The patient should report these to their general practitioner. Patients on a large dose of steroids should have their urine tested for any presence of sugar. Elderly patients on a moderate to large dose of steroids should be aware of any eye complaints, such as glaucoma and cataract.

Patients who are receiving large doses of steroids as immunosuppressant therapy, to reduce the risk of tissue rejection following transplant, should be advised to avoid situations that could easily put them at risk of catching an infection (such as being in a large crowd).

It is also important for the nurse to be aware of patients who may be at risk from infection, especially those who are being treated for various cancers (for example, the leukaemias). Strict hygiene should be maintained at all times to avoid cross infection.

Precautions should be taken when preparing steroid solutions for administration to the patients. It is therefore important to wear gloves and to avoid spillage on the eyes and the skin. The nurse must adhere to the policy/procedure of the health authority.